T0094217

The Patellofemoral Joint in the Athlete

Robin V. West • Alexis C. Colvin
Editors

The Patellofemoral Joint in the Athlete

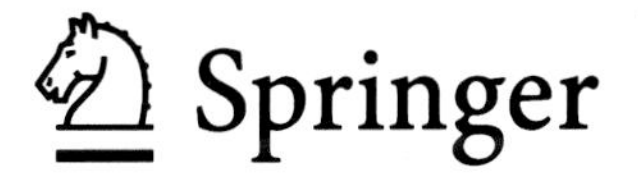

Editors
Robin V. West, M.D.
Associate Professor
Department of Orthopedic Surgery
Center for Sports Medicine
School of Health and Rehabilitation Sciences
University of Pittsburgh
Pittsburgh, PA, USA

Alexis C. Colvin, M.D.
Assistant Professor
Department of Orthopedic Surgery
Mount Sinai School of Medicine
New York, NY, USA

ISBN 978-1-4614-4156-4 ISBN 978-1-4614-4157-1 (eBook)
DOI 10.1007/978-1-4614-4157-1
Springer New York Heidelberg Dordrecht London

Library of Congress Control Number: 2013946417

Printed on acid-free paper

Springer is part of Springer Science+Business Media (www.springer.com)

Preface

Patellofemoral pain and instability can be challenging to treat, especially in the athlete. We are pleased to present this reference with contributions from the leaders in the field and have included topics that are critical to the treatment of patellar pathology.

We begin with chapters on the anatomy and function of the patellofemoral joint followed by the pertinent physical exam findings and imaging studies. Since many of these problems can be addressed nonoperatively, we have included a comprehensive chapter on rehabilitation. Next, we review the surgical treatments for the spectrum of patellar problems, including instability in both skeletally immature and mature athletes, cartilage procedures, osteotomies, and patellofemoral resurfacing. Finally, we have included a surgical decision-making chapter that will help to guide the orthopedic surgeon's treatment.

We believe that this book provides a comprehensive text on the treatment of patellofemoral disorders in the athlete and will become your "one-stop" guide.

Pittsburgh, PA, USA — Robin V. West
New York, NY, USA — Alexis C. Colvin

Acknowledgment

We would like to thank the contributing authors for sharing their expertise with us, our families for their love and support, our colleagues for their camaraderie, and, finally, all of our mentors who have inspired us throughout our medical and orthopedic surgery training.

Contents

Contributors

Elizabeth A. Arendt, M.D. Department of Orthopaedic Surgery, University of Minnesota, Minneapolis, MN, USA

Matthew Bollier, M.D. Department of Orthopaedic Surgery, University of Iowa Hospitals and Clinics, Iowa City, IA, USA

James P. Bradley, M.D. Burke and Bradley Orthopedics, Pittsburgh, PA, USA

Nicolas Brown, M.D. Rush University Medical Center, Chicago, IL, USA

Brian J. Cole, M.D., M.B.A. Rush University Medical Center, Chicago, IL, USA

Matthias Cotic, M.Sc. Department of Orthopedic Sports Medicine, Technical University Munich, Munich, Germany

Diane L. Dahm, M.D. Orthopaedic Surgery, Sports Medicine, Mayo Clinic, Rochester, MN, USA

Cory Edgar, M.D., Ph.D. Department of Orthopedic Surgery, University of Connecticut, Farmington, CT, USA

Jack Farr II, M.D. Orthopaedic Surgery, Cartilage Restoration Center of Indiana, Greenwood, IN, USA

John P. Fulkerson, M.D. Department of Orthopedic Surgery, Orthopedic Associates of Hartford, P.C., Farmington, CT, USA

University of Connecticut Medical School, Farmington, CT, USA

Ronald P. Grelsamer, M.D. Patellofemoral Reconstruction, Mount Sinai Medical Center, New York, NY, USA

Kyle E. Hammond, M.D. Orthopaedic Surgery, Sports Medicine, Emory University, Atlanta, GA, USA

William L. Hennrikus, M.D. Orthopaedics Department, Penn State College of Medicine, Hershey, PA, USA

Andreas B. Imhoff, M.D. Department of Orthopedic Sports Medicine, Technical University Munich, Munich, Germany

Mininder S. Kocher, M.D., M.P.H. Orthopaedic Surgery, Sports Medicine, Children's Hospital Boston, Harvard Medical School, Boston, MA, USA

Christopher M. LaPrade, B.A. Department of Biomedical Engineering, Steadman Philippon Research Institute, Vail Valley Medical Center, Vail, CO, USA

Robert F. LaPrade, M.D., Ph.D. The Steadman Clinic, Steadman Philippon Research Institute, Vail Valley Medical Center, Vail, CO, USA

Department of Orthopaedic Surgery, University of Minnesota, Minneapolis, MN, USA

Jeffrey Macalena, M.D. Department of Orthopaedic Surgery, University of Minnesota, Minneapolis, MN, USA

Jenny McConnell, B. App. Sci. (Phty), Grad. Dip. Man. Ther., M. Biomed. Eng., F.A.C.P. Center for Sports Medicine, Melbourne University, Melbourne, VIC, Australia

J. Lee Pace, M.D. Surgery Department, Orthopaedic Surgery, Children's Hospital Los Angeles, Los Angeles, CA, USA

Orthopaedic Surgery Department, Keck School of Medicine, University of Southern California, Los Angeles, CA, USA

Matthew T. Rasmussen, B.S. Department of Biomedical Engineering, Steadman Philippon Research Institute, Vail Valley Medical Center, Vail, CO, USA

Matthew J. Salzler, M.D. Orthopaedic Surgery, Sports Medicine, University of Pittsburgh Medical Center, Pittsburgh, PA, USA

Philip B. Schoettle, M.D. Isar Medical Center, Munich, Bavaria, Germany

Geoffrey S. Van Thiel, M.D., M.B.A. Sports Medicine Division, Department of Orthopedics, Rush University Medical Center, Chicago, IL, USA

Rockford Orthopedic Associates, Rockford, IL, USA

Willem M. van der Merwe, M.D. Orthopaedics Division, Sport Science Institute, University of Cape Town, Cape Town, South Africa

John Wechter, M.D. Department of Orthopaedic Surgery, University of Minnesota, Minneapolis, MN, USA

Anatomy of the Patellofemoral Joint

1

Christopher M. LaPrade, Matthew T. Rasmussen, and Robert F. LaPrade

Abbreviations

RF	Rectus femoris
VL	Vastus lateralis
VLO	Vastus lateralis obliquus
VM	Vastus medialis
VMO	Vastus medialis obliquus
LPFL	Lateral patellofemoral ligament
MPFL	Medial patellofemoral ligament
MPTL	Medial patellotibial ligament
LPTL	Lateral patellotibial ligament
ITB	Iliotibial band
IPB	Iliopatellar band
FCL	Fibular collateral ligament
ACL	Anterior cruciate ligament
PCL	Posterior cruciate ligament
MCL	Medial collateral ligament
QT	Quadriceps tendon
PT	Patellar tendon
AMT	Adductor magnus tendon

C.M. LaPrade, B.A. • M.T. Rasmussen, B.S.
Department of Biomedical Engineering,
Steadman Philippon Research Institute,
Vail Valley Medical Center, Vail, CO, USA

R.F. LaPrade, M.D., Ph.D. (✉)
The Steadman Clinic, Steadman Philippon
Research Institute, Vail Valley Medical Center,
181 W. Meadow Drive Suite 400, Vail,
CO 81657, USA

Department of Orthopaedic Surgery,
University of Minnesota, Minneapolis, MN, USA
e-mail: drlaprade@sprivail.org

Introduction

The patellofemoral joint is a very complex and often misunderstood region of the knee. The anatomy consists of a variety of important structures—such as the numerous muscles, bones, ligaments, tendons, blood vessels, nerves, and bursa sacs—that contribute to the functionality of the knee joint. Comprehensive joint functionality is critical for athletes, and each structure has a very important role in allowing for a stable knee and preventing patellofemoral-related pain [1, 2].

Knowledge about the anatomy of this joint is still constantly evolving [3–5], and this knowledge is extremely important for finding improved methods to better treat patients with patellofemoral joint pathology and to prevent pain from developing in the first place. The surgically relevant anatomy for these patellofemoral joint structures will be discussed.

Anatomy

Primary Supporting Muscles of the Patellofemoral Joint

Rectus Femoris

The rectus femoris is the most superficial muscle of the quadriceps muscle group [6], and it courses over the anterior portion of the thigh deep to the sartorius muscle [7]. It originates from the ileum, where it has anterior and posterior attachments [7],

R.V. West and A.C. Colvin (eds.), *The Patellofemoral Joint in the Athlete*,
DOI 10.1007/978-1-4614-4157-1_1, © Springer Science+Business Media New York 2014

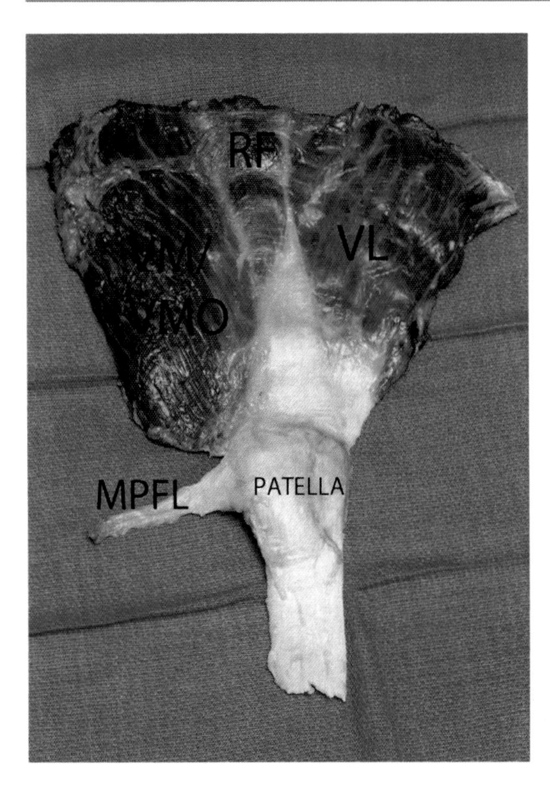

Fig. 1.1 A photograph of a *left knee* depicting the vastus medialis (VM)/vastus medialis obliquus (VMO) (*left*), rectus femoris (RF) (*center*), and vastus lateralis (VL) (*right*) combining to form the quadriceps tendon, which then inserts into the patella. The attachment of the medial patellofemoral ligament (MPFL) is also seen in the photo

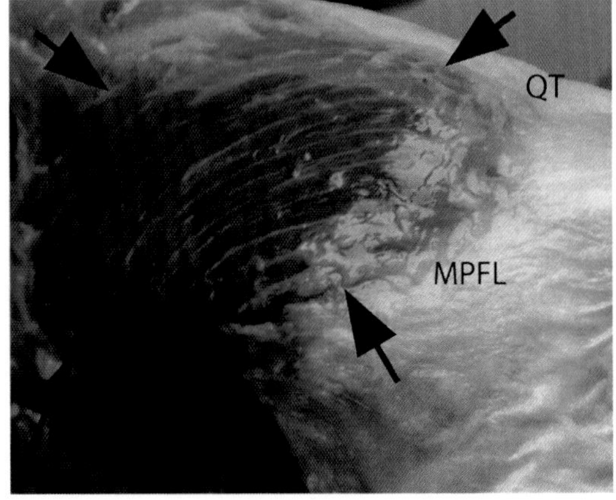

Fig. 1.2 *Arrows* define the outline of the vastus medialis obliquus (VMO), and its obliquely orientated muscle fibers can be seen in this intact *left knee*. The relation of the quadriceps tendon (QT) to the VMO and end of the VMO at the medial patellofemoral ligament (MPFL) is also seen

and inserts on the proximal aspect and superior third of the anterior surface of the patella after joining the quadriceps tendon about 3–5 cm proximal to the patella (Fig. 1.1) [6–9].

Vastus Lateralis

The vastus lateralis originates from the lateral aspect of the femur and centrally unites with the vastus medialis to insert into the proximal base of the patella (Fig. 1.1) [9]. Laterally, the vastus lateralis ends in an aponeurosis that combines with the lateral side of the rectus femoris [7, 9]. This expansion then becomes part of the lateral retinaculum and blends into the quadriceps tendon about 3 cm proximal to the superolateral region of the patella [7, 9]. The vastus lateralis also has an anatomically distinct group of fibers called the vastus lateralis obliquus (VLO) that has been reported to be separated from the main portion of the muscle by a thin layer of fat or fascia [9]. Historically, little attention has been given to the VLO due to the difficulty in identifying the divergent fibers [9]. These fibers attach more laterally to the patella than the longitudinal vastus lateralis fibers [9].

Vastus Medialis

The vastus medialis originates from the superomedial region of the femur and centrally unites with the vastus lateralis to insert into the base of the patella just posterior to the insertion of the rectus femoris (Fig. 1.1) [9]. Medially, the vastus medialis ends in an aponeurosis that combines with the rectus femoris to both attach to the superomedial aspect of the patella and reinforce the medial retinaculum with its distal fibers [9]. The vastus medialis also contains the vastus medialis obliquus (VMO), which has obliquely oriented fibers and is the most distal portion of the vastus medialis (Fig. 1.2) [6, 7, 9]. The VMO originates from the adductor magnus tendon and ends on the medial patellofemoral ligament [6, 10]. The VMO has considerable variability in regard to the presence of a thin layer of fat, fascia, or nerve branch that separates the VMO from the longitudinal head of the vastus medialis, and therefore, it can be difficult to discriminate between the two [9].

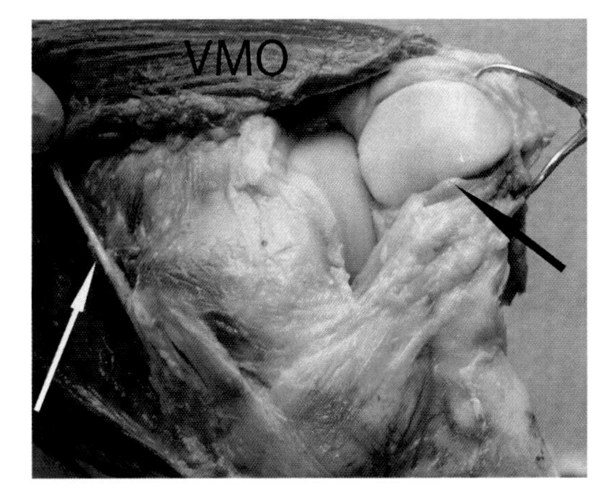

Fig. 1.3 The articular surface of the patella (*black arrow*) reflected from a *left knee* is shown. The medial and lateral facets are present on the posterior aspect of the patella. The adductor magnus tendon is shown with the *white arrow*, and the VMO is also labeled

Vastus Intermedius

The vastus intermedius lies deep to the other quadriceps muscles. It attaches proximally to the anterolateral upper two-thirds of the femur and runs anterior to the femur until its tendinous fibers combine with the vastus medialis and vastus lateralis to insert distally into the superior border of the patella [7].

Pertinent Bony Anatomy of the Patellofemoral Joint

Patella

The patella is the largest sesamoid bone in the body [6, 11, 12] and provides a mobile attachment for the quadriceps tendon and patellar tendon [6]. The patella is triangular, and it has a rounded and superior base that attaches to the quadriceps tendon [6]. It also has an inferior apex that points inferiorly and attaches to the patellar tendon [6]. The articular surface of the patella (Fig. 1.3) has been reported to have up to seven facets and is on the proximal two-thirds of the posterior aspect of the bone [7, 11]. Three medial facets (superior, middle, and inferior) and three lateral facets (superior, middle, and inferior) articulate with the femoral trochlear groove during knee flexion. The last medial facet, or odd facet, articulates with the medial femoral condyle in deep knee flexion [7, 11]. The medial facets are slightly smaller than the lateral facets [7, 11].

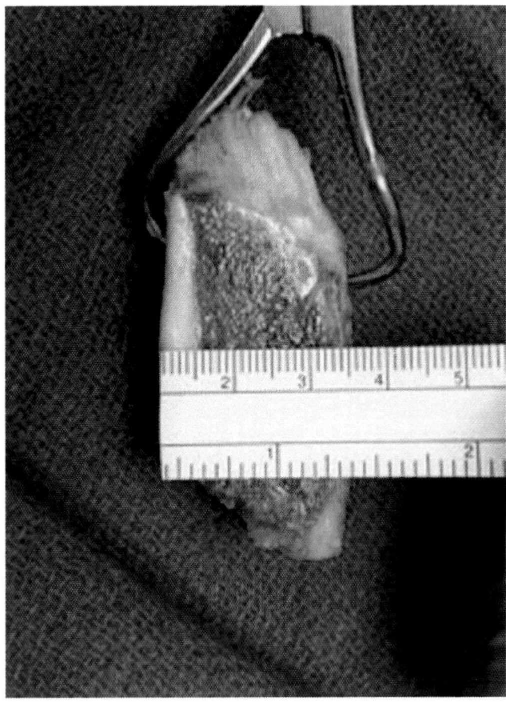

Fig. 1.4 A photograph demonstrates the cross section of a *right knee* patella. The thickness of the articular cartilage (about 6 mm) can be seen with the ruler

The articular cartilage covering the patella is one of the thickest in the body (Fig. 1.4), and the cartilage on the medial facet is thicker than the cartilage on the lateral facet [6]. The thickest part of the patellar articular cartilage has been reported to be about 6.4-mm thick and is on the median ridge of the patella [6].

Wiberg created a classification system for different patella shapes based on a generalized comparison of the medial facets to the lateral facets [13]. Type I has a prevalence of about 10 % and has equally sized, concave medial and lateral facets [7, 11]. Type II has normal lateral facets with considerably smaller medial facets that are mostly flat [7, 11]. This type accounts for approximately 65 % of patella types [7, 11]. Type III comprises the remaining 25 %, and it has normal lateral facets with smaller and convex medial facets [7, 11].

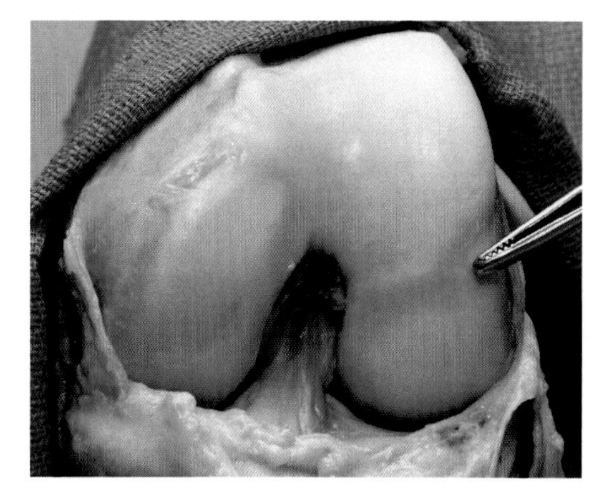

Fig. 1.5 The location of the sulcus terminalis, which separates the trochlea from the lateral femoral condyle, is shown with a hemostat in a *left knee*

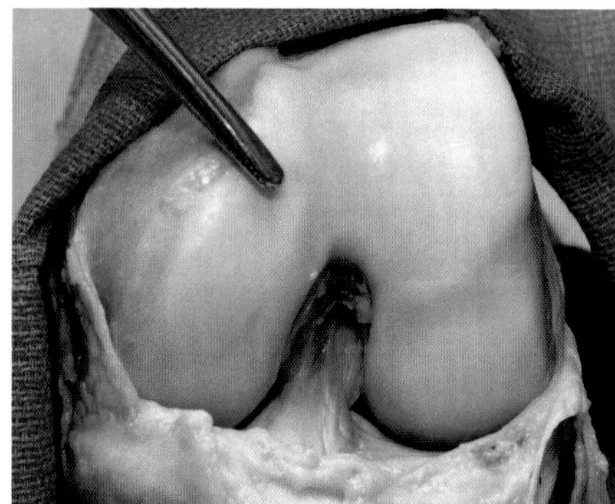

Fig. 1.6 A photograph illustrates a groove (forceps) that separates the trochlea from the medial femoral condyle in a *left knee*

Trochlea and Femoral Condyles

The other major articular surface of the patellofemoral joint is the trochlea, which consists of the lateral and medial facets of the femoral sulcus and is on the anterior, distal end of the femur [6, 11]. The anteroposterior trochlear groove is in the middle of the trochlea and divides it into the medial and lateral facets [6]. The lateral facet is larger and has a greater radius than the medial facet [6]. The trochlea deepens from proximal to distal, and it is not aligned perpendicular to the axis of femur to reflect how the distal articular surfaces of the femur are valgus in relation to the axis of the femur [8, 11]. This allows for the tibiofemoral joint to be horizontal to the ground while standing [8].

The trochlea joins the articular surface of the femoral condyles to help provide patellar tracking during knee flexion, and each femoral condyle is separated from the trochlea by a slight groove [11]. The sulcus terminalis separates the lateral femoral condyle from the trochlea (Fig. 1.5), while the medial femoral condyle has a less distinct notch (Fig. 1.6) [7]. The femoral condyles protrude only slightly anteriorly of the femoral shaft but protrude significantly posteriorly, and both anterior regions of the condyles are part of the articular area for the patella [6]. The femoral condyles are asymmetric with the lateral femoral condyle higher than the medial femoral condyle to help prevent lateral subluxation and keep the medial femoral condyle from extending further distally [7].

Tibial Tubercle

The tibial tubercle is the insertion point of the patellar tendon [14]. The tibial tubercle is a traction apophysis for the patellar tendon, and separation of the apophysis from the proximal end of the tibia results in the Osgood–Schlatter disease in adolescents (Fig. 1.7) [15].

Pertinent Ligaments and Tendons of the Patellofemoral Joint

Patellar Ligament (Tendon)

Although the patellar ligament is commonly referred to as the patellar tendon, its bone-to-bone attachments would classify it as a ligament. It courses from the lowest point of the patella to the tibial tubercle (Fig. 1.7) [7]. Multiple studies have determined the length of the patellar tendon to be between 40 and 55 mm [7, 14]. At its tibial tubercle insertion, it has been reported to have a width of 26.1 ± 2.8 mm [14].

Lateral Patellofemoral Ligament

Another important contributor to patellar stability is the lateral patellofemoral ligament (LPFL). The LPFL is a noticeable thickening of the lateral joint capsule, which connects the lateral edge of

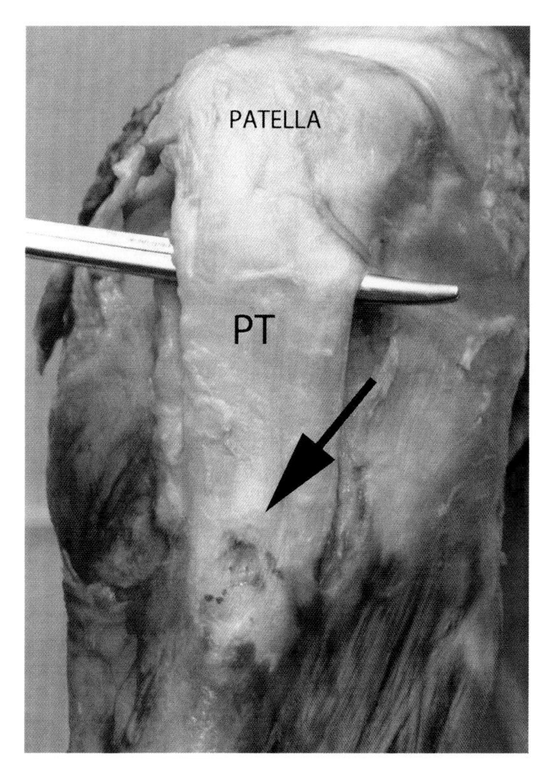

Fig. 1.7 The patellar tendon (PT) in a *left knee* is shown in relation to the patella. A bony protuberance due to Osgood–Schlatter disease can be seen near its insertion into the tibial tubercle (*arrow*)

the patella to the femur [16], and increased tension of the LPFL can cause patellar subluxation or lateral dislocation [16]. The LPFL resides in the deep layer of the lateral retinaculum [16], but it is smaller and more difficult to define than the medial patellofemoral ligament (MPFL) [9]. Some studies report that the LPFL might not be present in all knees [9, 17, 18], including reports of its presence in only two-thirds of knees [18]. The width of the LPFL has been reported to be an average of about 16 mm, and the length has been reported to be an average of about 42.1 mm [16]. A correlation between the length of the LPFL and the width of the lateral patellar facet has been reported, with shorter LPFLs correlating with wider lateral patellar facets [16].

Medial Patellofemoral Ligament

One of the most important and critical structures within the patellofemoral joint is the medial

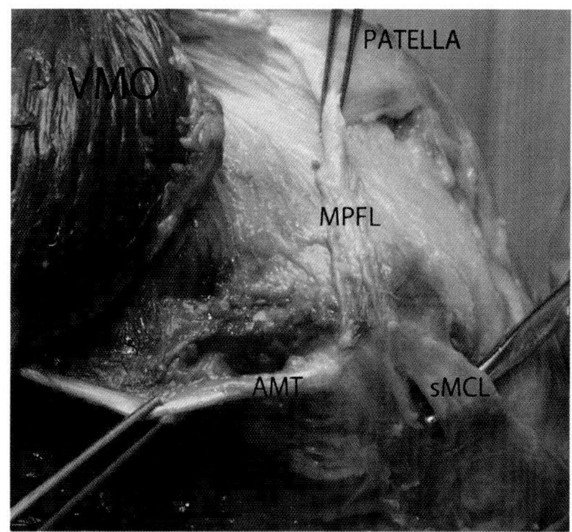

Fig. 1.8 The MPFL is shown (*top*) in relation to the attachments of the adductor magnus tendon (AMT) (*left*) and proximal superficial medial collateral ligament (sMCL) (*right*)

patellofemoral ligament (MPFL). Contrary to the presumption that the MPFL attaches at the femoral medial epicondyle, LaPrade et al. [10] provided measurable locations of the MPFL attachment in relation to the medial epicondyle and adductor tubercle (Fig. 1.8). They reported that the attachment site was an average of 10.6 mm proximal and 8.8 mm posterior to the medial epicondyle and 1.9 mm anterior and 3.8 mm distal to the adductor tubercle [10]. To improve noninvasive identification of the MPFL, a radiographic study reported on anteroposterior radiographs that the MPFL attached 13.3 ± 2.4 mm proximal to the medial epicondyle, 6.2 ± 1.5 mm distal to the adductor tubercle, 3.1 ± 1.0 mm proximal to the gastrocnemius tubercle, and 42.3 ± 2.1 mm proximal to the femoral joint line [19]. Through the use of two-dimensional lateral radiographs, the MPFL was determined to be 15.9 ± 3.2 mm from the medial epicondyle, 8.9 ± 2.0 mm from the adductor tubercle, 12.5 ± 3.0 mm from the gastrocnemius tubercle, 8.8 ± 5.3 mm anterior to the posterior femoral cortex extension line, and 2.6 ± 2.1 mm proximal to the perpendicular line at the posterior aspect of the Blumensaat's line [19]. The MPFL has an average length of 65.2 mm and attaches at the superomedial aspect of the medial border of

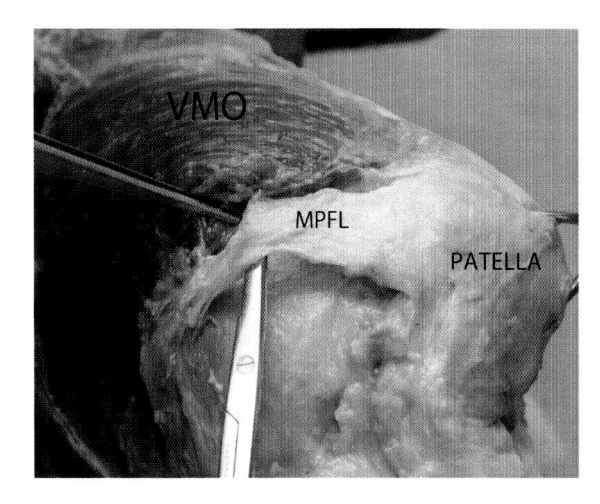

Fig. 1.9 The medial patellofemoral ligament (MPFL) is depicted in relation to the vastus medialis obliquus (VMO) and the patella in a *left knee*

the patella [8, 10]. The proximal edge is bounded, without tight adhesion, by the distal aspect of the VMO (Fig. 1.9) [10, 20]. The distal aspect is more or less a thickening within the fascial layer with some of the distal fibers intertwined with the deep layer of the medial retinaculum, which attaches to the patellar ligament [10, 20].

Medial Patellotibial Ligament

The medial patellotibial ligament (MPTL) helps to resist lateral translation of the patella. It originates inferiorly and medially on the patella and courses obliquely, as a condensation of the medial retinaculum, to its insertion approximately 1.5 cm distal to the joint line on the anteromedial region of the tibia (Fig. 1.10) [1, 21, 22].

Lateral Patellotibial Ligament

The lateral patellotibial ligament (LPTL) originates from the inferior aspect of the iliopatellar band and inserts anterior to Gerdy's tubercle (Fig. 1.11) [23]. The LPTL forms an anterior boundary for the superficial layer and connects the iliopatellar band and iliotibial tract [23].

Ligamentum Mucosum and Infrapatellar Fat Pad

The ligamentum mucosum, or infrapatellar plica (the thickened ligamentum mucosum), is another ligamentous structure in the patellofemoral joint [24]. It stretches from the top of the intercondylar notch of the femur to the infrapatellar fat pad anteriorly (Fig. 1.12) and lies anterior to the ACL [24, 25]. Additionally, some knees also have a ligamentum mucosum that is continuous with the ACL [24].

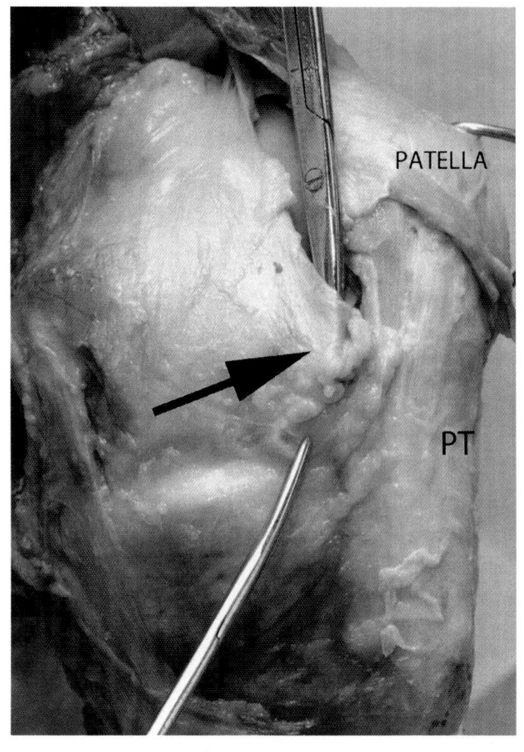

Fig. 1.10 A photograph illustrates the medial patellotibial ligament (MPTL) (*arrow*) in relation to the patella and patellar tendon (PT) in a *left knee*

The infrapatellar, or retropatellar, fat pad is an intracapsular, extrasynovial structure of the anterior aspect of the knee. The fat pad attaches to the ligamentum mucosum, proximal part of the patellar tendon, inferior aspect of the patella, anterior intermeniscal ligament, lateral meniscal horns, lateral retinaculum, and periosteum of the tibia [24, 26].

It can become inflamed in some patients after injury, but more commonly, it can become scarred and fibrosed after arthroscopic surgery and should be examined in all patients as a potential cause of anterior knee pain [24].

Quadriceps Tendon

The muscles of the rectus femoris, vastus lateralis, vastus medialis, and vastus intermedius join to form the quadriceps tendon in a trilaminar

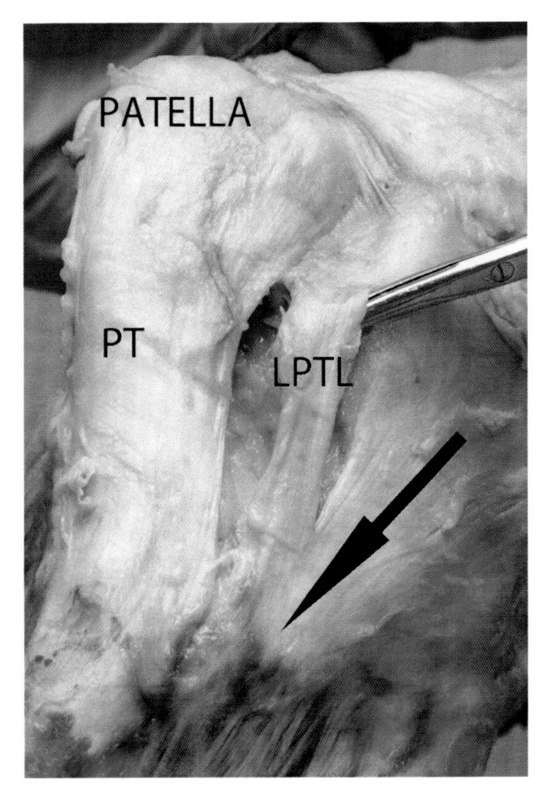

Fig. 1.11 The lateral patellotibial ligament (LPTL) is shown in relation to the patella and patellar tendon (PT) in a *left knee*. The insertion of the LPTL to Gerdy's tubercle is shown with an *arrow*

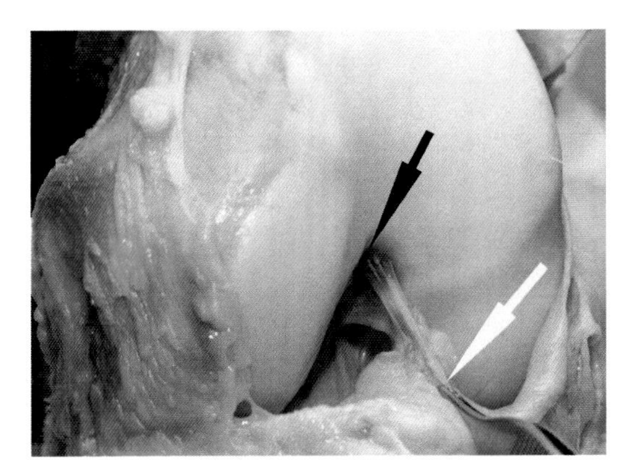

Fig. 1.12 A photograph of the ligamentum mucosum and its attachments to the infrapatellar fat pad (*white arrow*) and intercondylar notch (*black arrow*) in a *left knee* is shown

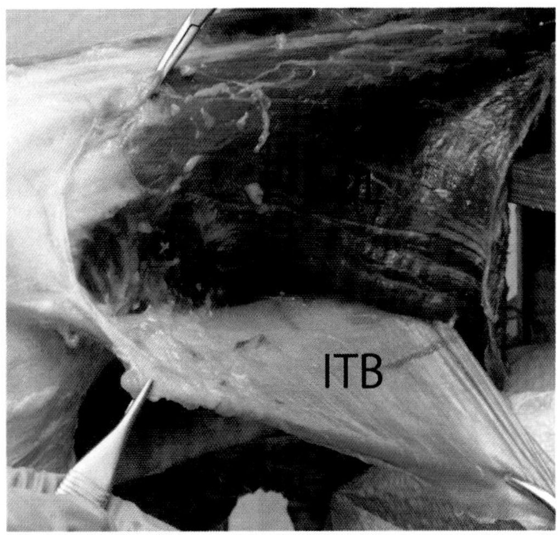

Fig. 1.13 A photograph displays the iliotibial band (ITB) reflected in a *left knee*. The vastus lateralis (VL) muscle is shown deep

fashion about 2 cm proximal to the patella (Fig. 1.1) [7, 9]. The quadriceps tendon extends over the anterior surface of the patella and combines distally with the patellar tendon [7]. The quadriceps tendon is reported to be approximately twice the thickness of the patella tendon at a mean length of 7 mm and a mean width of 27 mm [27, 28]. It also has a broader tendinous insertion into the patella [28]. Additionally, the quadriceps tendon is reported to have over 6 cm of common tendon length with increasing length of up to 2 cm when the rectus femoris and vastus intermedius tendons are included [27].

Pertinent Connective Tissue of the Patellofemoral Joint

Iliotibial Band and Iliopatellar Band

The iliotibial band (ITB), or iliotibial tract, is a prominent and complex structure on the lateral aspect of the knee (Fig. 1.13). The ITB originates from the tensor fascia femoris, gluteus medius, and gluteus maximus and then attaches to the linea aspera of the femur [23]. It then courses distally towards the knee, where it separates into

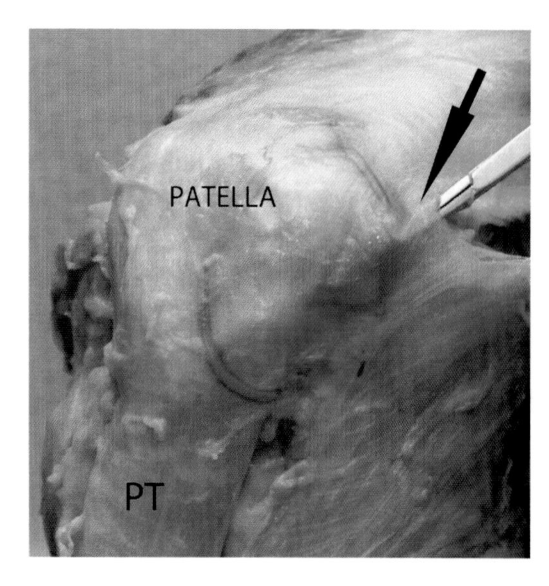

Fig. 1.14 A photograph is shown of the proximal aspect of the iliopatellar band (*arrow*) in relation to the patella and patellar tendon (PT) in a *left knee*

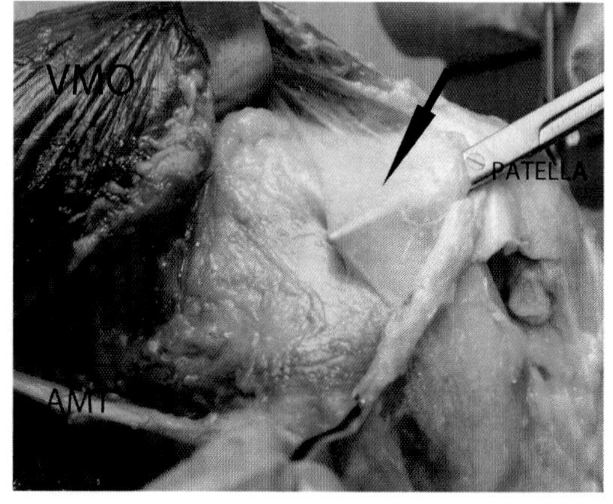

Fig. 1.15 The medial retinaculum (*arrow*) in a *left knee* is shown in relation to the vastus medialis obliquus (VMO), patella, and adductor magnus tendon (AMT)

two portions: the ITB and iliopatellar band (IPB) [23]. The iliopatellar band connects the anterior region of the iliotibial band and femur to the patella (Fig. 1.14) [23].

The iliotibial and iliopatellar bands consist of several anatomic layers: the aponeurotic layer, superficial layer, middle layer, deep layer, and capsulo-osseous layer [23]. The aponeurotic layer is the most superficial layer and consists of arciform fibers and the fascia that covers the vastus lateralis and biceps femoris [23]. It crosses over both the patella and patellar tendon at the anterior aspect and connects with the sartorius from the medial side [23].

Below the aponeurotic layer resides the superficial layer, which consists of the vastus lateralis, iliopatellar band, lateral patellotibial ligament, iliotibial tract, and biceps femoris [23]. The superficial layer inserts on the tibia at Gerdy's tubercle, and it is bounded anteriorly by the patella and lateral patellotibial ligament and posteriorly by the biceps femoris [23, 29]. The middle layer is rather simplistic and purely identified by a different orientation in its fibers in comparison to the superficial layer [23].

The deep layer has a three-dimensional orientation with an anterior border of the vastus lateralis and patella, posterior boundary of the biceps femoris, and distal boundary of the tibia [23]. It thickens and strengthens the superficial layer of the iliotibial tract and iliopatellar band laterally [23].

The capsulo-osseous layer originates from the fascia covering the plantaris and lateral gastrocnemius muscles and inserts just posterior to Gerdy's tubercle on the lateral tibial tubercle [23]. The short head of the biceps femoris muscle also inserts into the capsulo-osseous layer during its course [23].

Medial Retinaculum

The medial retinaculum (Fig. 1.15), or medial joint capsule, is an aponeurotic expansion from the vastus medialis that combines with the superficial medial collateral ligament (MCL) and the medial patellar tendon [6]. The medial retinaculum is much thinner than the lateral retinaculum [12]. The medial retinaculum consists of three ligaments: the medial patellofemoral ligament (MPFL), medial patellotibial ligament (MPTL), and medial patellomeniscal ligament [12]. These ligaments combine to be the main soft-tissue restraint to lateral patellar displacement [30].

Lateral Retinaculum

The lateral retinaculum is an aponeurotic expansion from the vastus lateralis that has been reported to be richly innervated [6]. It consists of two main layers: the superficial oblique layer and the deep transverse layer [6, 12]. The superficial oblique layer is comprised of the combination of the patellar tendon, vastus lateralis, and iliotibial band [12] and provides minimal support to patellar stability [6]. The deep transverse layer has three main structures: the lateral patellofemoral ligament (LPFL), the lateral patellotibial ligament (LPTL), and the patellotibial band [6, 12]. The LPFL is in the superior border of the deep transverse layer and connects the patella to the lateral epicondyle to provide superolateral support to the patella [6, 12]. The LPTL is located in the inferior border of the deep transverse layer and anchors the patella to the anterolateral tibia to provide lateral support to the patella [6, 12]. The patellotibial band is the deepest part of the deep transverse layer and runs obliquely from the distal lateral patella to the tibia, while parallel to the patella, to provide inferolateral support to the patella [6].

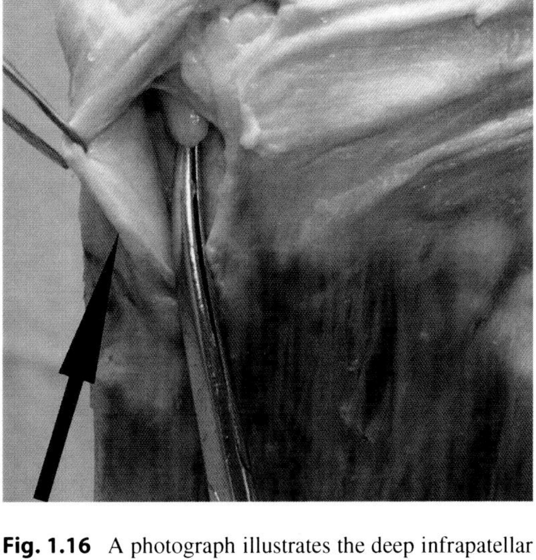

Fig. 1.16 A photograph illustrates the deep infrapatellar bursa in relation to the patella and patellar tendon (PT) in a *left knee*. The apron-like projection of fat can be seen inside the bursa (curved hemostat). The *arrow* shows the patellar tendon reflected

Primary Bursa of the Patellofemoral Joint

Deep Infrapatellar Bursa

The deep infrapatellar bursa is located posterior to the patellar tendon and just proximal to the tibial tubercle [14]. The bursa is slightly wider than the patellar tendon at its insertion site [14]. The deep infrapatellar bursa consists of two main portions: the posterior compartment and an apron-like projection of fat (Fig. 1.16) [14]. The posterior compartment is deeper and forms a trapezoidal shape between the proximal part of the tibial tubercle and the distal attachment of the retropatellar fat pad to the proximal tibia [14]. The lateral side of the base is wider than the medial side [14]. The apron-like projection of fat is anterior to the posterior compartment of the deep infrapatellar bursa and covers most of the posterior compartment [14].

Pes Anserine Bursa

The pes anserine bursa is located between the medial aspect of the tibia and the distal attachment of the superficial medial collateral ligament (MCL) and the conjoined tendons of the sartorius, semitendinosus, and gracilis (Fig. 1.17) [31]. This bursa does not communicate with the knee joint [31].

Semimembranosus Bursa

The semimembranosus bursa is located around the semimembranosus tendon on the posteromedial aspect of the tibia [32]. Its distal border is along the proximal edge of the tibial attachment of the direct arm of the semimembranosus tendon [10]. The bursa continues medially to where the anterior arm of the semimembranosus tendon attaches to the bone on the posteromedial aspect of the tibia (Fig. 1.18) [10]. The semimembranosus bursa has both deep and superficial pockets that connect along their posterosuperior aspect to give the shape of an inverted "U" [32].

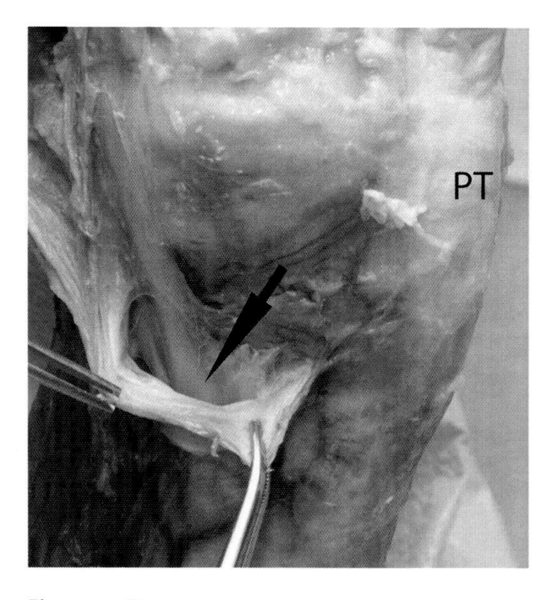

Fig. 1.17 The pes anserine bursa is shown in relation to the patellar tendon (PT) in a *left knee*. The attachment of the distal insertion of the superficial MCL (*arrow*) and the reflection of pes anserine tendons (curved hemostat and forceps) can also be seen

Biceps Femoris Bursa

The biceps femoris bursa, or fibular collateral ligament (FCL) bursa, is positioned laterally and anterior-anteromedially to the distal part of the FCL and just proximal to the FCL insertion on the fibular head [33]. Its lateral wall touches the anterior arm of the long head of the biceps femoris muscle [33]. The biceps femoris bursa forms an inverted "J" shape around the lateral, anterior, and anteromedial regions of the FCL (Fig. 1.19) [33]. The biceps femoris has been reported to have a mean length of 18 mm and a mean width at its midportion of 8.4 mm [33].

Prepatellar Bursa and Superficial Infrapatellar Bursa

The prepatellar bursa is located anterior to the patella in the subcutaneous tissue [34]. It is generally centered anterior to the patella, and it has been reported to have three compartments—superficial, intermediate, and deep—separated by two thin septa [31, 34]. The superficial compartment is located between the subcutaneous tissue and the transverse superficial fascia [31, 34].

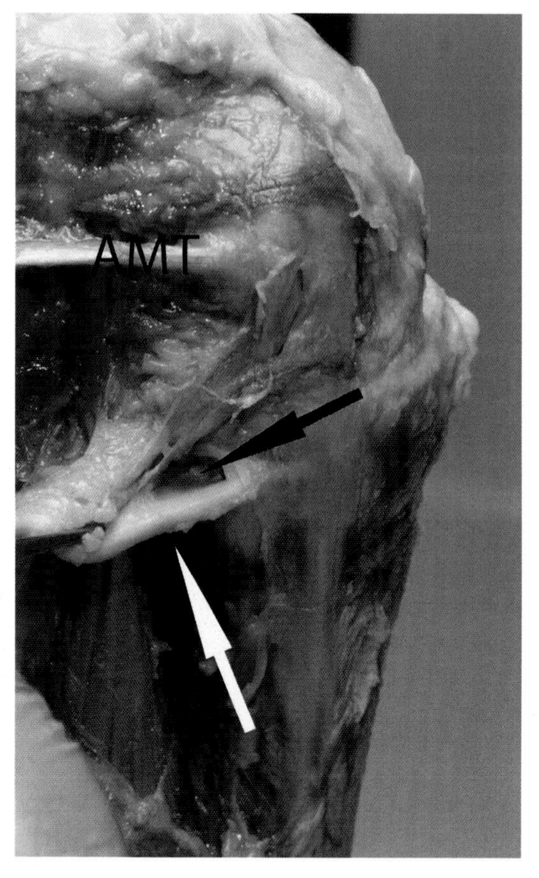

Fig. 1.18 A photograph shows the semimembranosus bursa (*black arrow*) in relation to the adductor magnus tendon (AMT) and semimembranosus tendon (*white arrow*) in a *left knee*

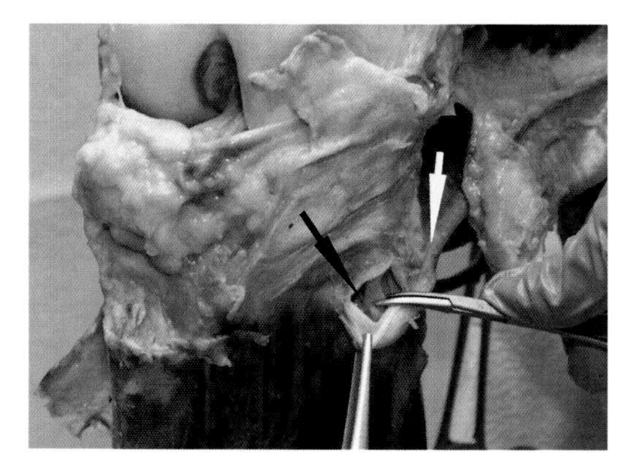

Fig. 1.19 A photograph illustrates the biceps femoris bursa (*black arrow*) and biceps femoris tendon (*white arrow*) in a *left knee*. The fibular collateral ligament (FCL) can also be seen inside of this bursal space (held in curved hemostat)

The intermediate compartment is located between the transverse superficial fascia and intermediate oblique fascia [31, 34]. The deep compartment is situated between the intermediate oblique fascia and the deep longitudinal fibers of the rectus femoris tendon [31, 34].

The superficial infrapatellar bursa is located anterior to the patellar tendon [35]. It is situated in the soft tissue of the anterodistal third of the patellar tendon [35]. In some cases, the bursa can be located directly anterior to the tibial tubercle [35].

Primary Arterial Supply for the Patellofemoral Joint

Geniculate Arteries

The blood supply to the knee is accomplished by an anastomosis of five major arteries: the superomedial, superolateral, middle, inferomedial, and inferolateral genicular arteries [7, 12]. This circumpatellar anastomosis occurs between the anterior tibial recurrent artery and all of the genicular arteries, except for the middle genicular artery [12]. The circumpatellar anastomosis provides a blood supply for the superficial and deep bone, synovium, capsule, retinaculum, and subcutaneous fascia [12].

The superomedial genicular artery arises from the popliteal artery just above the tibial joint line and then travels medially and anteriorly to join the circumpatellar anastomosis [12]. It is located anterior to the semimembranosus and semitendinosus muscles [12].

The superolateral genicular artery divides from the popliteal artery just above the tibial joint line and then travels laterally and anteriorly to anastomose with the descending lateral collateral femoral artery [7, 12]. The superolateral genicular artery supplies the vastus lateralis, vastus intermedius, and branches of the femoral nerve [7, 12].

The middle genicular artery travels anterior to the joint line and into the posterior joint capsule, where it supplies the anterior cruciate ligament (ACL) and posterior cruciate ligament (PCL) [12]. The middle genicular artery is the only artery that does not make a contribution to the circumpatellar anastomosis [12].

The inferomedial genicular artery divides from the popliteal artery just below the tibial joint line and travels anteromedially along the side of the tibial metaphysis to provide the medial collateral ligament (MCL) with blood supply [7, 12]. It then anastomoses with the saphenous branch of the descending genicular branch and anterior tibial recurrent artery [7, 12]. The inferomedial geniculate artery is the most inferior of genicular arteries [7].

The inferolateral genicular artery arises from the popliteal artery just below the tibial joint line and travels anteriorly along the lateral joint line next to the lateral meniscus [7]. It then forms an anastomosis with the anterior tibial recurrent artery and supplies the fibular collateral ligament (FCL) [12].

Primary Sensory Innervation of the Patellofemoral Joint

Infrapatellar Branch of Saphenous Nerve

The infrapatellar branch of the saphenous nerve is a sensory nerve that innervates the anterior aspect of the knee [36]. The nerve is superficial to the sartorius and curves anteroinferiorly below the patella to supply the skin and fascia over the anterior and medial knee [37]. The nerve has also been reported to have two main trunks, the superior and inferior branches, that are very distinct and course laterally and distally after dividing from the main saphenous nerve [37]. In knee extension, the superior branch has been reported to be a mean of approximately 4.5 cm distal to the medial border of the patella and 2.4 cm distal to the inferior pole of the patella [36]. The inferior branch has been reported to be a mean of about 7.5 cm distal to the medial border of the patella and 5.9 cm distal to the inferior pole of the patella [36].

References

1. Arendt EA. Medial side patellofemoral anatomy: surgical implications in patellofemoral instability. In: Arendt EA, Dejour D, Zaffagnini S, editors. Patellofemoral pain, implications, and arthritis. New York, NY: Springer; 2010. p. 149–53.
2. Fulkerson JP. Diagnosis and treatment of patients with patellofemoral pain. Am J Sports Med. 2002; 30(3):447–56.
3. Baldwin JL. The anatomy of the medial patellofemoral ligament. Am J Sports Med. 2009;37(12): 2355–61.
4. Nomura E, Inoue M, Osada N. Anatomical analysis of the medial patellofemoral ligament of the knee, especially the femoral attachment. Knee Surg Sports Traumatol Arthrosc. 2005;13:510–5.
5. Philippot R, Chouteau J, Wegrzyn J, Testa R, Fessy MH, Moyen B. Medial patellofemoral ligament anatomy: implications for its surgical reconstruction. Knee Surg Sports Traumatol Arthrosc. 2009;17: 475–9.
6. O'Brien M. Clinical anatomy of the patellofemoral joint. Int J Sports Med. 2001;2(1):1–8.
7. Tria AJ, Alicea JA. Embryology and anatomy of the patella. In: Scuderi GR, editor. The patella. New York, NY: Springer; 1995. p. 11–23.
8. Amis AA. Current concepts on anatomy and biomechanics of patellar stability. Sports Med Arthrosc. 2007;15:48–56.
9. Waligora AC, Johanson NA, Hirsch BE. Clinical anatomy of the quadriceps femoris and extensor apparatus of the knee. Clin Orthop Relat Res. 2009;467: 3297–306.
10. LaPrade RF, Engebretsen AH, Ly TV, et al. The anatomy of the medial part of the knee. J Bone Joint Surg Am. 2007;89(9):2000–10.
11. Tecklenburg K, Dejour D, Hoser C, Fink C. Bony and cartilaginous anatomy of the patellofemoral joint. Knee Surg Sports Traumatol Arthrosc. 2006;14: 235–40.
12. Waryasz GR, McDermott AY. Patellofemoral pain syndrome (PFPS): a systematic review of anatomy and potential risk factors. Dyn Med. 2008;7:9.
13. Wiberg G. Roentgenographic and anatomic studies on the femoro-patellar joint. Acta Orthop Scand. 1941; 12:319–410.
14. LaPrade RF. The anatomy of the deep infrapatellar bursa of the knee. Am J Sports Med. 1998;26(1): 129–32.
15. Antich TJ, Brewster CE. Osgood-Schlatter disease: review of literature and physical therapy management. J Orthop Sports Phys Ther. 1985;7(1):5–10.
16. Navarro MS, Beltrani Filho CA, Akita Junior J, Navarro RD, Cohen M. Relationship between the lateral patellofemoral ligament and the width of the lateral patellar facet. Acta Ortop Bras. 2010;18(1):19–22.
17. Merican AM, Sanghavi S, Iranpur F, Amis AA. The structural properties of the lateral retinaculum and capsular complex of the knee. J Biomech. 2009;42(14): 2323–9.
18. Reider B, Marshall JL, Koslin B, Ring B, Girgis FG. The anterior aspect of the knee joint. J Bone Joint Surg Am. 1981;63-A(3):351–6.
19. Wijdicks CA, Griffith CJ, LaPrade RF, et al. Radiographic identification of the primary medial knee structures. J Bone Joint Surg Am. 2009;91(3): 521–9.
20. Mochizuki T, Nimura A, Tateishi T, Yamaguchi K, Muneta T, Akita K. Anatomic study of the attachment of the medial patellofemoral ligament and its characteristic relationships to the vastus intermedius. Knee Surg Sports Traumatol Arthrosc. 2013;21: 305–10.
21. Conlan T, Garth WP, Lemons JE. Evaluation of the medial soft-tissue restraints of the extensor mechanism of the knee. J Bone Joint Surg Am. 1993; 75-A(5):682–92.
22. Hautamaa PV, Fithian DC, Kaufman KR, Daniel DM, Pohlmeyer AM. Medial soft tissue restraints in lateral patellar instability and repair. Clin Orthop Relat Res. 1998;349:174–82.
23. Terry GC, Hughston JC, Norwood LA. The anatomy of the iliopatellar band and iliotibial tract. Am J Sports Med. 1986;14(1):39–45.
24. Dragoo JL, Johnson C, McConnell J. Evaluation and treatment of disorders of the infrapatellar fat pad. Sports Med. 2012;42(1):51–67.
25. Tingstad EM. The knee. In: McGinty JB, editor. Operative arthroscopy. Philadelphia, PA: Lippincott Williams & Wilkins; 2003. p. 178–86.
26. Nelson EW, LaPrade RF. The anterior intermeniscal ligament of the knee. Am J Sports Med. 2000;28(1): 74–6.
27. Harris NL, Smith DA, Lamoreaux L, Purnell M. Central quadriceps tendon for anterior cruciate ligament reconstruction. Part I: morphometric and biomechanical evaluation. Am J Sports Med. 1997;25(1): 23–8.
28. Stäubli HU, Schatzmann L, Brunner P, Rincón L, Nolte LP. Quadriceps tendon and patellar ligament: cryosectional anatomy and structural properties in young adults. Knee Surg Sports Traumatol Arthrosc. 1996;4:100–10.
29. Terry GC, LaPrade RF. The posterolateral aspect of the knee: anatomy and surgical approach. Am J Sports Med. 1996;24(6):732–9.
30. Feller JA, Amis AA, Andrish JT, et al. Surgical biomechanics of the patellofemoral joint. Arthroscopy. 2007;23(5):542–53.
31. Hirji Z, Hunjun JS, Choudur HN. Imaging of the bursae. J Clin Imaging Sci. 2011;1(1):22–8.
32. Demeyere N, De Maeseneer M, Van Roy P, Osteaux M, Shahabpor M. Imaging of semimembranosus bursitis: MR findings in three patients and anatomical study. JBR-BTR. 2003;86(6):332–4.

33. LaPrade RF, Hamilton CD. The fibular collateral ligament-biceps femoris bursa: an anatomic study. Am J Sports Med. 1997;25(4):439–43.
34. Aguiar RO, Viegas F, Fernandez RY, Trudell D, Haghighi P, Resnick D. The prepatellar bursa: cadaveric investigation of regional anatomy with MRI after sonographically guided bursography. AJR Am J Roentgenol. 2007;188:W355–8.
35. Viegas FC, Aguiar ROC, Gasparetto E, Marchiori E, Trudell DJ, Haghighi P, Resnick D. Deep and superficial infrapatellar bursae: cadaveric investigation of regional anatomy using magnetic resonance after ultrasound-guided bursography. Skeletal Radiol. 2007;36:41–6.
36. Tifford CD, Spero L, Luke T, Plancher KD. The relationship of the infrapatellar branches of the saphenous nerve to arthroscopy portals and incisions for anterior cruciate ligament surgery. Am J Sports Med. 2000; 28(4):562–7.
37. Arthornthurasook A, Gaew-Im K. Study of the infrapatellar nerve. Am J Sports Med. 1988;16(1): 57–9.

Lateral Patella Dislocations: History, Physical Exam, and Imaging

2

John Wechter, Jeffrey Macalena, and Elizabeth A. Arendt

Introduction

Most sports medicine physicians today consider lateral patella dislocations in the differential diagnosis of an acute knee injury in an athlete. In the recent past, this was not necessarily the case. Hughston, in 1964, felt that an athlete's report of a knee giving way was almost never attributable to a patellar dislocation [1]. Rather he opined "[these] immediate impressions are due to the unfortunate and erroneous idea that subluxation of the patella occurs predominantly in the female and is absent in the athlete." To this effect, acute first-time [primary] patellar dislocations have been shown to occur nearly equally across sexes, with greater than 60 % usually attributed to athletic activity [2–4].

Acute, primary lateral patellar dislocations occur primarily in the second decade of life [4, 5] at a rate of 29 per 100,000 [4]. They are associated with significant disability including pain or feelings of instability in 30–50 % of people [6, 7]. Associated injuries frequently occur, including medial patellofemoral ligament injuries in over 80 % of patients and associated ligamentous or meniscal injury in 31 % [8]. Though osteochondral fractures in over 50 % [7, 9–11] have been reported in the literature for primary and recurrent dislocations literature, a recent systemic review noted 24.7 % of patients had chondral and osteochondral damage in primary patella dislocations [12].

Recurrent patellar dislocation is a significant problem, reported in 15–44 % of patients treated nonsurgically [3, 6, 13, 14]. A prior dislocation is, in itself, a significant risk factor for having a recurrent dislocation, and risk progressively increases with subsequent dislocations. Fithian reported that patients with multiple dislocations, either ipsilateral or contralateral, had more than double the incidence of a future instability episode in comparison to first-time dislocators. Sex and positive family history also have a high correlation to recurrence risk. While first-time dislocations occur equally across sexes, recurrent dislocators tended to be female and tend to have a positive family history of patellar instability [4]. In addition, certain anatomic features have a high prevalence in patients with symptomatic patellar instability. These include trochlear dysplasia (>85 %), an increased tibial tubercle to trochlear groove (TT–TG) horizontal distance (56 %), patella alta (24 %), and patellar tilt (>70 %) of patients with instability [3, 5, 15, 16].

The history, physical exam, and imaging after an acute patellar dislocation should therefore be performed with the goals of (1) diagnosing the patellar dislocation, (2) recognizing associated

J. Wechter, M.D. • J. Macalena, M.D. (✉)
E.A. Arendt, M.D.
Department of Orthopaedic Surgery, University of Minnesota, 2450 Riverside Avenue, Suite R200, Minneapolis, MN, 55454, USA
e-mail: jwechter@umn.edu; maca0049@umn.edu; arend001@uwn.edu

R.V. West and A.C. Colvin (eds.), *The Patellofemoral Joint in the Athlete*,
DOI 10.1007/978-1-4614-4157-1_2, © Springer Science+Business Media New York 2014

injuries, and (3) recognizing any historical, congenital, or anatomic risk factors for recurrent dislocation.

History

Mechanism

The patient nearly always describes an indirect mechanism, where the limb and torso is internally rotated on a fixed tibia as the knee is held in a position of flexion and valgus. This knee position creates a strong lateral force on the patella. Less commonly, patients may report a dislocation after a direct blow to the patella [6, 7, 13, 17]. As the patella dislocates, patients experience a sudden giving way of the knee. Reduction of the patella is usually spontaneous and occurs as the patient contracts the quadriceps and straightens the knee. A manual reduction, when required, is usually accomplished by passively extending the knee and manipulating the patella medially. In very rare instances, the patella may impact into the lateral aspect of the lateral femoral condyle, requiring an open reduction [18].

Associated Injuries

The location and nature of the pain may help identify underlying injuries. Though the patella is dislocated laterally, pain is predominantly medially based due to the injury to the medial patella soft tissue structures. Pain located medially near the adductor tubercle of the distal femur may signify MPFL avulsion from its femoral insertion. The most common site of injury has varied in the literature; however, a recent review has shown the incidence to be patella attachment 54 % (range 13–75 %), midsubstance tears 12 % (range 0–30 %), and femoral attachment site 34 % (range 12–66 %) [19]. Further, pain described along either the lateral femoral condyle or medial patella may correlate with chondral injury sustained during patella relocation. Mechanical symptoms such as locking or catching suggest an obstruction to movement, such as loose bodies or a displaced meniscal tear.

Differential Diagnosis

The diagnosis of patella dislocation is most apparent when the patient actually describes the patella subluxing or dislocating. Other descriptions of the incident may be confounding. For example, twisting of the knee with sudden giving way and swelling is also seen with ACL injuries. Reports of the knee "giving out" is nonspecific and can be seen with other entities such as meniscal pathology, loose bodies or chondral injuries, or simply patellofemoral (PF) pain with bent knee activities. Patients may report feelings of instability with pain and crepitus, such as with descending stairs, without movement of the patella from its groove.

Physical Exam

The focused physical exam of the PF joint should be approached with the goal of establishing the diagnosis of patellar instability and identifying associated injuries and anatomic risk factors for instability. One should use a systematic approach including inspection; palpation; testing for laxity; assessing patellar position, stability, and tracking; and identification of cartilage injury. In addition to the PF exam, a comprehensive knee exam should also be performed (meniscal provocative maneuvers, measurement of range of motion, and varus-valgus, anterior-posterior knee stability, extensor mechanism integrity) to rule out concomitant injuries.

Inspection

Inspection of the knee should be performed in a standing, seated, and supine position. In the standing position, note whether the knees are directed straight forward. Knees turned inward may represent an underlying internal femoral torsion or external tibial torsion, one or both which may contribute to lateral tracking of the patella. Coronal plane alignment such as excessive *genu valgum* may also be observed, though is better evaluated with long leg standing alignment radiographs.

In a seated position, calculate the tubercle-sulcus angle, a measure of the relationship between the tibial tubercle and the trochlear sulcus. Described by Kolowich et al., the test assesses the distal force vector acting on the patella. With the knee flexed at 90°, a vertical line drawn downward from the center of the patella (which represents the center of the trochlear groove) should intersect the tibial tubercle in asymptomatic individuals. Though an exact upper value of normal has not been establish, a tibial tubercle lateral to this line, particularly if greater than 10°, may contribute to an increased lateral pull on the patella [20].

In a supine position, evaluate the skin for prior incisions and signs of trauma. The presence of an effusion is important to note. Typically a primary lateral patella dislocation is associated with dramatic swelling with disruption of the medial capsule and extracapsular extension.

Palpation

In systematic fashion, palpate all relevant patellofemoral joint structures and stabilizers, including the MPFL, tibial tubercle, patellar tendon, quadriceps tendon, and the patella itself. Pain or palpable defects should be correlated with injury mechanism and imaging findings. Next, apply compressive force to the patella, at different angles to concentrate the force on various regions of the patella and trochlea. Feel anteriorly for patellar crepitus during knee flexion and extension. Pain and/or crepitus, though not exacting in its relationship to underlying pathology [21, 22], should be correlated with imaging to rule out localized chondral injury.

Patellar Stability and Tracking

Patellar Apprehension Test: The patellar apprehension test is typically performed with the knee in full extension. A lateral directed force is applied to the patella. A positive test is confirmed by the presence of patient verbal reported apprehension and pain or a strong quadriceps muscle contraction resisting lateral patella translation. This is always compared to the contralateral (usually uninvolved) side for comparison. Ahmad modified the apprehension test and renamed it the "moving patellar apprehension test" (MPAT), where the second portion of the exam involved medial-directed pressure (rather than lateral), with a positive result defined as the patient expressing a sense of relief. He compared his results to the ability to dislocate the same patellae under anesthesia. He found a positive MPAT to be highly sensitive (100 %) and specific (88.4 %) for detecting patellar instability under anesthesia [23, 24].

Patellar Glide: Restraint of the patella to lateral translation is dependent on both bony and soft tissue structures as well as the degree of knee flexion (dictating patellar position in the trochlea) [17, 25, 26]. Of the soft tissue structures, the MPFL was found to provide 53 % and 60 % of the total restraint to lateral patellar translation in two biomechanical studies [25, 26]. The high rate of MPFL tears after patellar dislocations warrants evaluation of the medial restraints via lateral patellar glide. The exam is performed by grasping the patella and shifting it laterally, quantifying the maximum translation in number of patellar quadrants that are lateral to the lateral trochlear ridge (Fig. 2.1) [20].

Translation less than two quadrants is considered normal while two or more quadrants represent laxity of the medial restraints. When this is unilateral and associated with an acute injury, it likely represents an MPFL injury. More important than the absolute translation is the comparison to the opposite (uninjured) knee, whether there is a firm or soft endpoint, and the presence of an apprehension sign with this test.

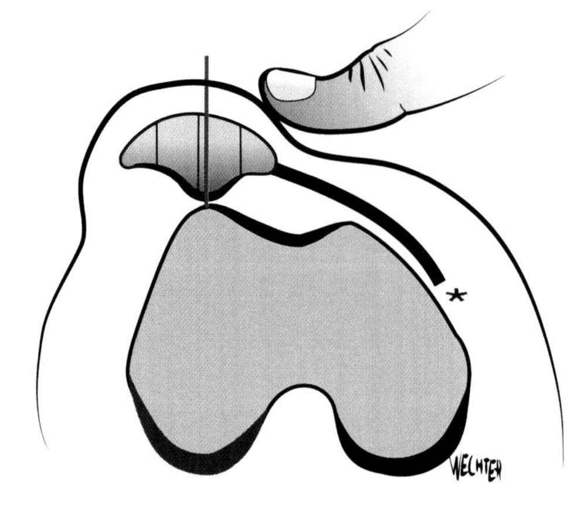

Fig. 2.1 Patellar glide: greater than two quadrants of lateral patellar translation, in relation to the lateral. Published with kind permission of John Wechter 2013. All rights reserved

Medial translation is assessed in similar fashion. Less than one quadrant of medial translation signifies a tight lateral retinaculum [20].

Patellar Tilt: Lateral tilt of the patella as assessed on overlapping CT images is seen in 83 % of patients with symptomatic patellofemoral instability [16]. On physical exam, the diagnosis is made by lifting the lateral patellar edge, attempting to manually restore it to a normal horizontal position. Inability to do so signifies the presence of a tight lateral retinaculum [27].

Patellar Tracking: In a supine position, the patient elevates their leg against gravity, then actively flexes and extends the knee slowly. As the knee nears full extension, the patella is normally seen to track slightly lateral with a smooth progression. More pronounced lateral movement of the patella in terminal knee extension has been termed "J-tracking" or the "J-sign." This phenomenon is not clearly understood [28] but is likely due to a combination of factors, most prominently the morphology of the trochlea and sagittal position of the patella in terminal extension (dictated by patella height and trochlear length) [29].

Comprehensive Knee Exam

A patellar dislocation may be accompanied by additional injuries to the knee; therefore, a thorough physical exam of the knee should include range of motion, an evaluation of ligaments, strength testing, and neurovascular assessment.

Imaging

Imaging studies are obtained to confirm the diagnosis, recognize associated injuries, and identify anatomic abnormalities that may have predisposed the patient to a patellar dislocation. Objective measurements of patella position and trochlear morphology are used to guide surgical planning.

Preferred Studies

Standard office radiographs and magnetic resonance imaging (MRI) are usually sufficient in achieving the above stated goals and are the mainstay in the workup following a patella dislocation. A combination of radiographs and MRI are employed to identify anatomic risk factors for dislocation including patellar tilt, height and translation, trochlear morphology, and tibial tubercle-trochlear groove alignment. Computed tomography (CT) is less commonly used, though it can be useful when femoral or tibial version is suspected as an underlying bony risk factor. Importantly, the complexity of patellofemoral instability demands that assumptions and decisions not be based on any single radiologic finding or measurement. Rather, a combined assessment of all variables, in conjunction with the history and physical exam, will help the clinician better understand the injury pattern, risk for re-dislocation, and guide further treatment.

Radiographs

Essential radiographic views include (1) AP of bilateral knees, with bilateral hip-to-ankle standing coronal alignment films; (2) weight-bearing true lateral of both knees in 20–30° of flexion; and (3) axial views of both knees in a low flexion angle (20–30°).

AP Bilateral Knees, AP Hip-to-Ankle Alignment Films

AP radiographs should be obtained in weight bearing. The focused view of the knees may show asymmetric patella height or evidence of a patellar dislocation such as a vertical patella fracture, though these findings are better seen on other views. The long leg hip-to-knee alignment films are primarily used for evaluation of coronal knee alignment. The method described by Stevens et al. [30] may be the simplest. The mechanical axis is drawn from the center of the hip to the center of the ankle and should pass through the central one-third of the tibial plateau. Deviation medially or laterally is deemed *varus* or *valgus* malalignment [30]. The *Q*-angle, representing the lateral vector of pull between the quadriceps and patellar tendon, is the angle between a line from the anterior–superior iliac spine to the center of the patella and a line from the patella to the tibial tubercle. Some authors have attributed *genu valgum* or increased *Q*-angle to recurrent patella dislocations or to abnormal patellar congruence [31, 32]; however, this has been strongly contested [33–36].

Lateral Radiographs

The lateral radiograph is typically taken with the knee flexed 30° in full weight bearing, which tensions the patellar tendon and leads to a statistically significant difference in patellar height when compared to non-weight-bearing films [37, 38]. The bent knee stance is necessary to separate the image from the opposite knee. Some have chosen to have a single leg stance with the opposite hip flexed to 90°; this can be useful to determine patella height in full extension, with quadriceps muscle tension fully engaged.

The lateral view is helpful for identifying trauma incurred during a patellar dislocation, such as transverse patellar fractures from a direct impact, or proximal/distal patellar pole avulsions. It also allows evaluation of patellar instability risk factors, specifically patellar tilt, patella alta, and trochlear dysplasia.

Patellar Tilt on the Lateral Radiograph

Patellar tilt is present in greater than 70 % of patients with symptomatic patellar instability [5, 16]. While Dejour and Burmann measured patellar tilt on the CT scan, Malghem described a classification system based on the lateral radiograph, assessing the relationship of the central patellar ridge to the lateral facet. With increasing patellar tilt, the central patellar ridge will become superimposed on, and eventually anterior to, the lateral facet [39] (Fig. 2.2).

Femoral-Based Patellar Height Measurement

The *Biedert patellotrochlear index* [40] (Fig. 2.3) is based on sagittal MR images. It measures the percent of patellar articular surface which is overlapped by the trochlea cartilage. A trochlea–patella cartilage engagement of less than 12.5 % (index <0.125) signifies too little overlap and is labeled patella alta, while greater than 50 % overlap (index >0.5) indicates patella infera.

Tibial-Based Patellar Height Measurement (Fig. 2.4)

The Insall-Salvati (IS) index is calculated by dividing the patellar tendon length over the greatest longitudinal dimension of the patella. The normal range is 0.8–1.2 with values greater than 1.2 considered patella alta. Since the IS index uses the tibial tubercle, it should not be used in patients with prior tibial tubercle osteotomies or in preoperative planning for their osteotomy. Additionally, the IS index should not be used when a long distal non-articular patellar pole is present, as this may underestimate the height of the *articular* portion of the patella [41].

The modified Insall-Salvati (MIS) index [41] describes the location of the articular portion of the patella in relation to the tibial tubercle. It is useful when a large distal patellar pole is present, as the calculation ignores the distal non-articulating portion of the patella. Values greater than two are deemed patella alta. The cutoff value of two, chosen in order to simplify calculation, was unfortunately found to miss 22 % of patella alta cases when compared to other indices [41].

The Caton–Deschamps (CD) index [42] measures the distance from the anterior–superior border of the tibia to the distal aspect of the patellar articular surface and divides this by the

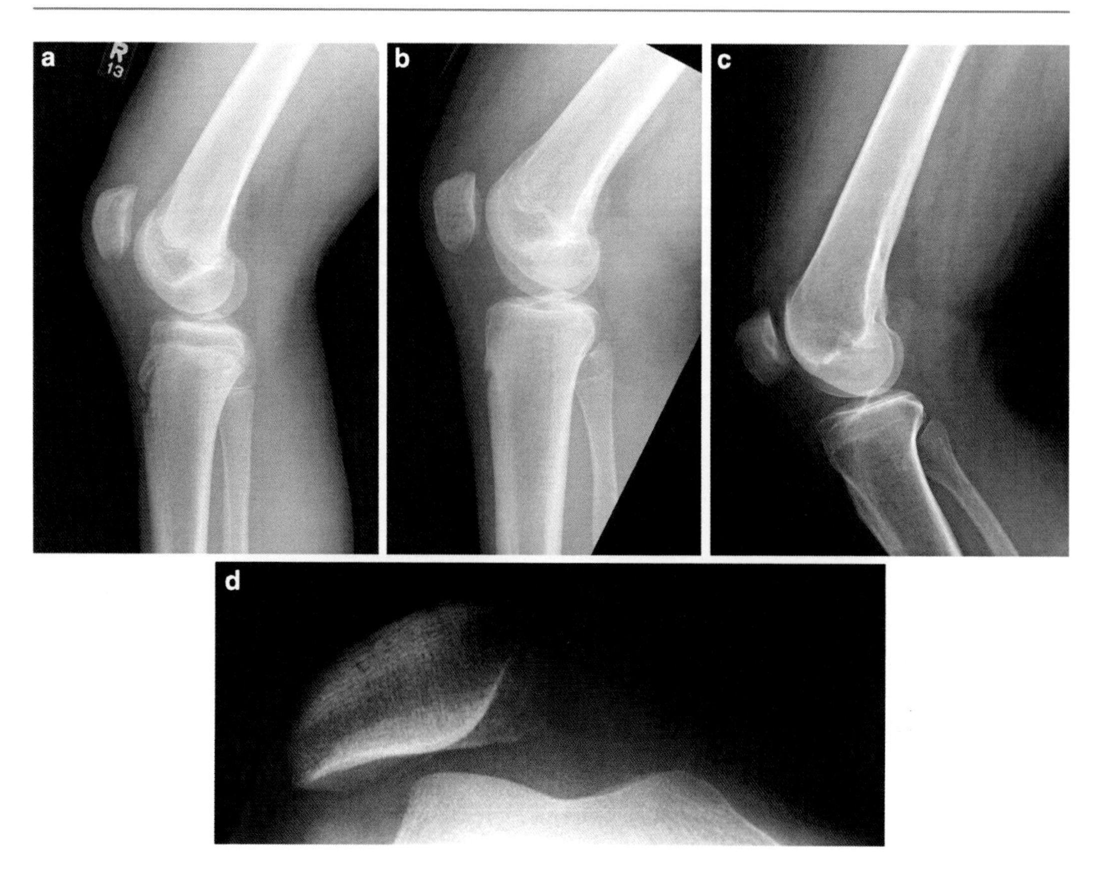

Fig. 2.2 Patella tilt evaluation as described by Malghem et al. [39]. (**a**) Position 1 normal position with the lateral facet artesior to the crest (median ridge). (**b**) Position 2 is mild tilt with the two lines (lateral facet and central ridge) superimposed; (**c**) Position 3 is major tilt with the lateral facet posterior to the crest; (**d**) Axial view of the patella at 45° that correcponds to image "c" (major tilt)

length of the patellar articular surface. The normal range is 0.6 and 1.2. Since the measurement does not use the tibial tubercle, this index can be used to evaluate patella height after a distalization of the tibial tubercle. Disadvantages include the occasional difficulty in identifying the anterior–superior portion of the tibia or the inferior margin of the patellar articular surface [24].

The Blackburne–Peel (BP) index [43] is calculated by first drawing a line along the tibial articular surface. The perpendicular distance from this line to the inferior margin of the patellar articular surface is divided by the length of the articular surface, with the normal range between 0.5 and 1.0. Dependence on the tibial plateau may be a downside, due to measurements being affected by tibial slope variations, as well the technical difficulty of obtaining an adequate lateral radiograph [24].

The most optimal patellar height index has not yet been established; however, certain generalizations can be made. First, for the sake of simplicity, tibial-based indices are more widely used than femoral-based indices, since they can be calculated at any degree of knee flexion, and calculations can be made on office acquired imaging. Understanding the strengths and limitations of these measurements may dictate which indices to use. For example, prior distalization of the tibial tubercle or abnormal morphology of the distal patellar pole limits the use of the IS ratio. For these instances, MIS may be used, though this was found to miss 22 % of patella alta as judged by other methods [41]. An overall comparison of

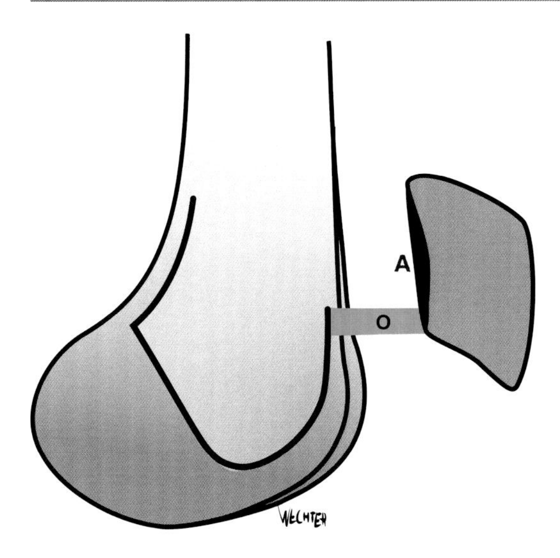

Fig. 2.3 *Biedert patellotrochlear index*: patellar–trochlear overlap (o)/patellar articular surface length (*A*) should be greater than 0.125 (12.5 %) [40]. Published with kind permission of John Wechter 2013.

the tibial-based indices was performed by Seil et al. [44]. He discovered a wide variation between the indices in classifying any given patella as alta, baha, or normal. He ultimately recommended the BP ratio since it was the most intermediate ratio in terms of frequency of diagnosing patella height as normal, alta, or baha. The best measurement may have yet to be developed. In 2011, Portner introduced a new tibial-based technique which may simplify the process [45]. He describes measuring the angle between a line drawn along the tibial plateau and the line from the inferior patellar articular margin to the posterior aspect of the plateau line [45].

Trochlear Dysplasia on the Lateral Radiograph

A true lateral radiograph of the knee (posterior condyles aligned) provides a thorough evaluation of the trochlea [37, 46] but requires an

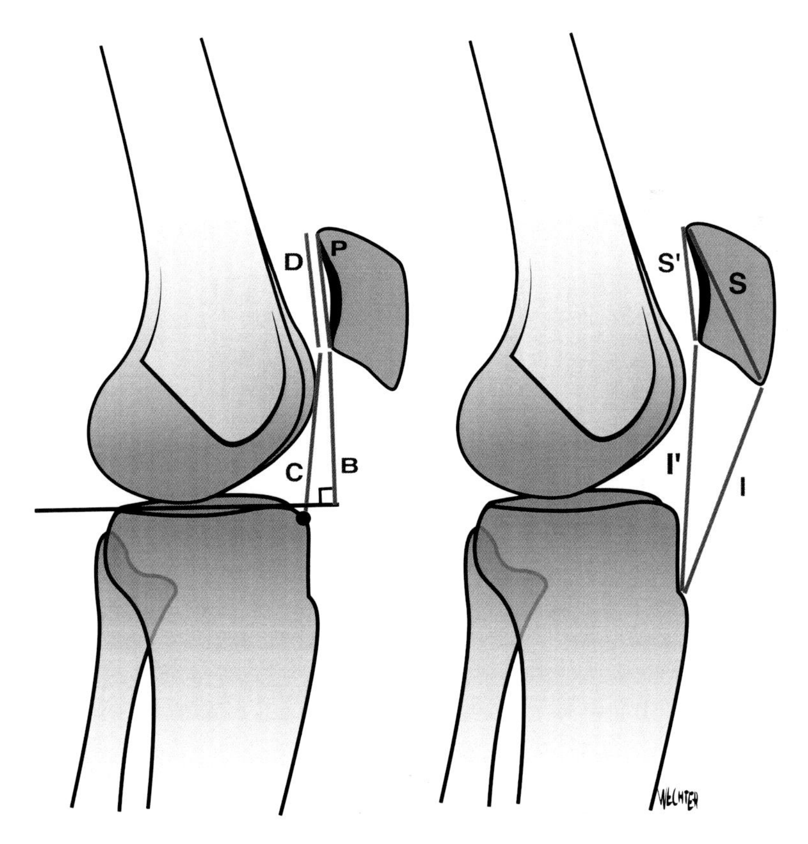

Fig. 2.4 Patellar height: measured on the lateral radiograph. *Bold line* = tibial surface. *Dot* = anterior–superior aspect of tibia. Caton–Deschamps index = *C*/*D*. Blackburne–Peel index = *B*/*P*. Insall–Salvati index = *I*/*S*. Modified Insall–Salvati = *I′*/*S′*. Published with kind permission of John Wechter 2013.

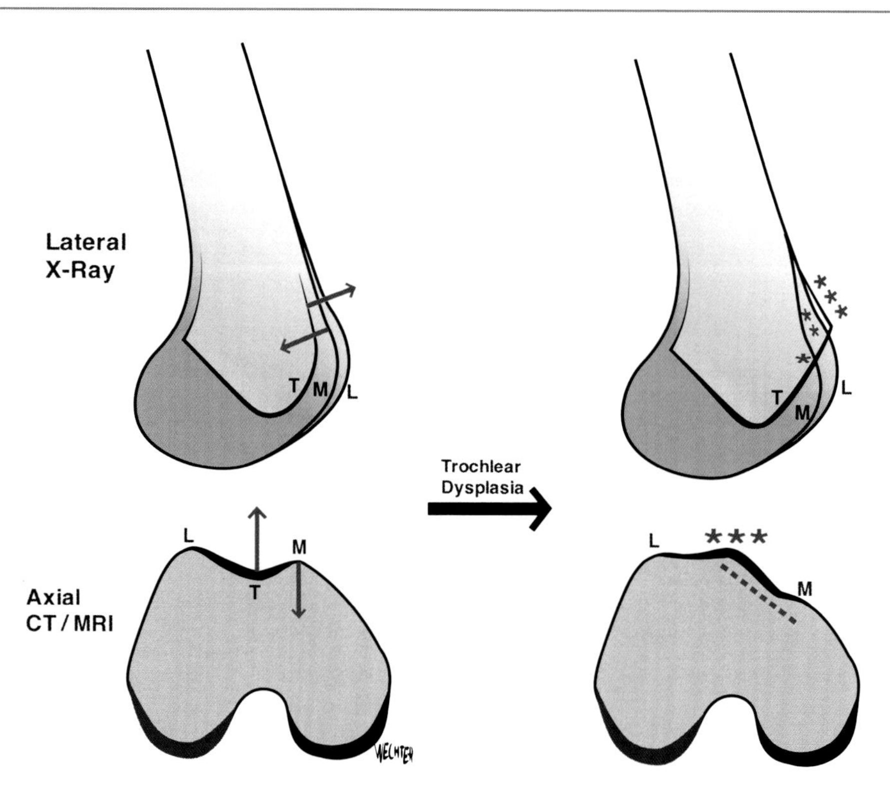

Fig. 2.5 Trochlear morphology [47]: the trochlear groove (T) should be posterior to the medial (M) and lateral (L) femoral condylar lines. In trochlear dysplasia, the trochlear groove is too prominent anteriorly (*anterior arrow*), which manifests as a "crossing sign" (*single star*) and sometimes a "supratrochlear" bump or "spur" (*triple star*). A hypoplastic medial femoral condyle (*posterior arrow*) manifests as a "double contour sign" (*double star*). A supratrochlear spur plus hypoplastic medial condyle creates a steep drop-off or "cliff sign" (*dotted line*) on the axial CT/MRI. Published with kind permission of John Wechter 2013. All rights reserved

understanding of the anatomy. With the femoral condyles superimposed at their distal and posterior aspects, the examiner follows three key lines from posterior to anterior, the lateral condylar line, medial condylar line, and trochlear groove line (Fig. 2.5).

Abnormal trochlear morphology is prevalent in >85 % of patients with symptomatic objective patellar instability [3, 5, 15, 16]. H. Dejour and his lyonnaise team were instrumental in describing markers of trochlear dysplasia as well as a classification system. He originally identified three classifications of trochlear dysplasia based on the level of the "crossing sign" on the lateral radiograph [48].

D. Dejour [49] later used the lateral radiograph in combination with the axial CT to introduce a four-grade classification of trochlear dysplasia [16] and ultimately included two new signs—the supertrochlear bump and double contour sign within this classification [49].

Figure 2.5 illustrates some of the radiographic signs of trochlea dysplasia, using two-dimensional imaging to describe a 3D process. These signs include a flattened or prominent trochlear groove, hypoplasia of the medial trochlear facet, the "crossing sign," a "supratrochlear spur sign," the "double contour sign," and the "cliff sign" (Fig. 2.5).

The crossing sign is found in 96 % of patients with a patellar dislocation and is pathognomonic of trochlea dysplasia. It is defined by a trochlear groove line which meets, or crosses anteriorly to, the medial facet line. This signifies that the trochlear groove is flat or even convex in relation to the medial trochlear facet [16].

The trochlear bump, or supratrochlear spur, is found in 66 % of patellar dislocations. It is defined by a trochlear groove line which is greater than 3 mm anterior to a line drawn along the anterior femoral cortex and represents a prominent trochlear groove [16]. This may contribute to instability by resisting patellar entrance into the proximal trochlea during early flexion [24].

The double contour sign is seen on the lateral radiograph as two separate lines, signifying a space between the medial and lateral trochlear facet lines on sagittal profile. This corresponds to a hypoplastic medial facet and was described by D. Dejour as occurring in high-grade trochlear dysplasia [15].

The "cliff sign" is seen on the axial MRI/CT. It is named due to the appearance of a prominent lateral trochlea in combination with a hypoplastic medial facet with a lack of cartilaginous continuity in the steep drop-off between the two condyles [47].

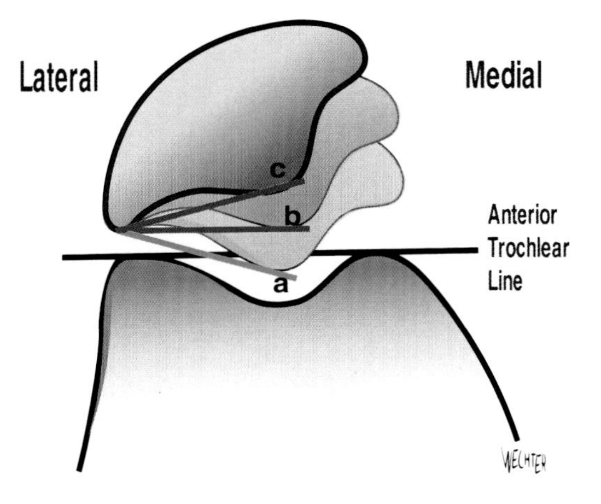

Fig. 2.6 Laurin's lateral patellofemoral angle [51]. Laterally, the anterior trochlear line should diverge from the lateral facet line (*line a*). With lateral patellar tilt, the two lines become parallel (*line b*) or converge laterally (*line c*). Published with kind permission of John Wechter 2013. All rights reserved

Axial Radiographs

Axial radiographs were first reported by Settegast in 1921 [50] and allowed analysis and measurement of patella position in relation to the trochlear groove. There are over a dozen methods described, with Laurin [51] and Merchant views [52] most used in the USA. Low angle of knee flexion becomes important when evaluating the trochlea, as lesser degrees of flexion will show the proximal portion of the trochlea, where dysplasia of the trochlea is most manifest. Axial views on plain radiographs have been criticized for image distortion and lack of reproducibility. With the advent of serial slicing on axial MRI and CT, which allows visualization of the posterior condylar line, more precision has been afforded for the measurement of tilt. Axial radiographs, however, have remained an easy and affordable clinical imaging test to include in the outpatient evaluation of PF disorders.

Axial Radiograph Techniques

Laurin's technique [51] describes the knee at 20° flexion, with the X-ray beam aimed proximally, parallel to the patellofemoral joint. The cassette is held 12 cm proximal to the knee, perpendicular to the X-ray beam, and is pushed into the thigh. In obese or muscular patients, the cassette may need to be moved more proximally or pushed more firmly into the thigh.

Merchant's technique [52] was originally described with the knee flexed at 45°, with the X-ray beam aimed distally and elevated 30° from the femur. The cassette is held over the anterior tibia, perpendicular to the beam. More recently, 30 and 60° of knee flexion with a similar beam angle have been analyzed and normal parameters of patella position described.

Patellar Tilt on Axial Radiograph

Laurin's lateral patellofemoral angle [53] (Fig. 2.6) is calculated on the 20° flexion view and consists of the angle between a line drawn across the anterior aspects of the trochlear facets and a second line drawn along the lateral patellar facet. Laurin found that 97 % of normal patients had lateral diversion of the lines, whereas all patients with patellar subluxation had either parallel or converging lines, implying increased lateral patellar tilt. A meta-analysis by Smith [54] found high heterogeneity across studies in the ability for this measurement to distinguish between normal controls and patients with patellar instability.

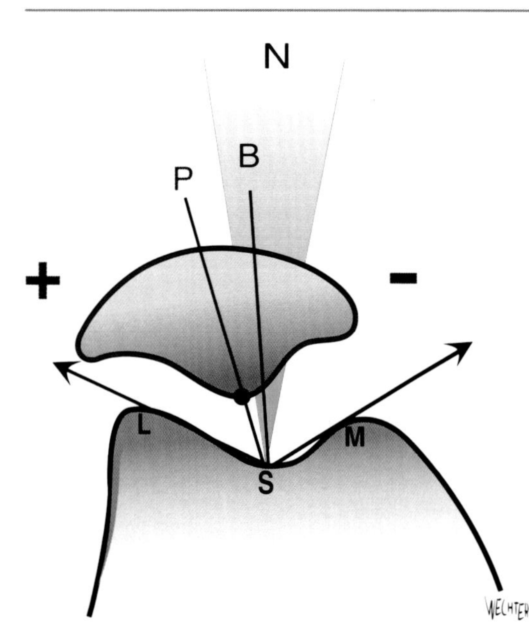

Fig. 2.7 Merchant's congruence angle [52]: quantifies medial (–) and lateral (+) patellar translation. The sulcus angle is drawn from the apices of the medial (*M*) and lateral (*L*) trochlear facets to the lowest point of the trochlear sulcus (*S*). Two lines are drawn upward from the sulcus apex, one which bisects the sulcus angle (*B*) and the other connecting to the central patellar ridge (*P*). The angle between *B* and *P* is the congruence angle. Normal (*N*) is –6° ± SD 11°. Published with kind permission of John Wechter 2013. All rights reserved

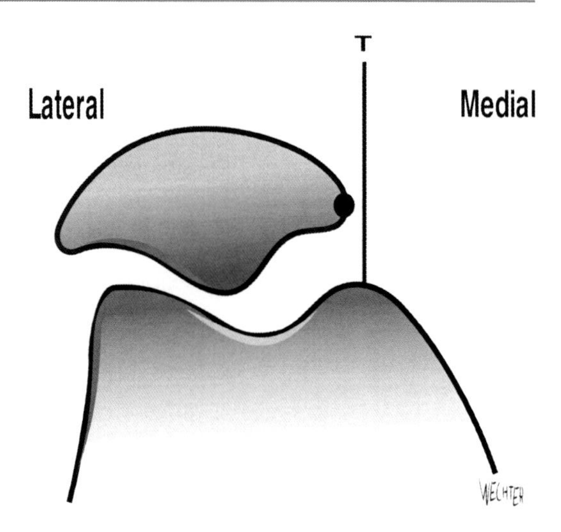

Fig. 2.8 Laurin's lateral displacement [51]. The medial edge of the patella (*dot*) should be even with or medial to the medial trochlear apex (*T*). Published with kind permission of John Wechter 2013. All rights reserved

Patellar Translation on Axial Radiograph

Merchant's congruence angle [52] (Fig. 2.7) is the angle between two lines drawn upward from the sulcus apex, one which bisects the sulcus angle and the other connecting to the central patellar ridge. Lateral and medial translation of the patellar ridge in relation to the sulcus is labeled in positive and negative degrees, respectively. Merchant found the average congruence angle in normal controls to –6° (SD 11°) compared to patellar instability patients who averaged +23°. Smith's meta-analysis [54], however, was unable to determine the reliability or validity of this measure, due to "recurrent methodologic limitations" across studies.

Lateral patellar displacement (Fig. 2.8) was defined by Laurin [51] as the relationship of the medial edge of the patella to the summit of the medial trochlear facet. They found that the medial patellar edge was lateral to the medial facet summit in 50 % of patients with lateral patellar instability compared to only 3 % of the normal controls.

Stress radiographs may be useful when there is a high clinical suspicion of lateral patellar instability despite the standard axial radiographs being normal. Teitge [55] applied 16 lb of laterally directed force to the patella and found that lateral patellar excursion >4 mm more than the contralateral knee was correlated with recurrent patellar dislocations.

Trochlear Morphology on Axial Radiograph

The sulcus angle is calculated as the angle between the apices of the medial and lateral trochlear facets and the deepest portion of the trochlear groove. Merchant, with the knee in 45° of flexion, found normal subjects to have a mean sulcus angle of 138° with a standard deviation of 6° [52]. Values greater than 144° represent a flattened trochlea groove. In a meta-analysis by Smith et al. [54], sulcus angle was able to discriminate well between healthy controls and patients with patellar instability. Another study showed higher sulcus angles (flatter sulcus) correlated well with other markers of trochlear dysplasia, in particular increased patellar tilt and patella alta [56].

Magnetic Resonance Imaging

Identifying Trauma

Evaluation of the trochlear cartilage, patellar cartilage, and medial and lateral aspects of the femoral condyles is performed on both the axial images and the coronal/sagittal reconstructions. The presence of reciprocal lesions of the lateral femoral condyle and medial patellar facet imply an impaction injury sustained during patellar relocation and are pathognomonic for a lateral patella dislocation. Evaluate the mid-substance of the MPFL as well as its patellar and femoral insertions to identify the site of injury. Sagittal and coronal images are inspected to identify injuries to the meniscus, tibio-femoral joint, cruciate ligaments, and tibial–collateral and fibular–collateral ligaments.

Trochlear Analysis on MRI

D. Dejour's four-grade classification was originally based upon radiographs and CT; however, today, MRI is widely used in place of CT. A 2012 study by Lippacher and D. Dejour comparing the MRI and lateral radiograph found fair inter- and intra-observer reliability in classifying dysplasia as A, B, C, or D and excellent reliability in classifying dysplasia as low grade (Type A) or high grade (Types B, C, D) [57].

Increasing emphasis is being placed on a more detailed description of trochlear morphology. Several measurements are used, all of which essentially examine the relationship of the height of the medial and lateral trochlea to the sulcus. These MRI measurement schemes include the following:

Trochlear groove depth (Fig. 2.9): A shallow trochlear groove is a radiographic characteristic of trochlear dysplasia and patellar instability [16, 58]. On MRI, groove depth is measured on the axial sequence. First, a line is drawn along the posterior aspect of the femoral condyles. Then, at a level 3 cm proximal to the tibiofemoral joint, three perpendicular lines are drawn extending anteriorly from the posterior condyle line, to the apices of the medial and lateral trochlear facets, and to the deepest point of the trochlear groove. The length of the trochlear groove line is subtracted from the average length of the facet lines, to yield the trochlear depth. A trochlear groove depth less than 3 mm on the MRI is highly correlative with the presence of trochlear dysplasia on the lateral radiograph [59, 60].

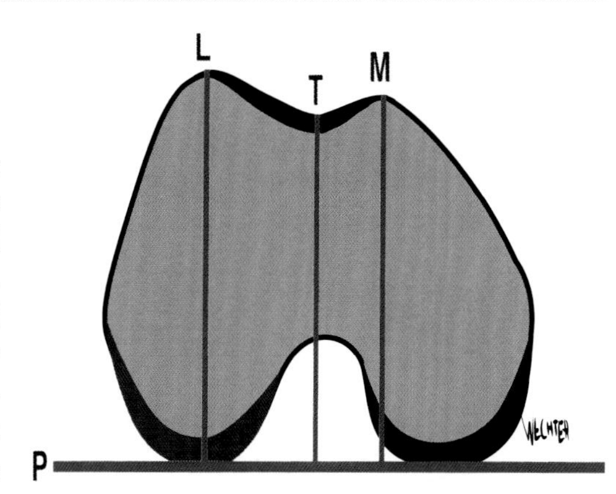

Fig. 2.9 Trochlear groove depth: $((L+M)/2)-T$. *P*—posterior condylar line; *L*—lateral facet height; *M*—medial facet height; *T*—trochlear groove height. Published with kind permission of John Wechter 2013. All rights reserved

Lateral trochlear inclination measures the angle of the lateral trochlear facet in relation to the posterior condylar line, while the *trochlear facet ratio* compares the widths of the medial and lateral trochlear facets at a level 3 cm proximal to the tibio-femoral joint. MRI studies by Diederichs and Pfirrmann found lateral trochlear inclination <11° and a disproportionately small medial trochlear facet (medial:lateral facet ratio <40 %) to correlate well with a trochlear bump >3 mm and a positive crossing sign, both which are established radiographic markers of trochlear dysplasia [59, 60].

The *sulcus angle* (Fig. 2.7), measured on radiographs as the high points of the trochlear facets to the deepest point of the sulcus, has an unclear role in MRI evaluation. While it has been found to correlate with patellar instability [10], one study found inconsistency between radiographic and MRI measurements of sulcus angle [61] and another found poor intra and inter-observer reliability [62]. Technique may play a factor, as the sulcus angle was found to be larger (flatter trochlea) when measurements were made along the articular cartilage as opposed to the subchondral bone [63].

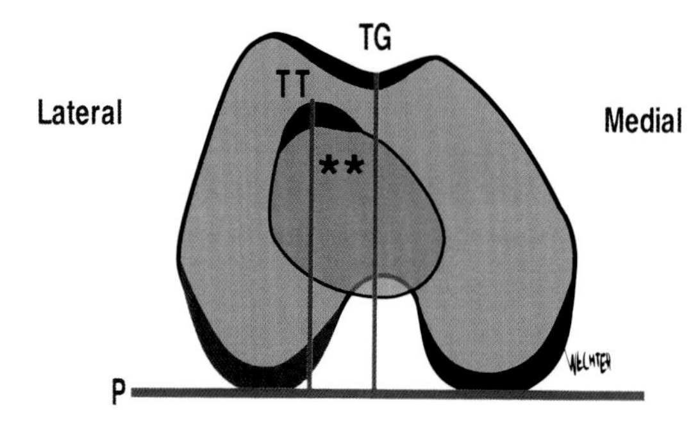

Fig. 2.10 Tibial tubercle to trochlear groove distance (TT–TG) [16]: the horizontal distance (*double asterisk*) between two perpendicular lines extended from the posterior condylar line (*P*); one to the anterior aspect of the tibial tubercle (TT) and the other to the deepest portion of the trochlear groove (TG). Published with kind permission of John Wechter 2013. All rights reserved

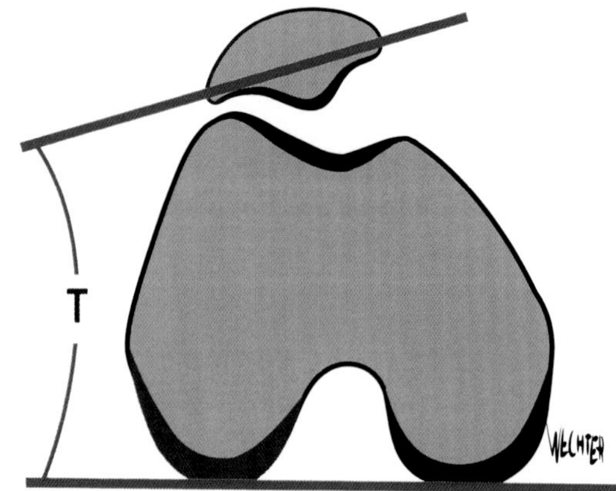

Fig. 2.11 Patellar tilt (MRI/CT): the angle between a line drawn along the posterior condyles and another drawn through the patellar axis. Published with kind permission of John Wechter 2013. All rights reserved

Alignment Evaluation on MRI

Tibial Tubercle to Trochlear Groove Distance (Fig. 2.10)

Increased TT–TG distance is a risk factor for patellar instability [16]. The measurement is made on a CT or MRI, using superimposed images. It is defined as the horizontal distance from the anterior aspect of the tibial tubercle to the deepest part of the proximal trochlear groove on the first axial image showing a complete cartilaginous trochlea [9, 64]. TT–TG values as low as 12.6 on MRI [9] and 14.4 on CT [64] and as high as 20 mm [16] have been deemed pathologic cutoffs, correlating with symptomatic patellar instability. One reason for this wide variation may be the wide heterogeneity in soft tissue and bony landmarks used for measuring the TT–TG distance [65]. One study found improved inter- and intra-observer reliability when using the center of the patellar tendon as the tibial landmark, rather than the anterior aspect of the tibial tubercle [65]. Patient body size should also be taken into account when interpreting TT–TG, since it is a distance rather than a ratio.

Patellar Position on MRI

Patellar Tilt (Fig. 2.11)

Lateral patellar tilt greater than 20° has been found to be disproportionately present in patients with symptomatic lateral patellar instability, when compared to normal controls [5, 16]. The angle is measured between a line drawn along the posterior condyles and a line through the patellar axis.

Referencing off the posterior condyles may be superior to the radiographic technique, where patellar tilt is measured in relation to a line drawn anteriorly across the trochlear facet apices. This is an area prone to variation in trochlear dysplasia, such as a hypoplastic facet or a prominent trochlear bump.

Patella Alta: A high riding patella is established as a contributing factor in lateral patellar instability and is typically calculated using the above described radiographic techniques: IS, CD, BP, and femoral-based indices (Figs. 2.3 and 2.4). These same indices can potentially be applied to the lateral MRI, with the advantage that anatomic landmarks, particularly the distal insertion of the patellar tendon, and the distal extent of the patellar articular surface, can be visualized better on the MRI. Interpretation should consider, however, that full knee extension and a relaxed quadriceps could cause the patellar tendon to "sag" [66] and potentially effect the measurement. One study compared the IS ratio using radiographs and MRI and found no significant difference [66]; however, another study found a small but significant decrease in patellar height when using MRI and CT, as compared to radiographs.

They recommended that when using the IS ratio, 0.13 and 0.10 should be added for the MRI and CT, respectively. For the BP ratio, 0.09 should be added for the MRI only [67].

Conclusion

Acute lateral patellar dislocations carry significant morbidity, due to pain and associated injuries, as well as the risk for recurrence. The history and physical exam are used in conjunction with radiographs and MRI to confirm the diagnosis and identify injuries to the patellofemoral joint and adjacent structures. Anatomical measurements, made on physical exam and via imaging studies, are helpful for predicting recurrence risk and for planning surgical treatment.

References

1. Hughston JC, Stone MM. Recurring dislocations of the patella in athletes. South Med J. 1964;57:623–8.
2. Atkin DM, Fithian DC, Marangi KS, Stone ML, Dobson BE, Mendelsohn C. Characteristics of patients with primary acute lateral patellar dislocation and their recovery within the first 6 months of injury. Am J Sports Med. 2000;28:472–9.
3. Cash JD, Hughston JC. Treatment of acute patellar dislocation. Am J Sports Med. 1988;16:244–9.
4. Fithian DC, Paxton EW, Stone ML, Silva P, Davis DK, Elias DA, White LM. Epidemiology and natural history of acute patellar dislocation. Am J Sports Med. 2004;32:1114–21.
5. Burmann R, Locks R, Pozzi J, Konkewicz E, Souza M. Avaliation of predisposing factors in patellofemoral instabilities. Acta Ortop Bras. 2011;19:37–40.
6. Hawkins RJ, Bell RH, Anisette G. Acute patellar dislocations: the natural history. Am J Sports Med. 1986;14:117–20.
7. Sallay PI, Poggi J, Speer KP, Garrett WE. Acute dislocation of the patella. A correlative pathoanatomic study. Am J Sports Med. 1996;24:52–60.
8. Kirsch MD, Fitzgerald SW, Friedman H, Rogers LF. Transient lateral patellar dislocation: diagnosis with MR imaging. AJR AM J Roentgenol. 1993;161:109–13.
9. Balcarek P, Jung K, Ammon J, Walde TA, Frosch S, Schuttrumpf JP, Sturmer KM, Frosch KH. Anatomy of lateral patellar instability: trochlear dysplasia and tibial tubercle-trochlear groove distance is more pronounced in women who dislocate the patella. Am J Sports Med. 2010;38:2320–7.
10. Balcarek P, Walde TA, Frosch S, Schuttrumpf JP, Wachowski MM, Sturmer KM, Frosch KH. Patellar dislocations in children, adolescents and adults: a comparative MRI study of medial patellofemoral ligament injury patterns and trochlear groove anatomy. Eur J Radiol. 2011;79:415–20.
11. Hawkins RJ, Switlyk P. Acute prosthetic replacement of severe fractures of the proximal humerus. Clin Orthop Relat Res. 1993;289:156–60.
12. Stefancin J, Parker R. First-time traumatic patellar dislocation: a systematic review. Clin Orthop Rel Res. 2007;455:93–101.
13. Cofield RH, Bryan RS. Acute dislocation of the patella: results of conservative treatment. J Trauma. 1977;17:526–31.
14. MacNab I. Recurrent dislocation of the patella. J Bone Joint Surg Am. 1952;34:957–67.
15. Dejour D, Reynaud P, Lecoultre B. Douleurs et instabilite rotulienne. Essai de classification. Medecine et Hygiene 1998.
16. Dejour H, Walch G, Nove-Josserand L, Guier C. Factors of patellar instability: an anatomic radiographic study. Knee Surg Sports Traumatol Arthrosc. 1994;2:19–26.
17. Arendt EA, Fithian DC, Cohen E. Current concepts of lateral patella dislocation. Clin Sports Med. 2002;21:499–519.
18. Hackl W, Benedetto KP, Fink C, Sailer R, Rieger M. Locked lateral patellar dislocation: a rare case of irreducible patellar dislocation requiring open reduction. Knee Surg Sports Traumatol Arthrosc. 1999;7:352–5.
19. Sillanpaa PJ, Maenpaa HM. First-time patellar dislocation: surgery or conservative treatment? Sports Med Arthrosc. 2012;20:128–35.
20. Kolowich PA, Paulos LE, Rosenberg TD. Lateral release of the patella: indications and contraindications. Am J Sports Med. 1990;18:359–65.
21. Hand CJ, Spalding TJ. Association between anatomical features and anterior knee pain in a "fit" service population. J R Nav Med Serv. 2004;90:125–34.
22. Johnson LL, van Dyk GE, Green 3rd JR, Pittsley AW, Bays B, Gully SM, Phillips JM. Clinical assessment of asymptomatic knees: comparison of men and women. Arthroscopy. 1998;14:347–59.
23. Ahmed AD. Radiological assessment of the patella position in the normal knee joint of adult Nigerians. West Afr J Med. 1992;11:29–33.
24. Zaffagnini S, Dejour D, Arendt E. Patellofemoral pain, instability and arthritis: clinical presentation, imaging, and treatment. Berlin: Springer; 2010.
25. Conlan T, Garth WP, Lemons JE. Evaluation of the medial soft-tissue restraints of the extensor mechanism of the knee. J Bone Joint Surg Am. 1993;75A:682–93.
26. Desio SM, Burks RT, Bachus KN. Soft tissue restraints to lateral patellar translation in the human knee. Am J Sports Med. 1998;26:59–65.
27. Fulkerson JP, Shea KP. Disorders of patellofemoral alignment. J Bone Joint Surg Am. 1990;72:1424–9.
28. Sheehan FT, Derasari A, Fine KM, Brindle TJ, Alter KE. Q-angle and J-sign: indicative of maltracking

subgroups in patellofemoral pain. Clin Orthop Relat Res. 2010;468:266–75.
29. Post WR. Clinical evaluation of patients with patellofemoral disorders. Arthroscopy. 1999;15:841–51.
30. Stevens PM, Maguire M, Dales MD, Robins AJ. Physeal stapling for idiopathic genu valgum. J Pediatr Orthop. 1999;19:645–9.
31. Kwak JH, Sim JA, Kim NK, Lee BK. Surgical treatment of habitual patella dislocation with genu valgum. Knee Surg Relat Res. 2011;23:177–9.
32. Omidi-Kashani F, Hasankhani IG, Mazlumi M, Ebrahimzadeh MH. Varus distal femoral osteotomy in young adults with valgus knee. J Orthop Surg Res. 2009;4:15.
33. Cooney AD, Kazi Z, Caplan N, Newby M, St Clair Gibson A, Kader DF. The relationship between quadriceps angle and tibial tuberosity-trochlear groove distance in patients with patellar instability. Knee Surg Sports Traumatol Arthrosc. 2012;20:2399–404.
34. Kummel B. Tibiofemoral incongruity in association with patellar instability. Clin Orthop Relat Res. 1981:97–104.
35. Sanfridsson J, Arnbjornsson A, Friden T, Ryd L, Svahn G, Jonsson K. Femorotibial rotation and the Q-angle related to the dislocating patella. Acta Radiol. 2001;42:218–24.
36. Smith TO, Hunt NJ, Donell ST. The reliability and validity of the Q-angle: a systematic review. Knee Surg Sports Traumatol Arthrosc. 2008;16: 1068–79.
37. Fulkerson JL, Hungerford DS. Patellar tilt/compression and the excessive lateral pressure syndrome (ELPS). In: Fulkerson JL, Hungerford DS, editors. Disorders of the patellofemoral joint. Baltimore, MD: Williams & Wilkins; 1990. p. 102–23.
38. Yiannakopoulos CK, Mataragas E, Antonogiannakis E. The effect of quadriceps contraction during weight-bearing on four patellar height indices. J Bone Joint Surg Br. 2008;90:870–3.
39. Malghem J, Maldague B, Lecouvet F, Koutaissoff S, Vande Berg B. [Plain radiography of the knee: the articular surfaces]. J Radiol. 2008;89:692–7. quiz708-10.
40. Biedert RM, Albrecht S. The patellotrochlear index: a new index for assessing patellar height. Knee Surg Sports Traumatol Arthrosc. 2006;14:707–12.
41. Grelsamer RP, Meadows S. The modified Insall-Salvati ratio for assessment of patellar height. Clin Orthop Relat Res. 1992;170–6.
42. Caton J, Deschamps G, Chambat P, Lerat JL, Dejour H. [Patella infera. Apropos of 128 cases]. Rev Chir Orthop Reparatrice Appar Mot. 1982;68:317–25.
43. Blackburne JS, Peel TE. A new method of measuring patellar height. J Bone Joint Surg Br. 1977;59: 241–2.
44. Seil R, Muller B, Georg T, Kohn D, Rupp S. Reliability and interobserver variability in radiological patellar height ratios. Knee Surg Sports Traumatol Arthrosc. 2000;8:231–6.
45. Portner O, Pakzad H. The evaluation of patellar height: a simple method. J Bone Joint Surg Am. 2011; 93:73–80.
46. Dejour H. La dysplasie de la trochlee femorale. Rev Chir Orthop. 1990;76:45.
47. Dejour H. La trochleoplastie creusement dans le traitement de l'instabilite rotulienne a propos de 33 cases. Lyon; 1994.
48. Dejour H. Terminologie classification des affections femoro-patellairet. In Journees Lyonnaise de chirurgie du Genou. Lyon; 1987.
49. Dejour D, Le Coultre B. Osteotomies in patellofemoral instabilities. Sports Med Arthrosc. 2007;15: 39–46.
50. Settegast J. Typische roentgenbilder von normalen meschen. Lehmanns Med Atlanten. 1921;5:211.
51. Laurin CA, Dussault R, Levesque HP. The tangential X-ray investigation of the patellofemoral joint: X-ray technique, diagnostic criteria and their interpretation. Clin Orthop. 1979;144:16–26.
52. Merchant AC, Mercer RL, Jacobsen RH, Cool CR. Roentgenographic analysis of patellofemoral congruence. J Bone Joint Surg Am. 1974;56:1391–6.
53. Laurin CA, Levesque HP, Dussault RG, Labelle H, Peides JP. The abnormal lateral patellofemoral angle: a diagnostic roentgenographic sign of recurrent patellar subluxation. J Bone Joint Surg Am. 1978;60: 55–60.
54. Smith TO, Davies L, Toms AP, Hing CB, Donell ST. The reliability and validity of radiological assessment for patellar instability. A systematic review and meta-analysis. Skeletal Radiol. 2011;40:399–414.
55. Teitge RA, Faerber W, Des Madryl P, Matelic TM. Stress radiographs of the patellofemoral joint. J Bone Joint Surg Am. 1996;78:193–204.
56. Davies AP, Costa ML, Shepstone L, Glasgow MM, Donell S. The sulcus angle and malalignment of the extensor mechanism of the knee. J Bone Joint Surg Br. 2000;82:1162–6.
57. Lippacher S, Dejour D, Elsharkawi M, Dornacher D, Ring C, Dreyhaupt J, Reichel H, Nelitz M. Observer agreement on the Dejour trochlear dysplasia classification: a comparison of true lateral radiographs and axial magnetic resonance images. Am J Sports Med. 2012;40:837–43.
58. Malghem J, Maldague B. Depth insufficiency of the proximal trochlear groove on lateral radiographs of the knee. Radiology. 1989;170:507–10.
59. Diederichs G, Issever AS, Scheffler S. MR imaging of patellar instability: injury patterns and assessment of risk factors. Radiographics. 2010;30:961–81.
60. Pfirrmann CW, Zanetti M, Romero J, Hodler J. Femoral trochlear dysplasia: MR findings. Radiology. 2000;216:858–64.
61. Salzmann GM, Weber TS, Spang JT, Imhoff AB, Schottle PB. Comparison of native axial radiographs with axial MR imaging for determination of the trochlear morphology in patients with trochlear dysplasia. Arch Orthop Trauma Surg. 2010;130:335–40.

62. Nicolaas L, Tigchelaar S, Koeter S. Patellofemoral evaluation with magnetic resonance imaging in 51 knees of asymptomatic subjects. Knee Surg Sports Traumatol Arthrosc. 2011;19:1735–9.
63. Toms AP, Cahir J, Swift L, Donell ST. Imaging the femoral sulcus with ultrasound, CT, and MRI: reliability and generalizability in patients with patellar instability. Skeletal Radiol. 2009;38:329–38.
64. Schoettle PB, Zanetti M, Seifert B, Pfirrmann CW, Fucentese SF, Romero J. The tibial tuberosity-trochlear groove distance; a comparative study between CT and MRI scanning. Knee. 2006;13:26–31.
65. Wilcox JJ, Snow BJ, Aoki SK, Hung M, Burks RT. Does landmark selection affect the reliability of tibial tubercle-trochlear groove measurements using MRI? Clin Orthop Relat Res. 2012;470: 2253–60.
66. Miller TT, Staron RB, Feldman F. Patellar height on sagittal MR imaging of the knee. AJR Am J Roentgenol. 1996;167:339–41.
67. Lee PP, Chalian M, Carrino JA, Eng J, Chhabra A. Multimodality correlations of patellar height measurement on X-ray, CT, and MRI. Skeletal Radiol. 2012;41:1309–14.

Rehabilitation Considerations for Nonoperative Management of Patellofemoral Conditions

3

Jenny McConnell

Patellofemoral pain is one of the common conditions presenting to clinicians involved in the management of sports injuries, accounting for 2–30 % of all presentations [1–8]. As patellofemoral pain is a multifactorial problem, the mechanism of symptom production is not always clear to the clinician. Thus, management of patellofemoral symptoms requires a thorough understanding not only of the anatomy and biomechanics of the patellofemoral joint but also the neural innervation of the various soft tissue structures around the knee and the effect of pain on muscle activation, so the clinician can effectively minimize the patient's symptoms and improve the lower limb mechanics.

This chapter will examine the relevant anatomy and biomechanics of the patellofemoral joint, outline the signs and symptoms of conditions of patellofemoral origin to assist in differential diagnosis, and provide assessment procedures and intervention strategies for the clinician.

J. McConnell, B. App. Sci. (Phty), Grad. Dip. Man. Ther., M. Biomed. Eng., F.A.C.P. (✉)
Center for Sports Medicine, Melbourne University, Melbourne, VIC, Australia

Center for Sports Medicine, Melbourne University, 4 Bond Street, Mosman, NSW 2088, Australia
e-mail: JennyMcConnell@bigpond.com

Anatomy

The patellofemoral joint is essentially a soft tissue joint, very much reliant on the soft tissue structures to determine the position of the patella on the femur. In fact, the patella has been likened to a tent with the surrounding soft tissue structures being the guy ropes [9].

Factors Influencing the Passive Stability of the Patellofemoral Joint

Femur

The Shape of the Trochlea

The lateral aspect of the femoral trochlea extends further anteriorly than the medial aspect, providing inherent stability once the patella is within the confines of the trochlea (from 20 to 30° knee flexion) [10, 11]. In a study on fresh frozen cadavers, Amis and colleagues found that abnormal trochlear geometry reduced the lateral stability of the patella by 70 % at 30° flexion. Trochlear dysplasia, which is a combination of decreased trochlear depth with a low lateral femoral condyle, is seen as an important risk factor for patellar instability as the patella cannot engage properly in the trochlea [12, 13]. The incidence of trochlear dysplasia in patellofemoral pain sufferers reported in the literature ranges from 0.7 to 2 % [13, 14].

R.V. West and A.C. Colvin (eds.), *The Patellofemoral Joint in the Athlete*,
DOI 10.1007/978-1-4614-4157-1_3, © Springer Science+Business Media New York 2014

Femoral Anteversion

Femoral anteversion is associated with numerous abnormalities in the spine and lower limb including spondylolisthesis, acetabular labral tears, and patellofemoral instability [15–17]. Femoral anteversion alters the position of the femur relative to the patella such that the patella starts in a relatively more laterally displaced position. The amount of anteversion can be estimated clinically by examining hip rotation range as well as measuring the *Q* angle. The *Q* angle, which represents the line of pull of the rectus femoris muscle, is influenced by both femoral and tibial positions, where external tibial torsion and/or lateral displacement of the tibial tubercle also increases the *Q* angle. A *Q* angle of >20°, which is more common in females, is associated with patellofemoral instability [9, 11]. Often individuals with an increased *Q* angle have "squinting" patellae and slight tibia vara because knee motion is occurring about a medially rotated axis.

The Patella

The Shape and Size of the Patella

The patella is a sesamoid bone located within the patellar ligament. Its posterior surface has five facets, which articulate with the femur: superior, inferior, medial, lateral, and odd. The geometry of the articular facets of the patella varies among individuals and may affect patellar tracking [18–20]. The inferior part of the posterior surface, representing 25 % of the patellar height, does not articulate with the femur but lies in close relationship to the highly nociceptive infrapatellar fat pad (IPFP) [9, 21, 22]. The articular cartilage of the central portion is the thickest in the body, reaching 4–5 mm [21]. Yet, despite the depth of the articular cartilage, it is susceptible to failure because of poor distribution of force through the joint.

The lateral facet is almost flat and lies at an angle of approximately 130° to the medial facet so it fits well with the lateral femoral condyle [23]. It is usually longer and broader than the medial facet. Radiographic and cadaveric studies have classified patellae into four types based on the size and shape of the medial and lateral facets [24, 25]. Type II is the most common patella shape while type III is the least common. Type III and type IV tend to be unstable, so are more likely to dislocate [26].

The Position of the Patella

The relationship between patella height and patella tendon length can determine how the patella seats in the trochlea. If an individual has a high sitting patella (patella alta), the patella will be unstable, as the patella will not engage well in the trochlea [27]. Patella alta is more common in females.

The Noncontractile Soft Tissue Structures

In the first 20° of knee flexion, there is no bony support for the patella, so passive stability is provided by the medial and lateral retinaculum and the joint capsule. Anteriorly, the capsule is very thin and loose to accommodate the large range of normal flexion. It stretches medially to laterally across the anterior surface to contribute to the patellar retinaculum [28]. Proximal excursion of the patella from the tibia is limited inferiorly by tension in the patellar tendon. The peripatellar retinaculum interdigitates with the tendon medially and laterally [9].

The lateral side of the knee is made up of various fibrous layers, forming the superficial and deep lateral retinaculum. The anterior portion of the superficial layer of the lateral retinaculum consists of the fibrous expansion of the vastus lateralis, running longitudinally along the lateral border and inserting into the patellar tendon [28]. Fibers from the iliotibial band interdigitate with fibers from the vastus lateralis and the patellar tendon to form the superficial oblique retinaculum (Fulkerson).

The deep layer, or deep transverse retinaculum, consists of three major components: the epicondylopatellar band (lateral patellofemoral ligament), which provides superolateral static support for the patella; the midportion, which is the primary support structure for the lateral patella, courses directly from the iliotibial band to the patella; and the patellotibial band which provides inferolateral stability for the patella [9]. As most of the lateral retinaculum arises from the iliotibial band, tightness of the band, which has its greatest influence at 20° of knee flexion, will contribute to lateral tracking and tilt of the patella. The retinacular support is stronger on the lateral side than it is on the medial side.

The medial retinaculum is thinner than the lateral retinaculum and was thought to play a lesser role in influencing patellar position or tracking. However, a recent study on eight cadaveric knees found that a ruptured medial retinaculum caused 49 % reduction in lateral stability at 0° flexion [29]. Three ligaments, the patellofemoral, patellomeniscal, and patellotibial, lie beneath the retinaculum and are palpable thickenings in the joint capsule [30, 31]. The medial patellofemoral ligament (MPFL) forms the primary restraint to lateral patellar translation, particularly at full extension, while the medial patellomeniscal and patellotibial ligaments are thought to be less important [32–35]. The MPFL is approximately 55 mm long and is reported to range from 3 to 30 mm in width, but although it is quite thin it has a tensile strength of 209 N. The distal part of the vastus medialis obliquus overlays MPFL where its fibers merge deep into the muscle. The medial and lateral retinacula are therefore affected by the active stabilizers; whereby not only the MPFL merges with the vastus medialis oblique (VMO) but a large proportion of the lateral retinaculum arises from the iliotibial band which provides both active, through the tensor fascia latae and gluteus maximus origins, and passive stabilization of the patella [35].

The anterior soft tissues around the hip can contribute to increasing the internal rotation of the hip, which can adversely affect the stability of the patellofemoral joint. These structures include the anterior hip joint capsule, iliofemoral and pubofemoral ligaments, and tendons of tensor fascia latae, rectus femoris, psoas, and adductor muscles.

Factors Influencing the Active Stabilization of the Joint

Local Stabilizers: Quadriceps

The primary active stabilization of the patella comes from the quadriceps. The main function of the quadriceps is to extend the knee and to control the rate of knee flexion during weight bearing. The most efficient extensor is the vastus intermedius, which is the deepest, inserting into the base of the patella, posterior to the other quadriceps insertions but anterior to the capsule. Acting alone it provides 12 % greater mean extensor force than the other quadriceps heads [36].

As the passive medial stability of the patella is poor, a great deal of medial patellar stability is obtained actively through the muscular attachment of the medial quadriceps into the patella. The vastus medialis is commonly divided into the oblique portion, the VMO, and the more vertical component, the vastus medialis longus (VML) [36–40]. While there is often difficulty accurately distinguishing the VMO and VML as separate entities, most authors agree that they act as two distinct functional units due to their fiber orientation and attachments and thus angle of force on the patella. The VMO is more obliquely aligned (50–55° medially in the frontal plane) than the VML (15–18° medially in the frontal plane) [36, 37, 41].

On the lateral side, the VL is oriented 12–15° laterally in the frontal plane with the obliquity of the distal fibers being greater. In a study by Hallisey and colleagues [42], it was noted that there was an anatomically distinct group of VL fibers separated from the main belly of the vastus lateralis by a thin layer of fat. They found that this part interdigitated with the lateral intermuscular septum before inserting into the patella. Vastus lateralis obliquus provides a direct lateral pull on the patella because of its interdigitation with the lateral intermuscular septum.

The vastus medialis obliquus (VMO) opposes the lateral vector force of the vastus lateralis (VL), allowing a more efficient extensor moment at the knee. In a recent cadaver study, Senavongse and Amis found that relaxation of VMO caused a

30 % reduction in lateral stability of the patella [29]. This is supported by studies of muscle fiber type, which indicate that vastus medialis functions more as a stabilizer than the VL. The mechanical advantage gained by the fiber orientation is required to counter the relatively larger cross-sectional area and thus force producing capacity of the VL. Although the VMO does not extend the knee, it is active throughout knee extension to keep the patella centered in the trochlea of the femur, thus enhancing VL efficiency during knee extension [36, 41, 43].

Thus, the synergistic relationship between the medial and lateral vastii is important in maintaining the alignment of the patella within the femoral trochlea. Electromyographic (EMG) studies have demonstrated that the muscle activity of VMO and VL in the normal population is relatively balanced in terms of activation magnitude and timing in a wide variety of static, dynamic, weight-bearing, and non-weight-bearing activities [44–49]. If the attachment points of VMO and VL are changed anatomically, then the retropatellar surface area of contact can be dramatically changed [50]. This has significant implications for patients undergoing plication and realignment procedures for patellofemoral problems. Symmetrical displacement of the insertion points of the VMO and the VL tendons, either proximally or distally, results in greater changes at larger flexion angles (>60°). If the insertion points are shifted in an asymmetrical manner, then the effect is greater at low flexion angles (<60°). At lower flexion angles the effect of a lateral imbalance manifests itself as a rotation of the patella in the coronal plane, while at higher flexion angles, the imbalance is more likely to produce a tilt of the patella in the sagittal plane [50].

The location and the orientation of the pressure zone on the retropatellar surface are particularly sensitive to the magnitude and direction of tension in the VMO [50]. A 50 % decrease in tension in the VMO may result in a significant displacement of the patella laterally, by 5 mm. If the VMO is deactivated or the tension in the VL is twice that of the VMO, then the pressure zone is almost entirely on the lateral facet. Pressure on the lateral facet will adversely affect the nutrition of the articular cartilage in the central and medial zones of the patella. Degenerative change will occur more readily in these areas. Therefore one of the aims of management of patellofemoral problems is to facilitate a balance between medial and lateral structures, so the load through the joint is distributed as evenly as possible.

The Proximal Stabilizers: The Gluteals

The control of the proximal segment, i.e., the thigh, by the pelvic muscles, particularly the gluteals, is critical for dynamically positioning the femur and hence the orientation of the trochlea. Subjects with patellofemoral pain have a delayed onset of gluteus medius relative to control subjects [51]. Strength of the gluteal muscles is also decreased in patellofemoral sufferers where hip abductor and external rotator strength is 26–36 % lower in females with patellofemoral pain than age and activity matched controls [52].

Functions of the Patella

The patella links the divergent quadriceps muscle to a common tendon. Its major function is to increase the extensor moment of the quadriceps muscle. The patella also protects the tendon from compressive stress and minimizes the concentration of stress by transmitting forces evenly to the underlying bone [9, 51–53].

The patella acts like a balance beam, adjusting the length, direction, and force of each of its arms, the quadriceps tendon and the patella tendon, at different degrees of flexion [18, 51, 54, 55]. When the knee is extending, the patellofemoral contact area moves from proximal to distal on the patella surface, so at terminal knee extension when the quadriceps muscle is at a mechanical disadvantage, it is functioning with a longer lever, thus minimizing the need to increase the muscle demand.

Patellar Excursion

The movement of the patella over the femoral trochlea and condyles is controlled by the complex geometries of all the surfaces, the muscles, and the soft tissue structures. As the patella glides cephalad and caudad on the femur during flexion and extension of the knee, it rotates about three orthogonal axes [23].

Sagittal Plane Movement

The prime movement of the patella is in the sagittal plane where the patella courses a proximal to distal path relative to the femoral condyles during flexion. The total excursion of the patella in this plane throughout the range of knee flexion is between 5 and 7 cm [56]. At full extension, the patella is not in contact with the femur but rests on the supratrochlear fat pad, so there is little compressive load [9, 26]. Between 0 and 10°, the inferior third of the patella starts to come in contact with the trochlea, whilst the superior two thirds remains in the supratrochlear fossa [26]. With increasing flexion, 10–20°, the articular surface of the patella comes into contact with the lateral femur through a small band of contact on the inferior patellar surface [23, 56]. In this position the patellofemoral joint is relatively unstable, as the tibia has de-rotated allowing the patella to move medial to be in contact with the trochlea.

From 30 to 60° the middle surface of the patella comes in contact with the middle third of the trochlea, with a broader band of contact. By 60–90°, the upper third of the patella has a broad band of contact deep within the trochlea [56]. Thus with increasing knee flexion, there is increased contact of the patella on the femur, which increases joint stability and decreases pressure experienced through the joint.

By 90° of flexion, the patella moves lateral again so the contact areas split into two smaller areas medially and laterally on the upper patellar surface, corresponding to areas of contact on the medial and lateral condyles of the femur. Although the patellofemoral contact area has diminished by this stage, there is extensive contact of the posterior surface of the quadriceps tendon with the trochlea. It is not until 135° of flexion that the medial (odd) facet of the patella makes contact with the trochlea. So at full flexion the lateral femoral condyle is completely covered by the patella, and the medial condyle is almost completely exposed [56].

Frontal Plane Movement

In the frontal plane the patella courses a concave lateral "C-"shaped curve. At full extension the patella sits lateral to the trochlea and rests on the supratrochlear fat pad. The "screw home" mechanism of the tibiofemoral joint during terminal extension causes the tibia to externally rotate in relation to the femur, thus lateralizing the tibial tubercle [9, 11]. When the knee is fully extended and the quadriceps are contracted, a valgus vector is produced as the patella is free from the confines of the trochlea. Lateral force at this stage is resisted by the medial retinaculum and the VMO. In the relaxed extended position, there is a mean displacement of the patella of approximately 22 mm, 12 in the medial direction and 10 in the lateral direction [57].

During the first 20° of flexion, the tibia derotates and the patella is drawn into the trochlear notch. The patella then remains in the trochlear notch until the knee has flexed to 90°. Beyond 90° the patella moves laterally over the lateral condyle so that at full flexion the lateral femoral condyle is completely covered by the patella and the medial condyle is, except for the lateral border, completely exposed. At this degree of flexion, the patella rotates around its vertical axis and shifts laterally, as it slips into the intercondylar notch [58].

Patellar motion during knee extension has been documented from cadaveric studies [58]. From 120° to 30° of knee flexion, there is a gradual medial shift of the patella reaching a maximum of 20 mm at 30°. Extension between 30 and 0° produces a slight lateral glide of the patella (2 mm). When the knee is flexed, slight changes in the rotation of the tibia have a significant effect on patellar rotation, because the patella is confined to the trochlea and the patellotibial band of the retinacula are taut. Small changes distally to the retinacula will affect patellar rotation [59].

The patella also has a pitching movement, which occurs around a transverse axis. As the knee flexes the contact area on the patella migrates proximally and the inferior pole of the patella rocks anteriorly in the sagittal plane [23]. As the knee extends, the inferior pole rocks posteriorly. Excessive posterior rocking of the inferior pole may irritate the IPFP and become a potent source of symptoms.

Biomechanical Considerations

The patellofemoral joint reaction force (PFJRF) is equal and opposite to the resultant of the quadriceps tendon tension and the patellar tendon tension. This force is a compressive force increasing with flexion, as the angle between the patellar tendon and the quadriceps becomes more acute. It changes from 0.5 × body weight during level walking, to 3–4 × body weight during stair ascent and descent, 7–8 × body weight when squatting, and 20 × body weight when jumping [9, 11, 51]. The increase in the PFJRF with knee flexion offers an explanation for the aggravation of patellofemoral symptoms experienced by individuals during bent knee activities. Joints are designed to handle compressive stress, by maximizing the surface area of contact. The therapist's objective should be to optimize the area of contact, rather than to decrease the force, as it will promote better nutrient exchange to the articular cartilage. Optimizing the area of contact will decrease the pressure experienced by the joint for the same amount of force, as pressure is proportional to force and inversely proportional to the area.

Sources of Pain

It has also been suggested that individuals with patellofemoral pain are outside their envelope of function and no longer in homeostasis [60]. These individuals demonstrate a failure of the intricate balance of the soft tissue structures around the joint, such that there may be an alteration of the pressure distribution from the patella to the femur. Many different causes of patellofemoral pain have been cited in the literature, but the mechanism of pain production is not fully understood.

The structures that may be the possible source of the actual PF pain are the synovium, lateral retinaculum, subchondral bone, and the IPFP, with the articular cartilage as it is aneural, providing only an indirect source, perhaps either through synovial irritation or increasing subchondral bone stress. Interestingly enough there is no correlation between amount of articular cartilage degeneration and pain experienced by patients with osteoarthritis (OA) of the knee, with many OA knee patients having episodic bouts of pain for years before requiring surgical intervention. The severity of OA knee pain is associated with bone marrow lesions (edema) with subarticular bone attrition [61, 62], synovitis/effusion, and degenerative meniscal tears, but it is not associated with presence of osteophytes or reduction in joint space [61, 63]. Hill and colleagues [61] followed 270 subjects with tibiofemoral (TF) and PF OA for 30 months finding no correlation between baseline synovitis and baseline pain score, but a decrease in synovitis at follow-up correlated with a reduction in pain. These investigators found synovitis in three locations, superior, medial, and inferior patella, with infrapatellar synovitis being most strongly correlated with pain severity. The synovitis was not associated with cartilage loss in either the TF or PF compartments [63].

Free nerve endings (IVa) are present in the synovium, [64] so peripatellar synovitis is a possible source of patellofemoral pain. Despite the evidence supporting the synovium as a potential pain source, histological changes in the synovium of patients with patellofemoral pain are only moderate [64]. However, there is evidence of histological changes in the lateral retinaculum with increased numbers of myelinated and unmyelinated nerve fibers, neuroma formation, and nerve fibrosis being found in some patients with patellofemoral pain [64–67]. Additionally, increased intraosseous pressure of the patella has been found in patients with PF pain who complain of pain when sitting with a bent knee ("movie goers knee"), possibly secondary to a transient venous outflow obstruction [67]. However, the structure that until recently has largely been ignored by the orthopedic community, even though it was first identified as a potent source of pain by Hoffa in 1904, is the IPFP [68].

The fat pad covers extra-articular part posterior patellar surface, merges superiorly with the peripatellar fold, extends into the ligamentum mucosum posteriorly, and is lined by synovium [69]. It attaches to the proximal patellar tendon, inferior pole of the patella, transverse meniscal ligament, medial and lateral meniscal horns, the retinaculum, and the periosteum of the tibia [69]. The fat pad is highly vascular and richly innervated, so is one of the most pain sensitive structures in the knee [21, 22]. The innervation of the fat pad is linked to the entire knee joint structure, so the fat pad may be affected by pathology in various knee joint components [22]. To simulate early knee OA change, Clements and colleagues [70] injected monoiodoacetate into the right knee of 150 rats and after 21 days of weight-bearing asymmetry found marked inflammatory changes in the fat pad, concluding that the IPFP contributed to the pain in the early stages of knee OA. Experimentally induced chemical irritation of the fat pad in asymptomatic individuals confirms that the pain is not just confined to the infrapatellar region but can refer to the proximal thigh as far as the groin [22]. In fact, the fat pad and medial retinaculum of PF pain patients contain a higher numbers of substance P nerve fibers than the same structures of individuals without PF pain [71, 72].

The fat pad facilitates distribution of synovial fluid, stabilizes the patella in the extremes of knee motion (that is less than 20° and greater than 100° of knee flexion), and increases tibial external rotation [73]. A total resection of the fat pad decreases patellofemoral contact area [73]. Inflammatory changes in the fat pad seen on MRI are most commonly the consequence of trauma and degeneration, with the commonest traumatic lesions following arthroscopy, where in 50 % of cases fibrous scarring can still be present 12 months later [74]. Impingement of the fat pad with diffuse edema occurs following patellar dislocation, often mimicking a loose body [75].

Effect of Pain

The presence of pain will certainly decrease muscle activity, timing, and endurance as well as alter movement patterns [76]. However, pain is a cortical experience, so extrinsic factors such as fear of pain, stress, and anxiety [77, 78] can amplify the pain experience for the patient, and the contribution of these factors must be understood if we are to satisfactorily improve the rehabilitation of individuals with PF pain. Hodges et al. [76] have found that inducing pain in the knee of asymptomatic individuals decreases both VMO and vastus lateralis (VL) activity, but when a painful electric shock is randomly and intermittently applied to the knee of the same individuals, mimicking the fear of pain state experienced by PF pain patients, only VMO activity is decreased. Exposure to fear and stress initiates the secretion of several hormones, including corticosterone/cortisol, catecholamines, prolactin, oxytocin, and renin, as part of the survival mechanism. Such conditions are often referred to as "stressors" and can be divided into three categories: external conditions resulting in pain or discomfort, internal homeostatic disturbances, and learned or associative responses to the perception of impending endangerment, pain, or discomfort [78]. Release of cortisol can be detrimental to a patient's recovery. In fact it has been found that stress-related hormones can alter inner ear fluid homeostasis and auditory function [77]. This could have implications for the balance of individuals exhibiting fear/avoidance behavior.

Factors Predisposing Individuals to PF Pain

Several factors predisposing an individual to patellofemoral pain have been identified, ranging from overuse and training errors to faulty biomechanics. Structural causes of patellofemoral pain are divided into intrinsic and extrinsic causes. Intrinsic structural factors are uncommon and relate to dysplasia of the patella or femoral trochlea and the position of the patella relative to the trochlea. Extrinsic structural faults are reported to cause a lateral tracking of the patella or an increase in the dynamic valgus vector force [9, 11, 58]. The extrinsic factors include increased *Q* angle, hamstrings and gastrocnemius muscle tightness, abnormal foot pronation, and quadriceps and gluteal muscle dysfunction.

The Q angle, representing the line of pull of the rectus femoris muscle, has long been the benchmark of orthopedic surgeons to indicate PF function. Its value is widely debated in the literature, with many authors questioning the diagnostic relevance of the static Q angle, suggesting the dynamic Q angle has greater relevance [9, 79, 80]. The dynamic Q angle is affected by the position of the hip from above and the foot below during weight-bearing activities. The alignment of the hip and the foot is particularly critical at 30° of knee flexion when the patella should be engaging in the trochlea.

Many individuals with patellofemoral pain have "squinting" patellae and an associated internal rotation of the femur, which has been hypothesized to cause tightness in the tensor fascia latae (TFL) muscle and weakness of the gluteus medius muscle. The pelvic muscle imbalance will cause faulty gait patterns, where these individuals demonstrate excessive medial rotation of the hip during the stance phase of gait, resulting in the pelvis dropping on the opposite side, giving a Trendelenburg appearance [80]. This altered hip movement will increase the dynamic Q angle [80] and hence increase the potential for patellofemoral pain. Subjects with patellofemoral pain have a delayed onset of gluteus medius relative to control subjects [51]. Strength of the gluteal muscles is also decreased in patellofemoral sufferers where hip abductor and external rotator strength is 26–36 % lower in females with patellofemoral pain than age and activity matched controls [52].

Soft tissue flexibility of various structures in the lower limb such as ITB, hamstrings, gastrocnemius, and anterior hip structures have also been implicated as being causative factors in PFP syndrome. A tight TFL, through its attachment into the ITB, will cause a lateral tracking of the patella, particularly at 20° of knee flexion when the band is at its shortest, affecting the engagement of the patella in the trochlea. Hamstrings and gastrocnemius tightness cause a lateral tracking of the patella, by increasing the dynamic Q angle [11, 80]. When individuals with tight hamstrings run, they land with greater knee flexion, so an increased amount of dorsiflexion is required to position the body over the planted foot. If the range of full dorsiflexion has already occurred at the talocrural joint, further range is achieved by pronating the foot, particularly at the subtalar joint. This causes an increase in the valgus vector force and hence increases the dynamic Q angle.

Abnormal foot biomechanics such as excessive, prolonged, or late pronation which alters tibial and even entire lower limb, rotation at varying times through range, has been proposed to adversely affect patellofemoral joint mechanics [81–84]. There are intrinsic and extrinsic causes of abnormal foot position. The intrinsic causes relate to static foot postures such as forefoot and rearfoot varus and valgus. The extrinsic causes relate to the foot being lateral to the weight-bearing line, such as genu valgus and internal rotation of the femur, or the weight being borne on the lateral aspect of the foot, such as tibial varum.

The most common cause of PFP cited in the literature is quadriceps muscle weakness particularly of the VMO. Ideally, the synergistic relationship between the VMO and VL should maintain the alignment of the patella in the femoral trochlea especially in the first 30° of knee flexion, before the patella is fully engaged in the trochlea. It has been proposed that this balanced activation of the VMO and VL is disrupted in patients with PFPS. The issue of whether the disruption is in part a motor control dysfunction has been investigated by Mellor and Hodges [85] who found that synchronization of motor unit action potentials is reduced in PFP subjects (38 %) compared with controls (90 %). However, the evidence to support an imbalance in the activation of the vastii (either decreased activation of VMO or enhanced activation of VL) is contentious [45, 86–93]. Differences in methodology (particularly with respect to the use of EMG) and the inherent heterogeneity in the PFPS population may account for some of the inconsistencies in study results.

While there is inconclusive evidence to support or refute an imbalance in the magnitude of vastii activation in patients with PFPS, disrupted activation of the vastii may take the form of delayed activation of the VMO relative to the VL. It has been hypothesized that the VMO, which has a smaller cross-sectional area than the VL, must receive a feedforward enhancement of its excitation level in order to track the patellar optimally [86, 87]. Many studies that have examined individuals with PFPS have supported this hypothesis, by demonstrating that the EMG activity and reflex onset time of the VMO relative to the VL is delayed, when compared with asymptomatic individuals [44, 87, 90, 91]. However, the issue is still controversial in the literature with some studies demonstrating no differences in EMG onsets [45, 48, 88, 89], but a more extensive study by Cowan and colleagues [44] found that although the majority of patellofemoral sufferers have a delayed onset of VMO relative to VL on a stair-stepping task (67 % concentrically, 79 % eccentrically), there were still some whose VMO preceded VL activation. Additionally, these investigators found that some of the control subjects (no history of PF pain) exhibited a delayed onset of the VMO relative to the VL (46 % concentrically and 52 % eccentrically) on the stair-stepping task. The study by Cowan et al. [44] may clarify some of the discrepancies found in the literature with regard to timing. The stratification of the groups only occurs when there are sufficient subject numbers to tease out the difference. Some of the earlier studies may not have a statistical significance because the power calculations had not been done and there were too few subjects.

Individuals with PFP not only demonstrate a delay in the onset of VMO relative to the VL but also relative to the prime mover (tibialis anterior) following postural perturbation where subjects were required to rock back on their heels in response to a light stimulus [91]. In control subjects the VMO preceded the prime mover and was activated with the VL [91]. This feedforward strategy used by the central nervous system to control the patella can be restored by physical therapy rehabilitation strategies directed at altering muscle recruitment in functional movements [92].

Examination

History

The initial part of the examination of the patient involves obtaining a detailed history, so a differential diagnosis can be proposed. The diagnosis is later confirmed or modified by the physical findings. In the history, the clinician needs to elicit the area of pain, the type of activity precipitating the pain, the history of the onset of the pain, the behavior of the pain, and any associated clicking, giving way, or swelling. This gives an indication of the structure involved and the likely diagnosis; for example, if the type of activity that precipitated the patient's pain is one that involves eccentric loading, such as jumping in basketball or increased hill work during running, patellar tendinopathy would be suspected [11, 69, 80]. On the other hand, if the athlete reports pain following tumble turning or vigorous kicking in the pool or on delivery of a fast ball in cricket, an irritated fat pad would be suspected [69]. In both these conditions the athlete complains of inferior patellar pain. The patient with an irritated fat pad is aggravated by straight leg raise exercises, so it is essential that the therapist recognizes the condition so appropriate management can be implemented to enhance, rather than impede, recovery. The clinical diagnosis of fat pad irritation may be confirmed on MRI on a T2-weighted image where inflammation of the fat pad may be visualized. Patellar tendinopathy can be confirmed on diagnostic ultrasound, particularly using color doppler or with MRI.

Symptoms of Patellofemoral Pain

The patient usually complains of a diffuse ache in the anterior knee, which is exacerbated by stair climbing [9, 11, 80]. For many, the knee will ache when they are sitting for prolonged periods with the knee flexed—the movie sign. However, patients with an irritated fat pad irritation have pain with prolonged standing rather than prolonged sitting.

Some patients will have crepitus, which is often a source of concern for them because they feel that the crepitus is indicative of "arthritis." However, the crepitus is mostly due to tight deep lateral retinacular structures and can be improved with treatment. Abernathy et al. [93] examined the knees of first year medical students ($n = 123$) and found that asymptomatic patellofemoral crepitus was present in 62 % of the students.

Some patients may experience "giving way" or a buckling sensation of their knee. This occurs during walking or stair climbing, i.e., movements in a straight line, and is a reflex inhibition of the quadriceps muscle. It must be differentiated from the giving way experienced when turning, which is indicative of an anterior cruciate deficient knee. Locking is another symptom, which must be differentiated from intra-articular pathology. Patellofemoral locking is usually only a catching sensation where the patient can actively unlock the knee, unlike loose body or meniscal locking, where the patient either is unable to unlock or can only passively unlock the knee [9, 11].

Mild swelling due to synovial irritation may also occur with patellofemoral problems. Mild swelling causes an asymmetric wasting of the quadriceps muscle, whereby the VMO is inhibited before the VL and RF [94, 95]. So an athlete, who has primary intra-articular pathology, such as a meniscal or ligamentous injury, may have great difficulty resolving the subsequent secondary patellofemoral problem, particularly if it is not identified.

When considering the possible differential diagnoses, the clinician must remember that the lumbar spine and the hip can refer symptoms to the knee. For example, the prepubescent male with a slipped femoral epiphysis may present with a limp and anterior knee pain so can initially be misdiagnosed as having patellofemoral pain [9].

Neural tissue may also be a source of symptoms around the patellofemoral joint. Lack of mobility of the L5 and S1 nerve roots and their derivatives can give rise to posterior or lateral thigh pain. Symptoms from neural tissue can be fairly easily differentiated from patellofemoral symptoms because the pain will be exacerbated in sitting, particularly when the leg is straight rather than in the classic movie sign position of a flexed knee. The slump sitting test will quickly verify the neural tissue as being a source of the symptoms [96]. Similarly, a peripheral nerve may scar down or become entrapped following arthroscopic surgery. The most common example is the infrapatellar branch of the saphenous nerve. Symptoms are sharp pain inferomedially with/without slightly altered sensation laterally. The symptoms are reproduced on deep bend and jumping so they are frequently confused with patellar tendonitis symptoms because of the proximity to the tendon. Pain is reproduced with the patient prone, flexing the knee, and externally rotating the tibia, to put the nerve on stretch [97].

Patellofemoral Instability

Patellofemoral instability or recurrent patellofemoral subluxation is a variant of patellofemoral pain syndrome, where there is actual subluxation of the patella. It is more common in females and tends to be associated with patella alta, a Q angle >20°, a high attachment of the VMO into the patella and dysplasias of the trochlea and patella [9, 11, 98]. Patients with patellofemoral instability will complain of a sensation of giving way on certain movements. This usually occurs when the femur internally rotates on a fixed externally rotated tibia [98]. When this happens acutely, there is usually swelling which appears within 12 h of the injury and if the fluid is aspirated, it is serosanguineous [98]. Whereas, with an acute rupture of the anterior cruciate ligament, which is often injured with the same cutting action as described above for patellofemoral subluxation, the swelling occurs within the first couple of hours and a hemarthrosis would be aspirated. It is important to image all acute knee problems to ensure that there has been no disruption to the lateral femoral condyle during the subluxation.

Patients with patellofemoral instability have the same predisposing factors as patellofemoral pain syndrome. They exhibit apprehension and sometimes pain on lateral movement of their patella. The apprehension sign confirms the diagnosis. Treatment is based on the same principles as those for patellofemoral pain management.

Other Causes of Knee Pain

Iliotibial Band Friction Syndrome

The athlete, particularly the distance runner and to a lesser extent the skier and the cyclist, who has increased the mileage or altered the terrain of the training or changed footwear can complain of quite specific knee pain over the lateral femoral epicondyle, where the iliotibial band is being frictioned [9, 11]. Iliotibial band friction syndrome accounts for 21 % of knee injuries in runners [2, 5]. These patients will have a tight iliotibial band as confirmed on a modified Ober's test, performed in side lying with the pelvis in a stable position. The test consists of hip extension, adduction, and slight external rotation; the knee is then flexed and extended where pain, and sometimes a clicking, is elicited. The individuals with iliotibial friction syndrome have faulty biomechanics, which predisposes them to the condition, so correction of the faulty biomechanics as well as correction of any training errors must be addressed in treatment.

Plica Syndrome

Anterior knee pain, particularly along the medial edge of the patella, may be due to an inflamed synovial plica [99–101]. The synovial plica is a redundant fold in the synovial lining of the knee joint, extending from the fat pad medially under the quadriceps tendon, superiorly to the lateral retinaculum. The plica is an embryonic remnant. The patients with an inflamed plica complain of pain in sustained flexed positions, which progressively improves with increased activity. Some patients may be aware of a significant pop or snap as they flex and extend their knee and present with a palpable thickening. It has been reported that as many as 60 % of examined knees have a palpable plica, but the large majority are asymptomatic [99, 101]. Plica problems are not common but are seen more often in elite cyclists. Arthroscopic resection of a thickened, inflamed plica in an athlete, who has failed conservative management, may be necessary at times [100, 101].

Apophysitis in the Adolescent Knee Pain Sufferer

The tibial tubercle or the inferior pole of the patella may be tender to palpation in the active, rapidly growing, usually male, adolescent, indicating that there is an excessive traction on the soft tissue apophysis at the proximal or distal attachment of the patellar tendon [102]. If pain is elicited on palpation of the tibial tubercle, the patient is diagnosed as having an Osgood–Schlatter disease, which is a more common condition than inferior pole apophysitis (Sinding–Larsen–Johansson syndrome). The diagnosis is a clinical diagnosis, so an X-ray is usually not necessary. However, X-ray may be indicated to exclude bony tumor, in cases, where the anterior knee pain is severe, and there is a large amount of associated swelling. Bone tumors are rare, but, in the 10–30-year-age-old group, the knee is the site of osteogenic sarcoma [9].

Both Osgood–Schlatter disease and Sinding–Larsen–Johansson syndrome are regarded as self-limiting conditions, that is, the pain subsides at the time of bony fusion which most clinicians suggest takes up to 2 years [9, 102]. The traditional treatment approach is modified activity and in extreme circumstances rest from sport [9, 102]. This is very difficult for active adolescents to do, because they are thoroughly enjoying their sport. Two years is a long time in the life of the adolescent and much skill development and maturation can be lost through lack of participation and practice. There is a great deal the therapist can do for these individuals such as decreasing the concentration of stress at the tibial tubercle by taping or use of a strap, specific muscle training, and ensuring adequate flexibility of the quadriceps, hamstrings, ITB, and gastrocsoleus. All these treatment strategies are aimed at reducing the symptoms while still allowing the adolescent to participate in sport.

Osteochondritis Dissecans in the Adolescent Knee Pain Sufferer

The patient with osteochondritis dissecans usually presents with intermittent pain and swelling of gradual onset. It must be differentiated from juvenile rheumatoid arthritis (Still's disease) and a partial discoid meniscus. In the acute situation, the patient with osteochondritis dissecans may have an extremely painful, locked, swollen knee. The swelling is a hemarthrosis and the locking is due to a loose body from a defect at the lateral aspect of the medial femoral condyle [9]. This is confirmed on X-ray and the patient requires an immediate orthopedic referral for either fixation of the loosened fragment or removal of the detached fragment [9, 102].

Physical Examination

The physical examination confirms the diagnosis and helps determine the underlying causative factors of the patient's symptoms so the appropriate treatment can be implemented. By examining the patient's standing position, the therapist has fair indication of how the patient will move. The therapist should observe the patient from the front, the side, and from behind. From the front, the therapist examines the femoral position, which is easier to see when the patient has the feet together (Fig. 3.1). A position of internal rotation of the femur is a common finding in patients with patellofemoral pain. The internal femoral rotation often causes a squinting of the patellae. The internal rotation of the femur is usually associated with a tight iliotibial band and poor functioning of the posterior gluteus medius muscle. This gives rise to poor control of the pelvis, causing an increase in the dynamic *Q* angle and increases the potential for patellofemoral pain. Moving down the leg to the knee the therapist can observe the bulk of the different heads of the quadriceps muscle, the tightness of the ITB attachment, and any swelling or puffiness about the knee. An enlarged fat pad, for example, is indicative that the patient is standing in hyperextension or a "locked back" position of their knees.

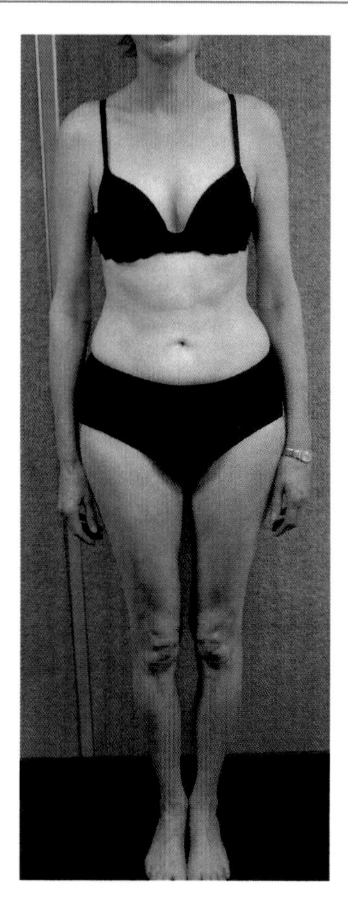

Fig. 3.1 Typical biomechanical alignment of an individual with PF pain—internally rotated femurs giving the squinting patellae appearance

From this the clinician can infer that the quadriceps control, particularly eccentric control, in inner range (0–20° flexion) will be poor. The position of the tibia relative to the femur (valgus/varus) is noted, and the presence or absence of torsion of the tibia is determined, as these bony malalignments can affect the way the foot hits the ground as well as the patellofemoral position.

The clinician should palpate the talus on the medial and lateral sides to check for symmetry of position. In relaxed standing, equal amounts of talus should be palpable on the medial and lateral sides of the foot. This is the mid-position of the subtalar joint. If the talus is more prominent medially (which is a common finding), then the patient has a midfoot collapse so their foot will remain pronated for too long a period of time, which increases the dynamic valgus vector force. The position of the talus from the front is correlated with the position of the calcaneum from behind. If the talus is prominent medially, the calcaneum should be sitting everted. If the calcaneum is sitting straight or inverted then the clinician can infer that the patient has a stiff subtalar joint and will pronate not at heel strike, but at mid-stance, thus exhibiting a midfoot collapse. The great toe and first metatarsal are examined for callus formation as well as position. If the patient has callus on the medial aspect of the first metatarsal or the great toe, or has a hallux valgus, then the therapist should expect the patient to have an unstable push-off in gait, which increases pelvic rotation. When examined prone, this patient will have a forefoot deformity.

From the side, the clinician checks the pelvic and lumbar spine position, to determine whether the pelvis has an anterior or a posterior tilt or whether the patient has a "sway back" posture. The pelvic position will affect the amount of available hip extension and rotation in walking. Knee hyperextension or a "locking back" is also seen from the side. From behind, the level of the PSIS is checked, to determine any leg length discrepancies, gluteal bulk is assessed, and the position of the calcaneum is observed.

Dynamic Examination

The aim of the dynamic examination is primarily to reproduce the patient's symptoms so the clinician has an objective reassessment activity to evaluate the effectiveness of the treatment. Additionally, the effect of muscle action on the limb mechanics can be evaluated. Any deviations from the anticipated give a great deal of information about the muscle control of the activity. The first dynamic activity examined is walking, as it is the least stressful activity for the PF joint. For example, if an individual stands in hyperextension of the knees, the quadriceps will not function well in inner range due to lack of practice, so the initial shock absorption at heel strike will be minimal. Initial shock absorption occurs with knee flexion of 10–15°, because the foot is supinated when the heel first strikes the ground. As soon as the heel hits the ground, the foot rapidly pronates, so if that same individual has a stiff subtalar joint, shock absorption must come from higher up in the body, in this case the pelvis. This patient will demonstrate a pelvic instability, which, depending on the tilt of the pelvis, will cause either an increase in pelvic and ultimately trunk rotation or lateral flexion. If the pelvis is anteriorly tilted, then the patient will exhibit an increase in pelvic rotation when walking, because that individual has a lack of hip extension and external rotation. If the pelvis is posteriorly tilted, the patient will present with a "Trendelenburg-like" gait, indicating weak gluteal musculature. The individual with a sway back posture walks with a combination of increased tilt and rotation. The optimal amount of pelvic movement is reported to be 10° for rotation, 4° for lateral tilt, and 7° for anteroposterior tilt [103].

The initial response, when evaluating a patient with abnormal pelvic motion, is to give that patient pelvic stability work to control the excessive motion. However, if this is the case, the patient, who is not shock absorbing at the knee or the foot and, now, no longer shock absorbing at the pelvis, must shock absorb even higher up, perhaps at the cervical spine. If stabilization work is given to a patient, the therapist must make sure the patient has some scope for movement elsewhere, so asking the patient to walk with the knees slightly flexed will improve the shock absorption and decrease the need for the excessive movement at the pelvis.

If the patient's symptoms have not been provoked in walking, then evaluation of more stressful activities, such as stair climbing, is performed. If symptoms are still not provoked, then squat and one leg squat may be examined and used as a reassessment activity. With athletes, however, these clinical tests are not strenuous enough to reproduce their symptoms, as longer duration activities, such as running 15 km, provoke symptoms. In this situation the clinician can evaluate the control of the one leg squat to determine the effect of treatment outcome.

Supine Examinatiovn

With the patient in supine lying, the clinician gains an appreciation of the soft tissue structures and begins to confirm the diagnosis. Gentle but careful palpation should be performed on the soft tissue structures around the patella. The joint lines are palpated to exclude obvious intra-articular pathology. The retinacular tissues are palpated to determine the parts of the retinaculum that are under chronic recurrent stress. If pain is elicited in the infrapatellar region on palpation, the clinician should shorten the fat pad by lifting it towards the patella. If on further palpation, the pain is gone, then the clinician can be relatively certain that the patient has a fat pad irritation. If the pain remains, then the patient has a patellar tendinopathy. The knee is passively flexed and extended with overpressure applied so the clinician has an appreciation of the quality of the end feel. If any of these maneuvers reproduce pain, they can be used as a reassessment sign [95]; for example, the symptoms of fat pad irritation can be produced with an extension overpressure maneuver.

Soft Tissue Flexibility

The hamstrings, iliopsoas, rectus femoris, tensor fascia latae, gastrocnemius, and soleus muscles are tested for length. Tightness of any of these muscles has an adverse effect on patellofemoral joint mechanics and will have to be addressed in treatment. The iliopsoas, rectus femoris, and tensor fascia latae may be tested using the Thomas test [45, 90]. To perform the Thomas test, the patient is standing with the ischia touching the end of the plinth. One leg is pulled up to the chest, to flatten the lumbar lordosis, then the patient lies down on the plinth, keeping the flexed leg close to the chest. The other leg should be resting such that the hip is in a neutral position (i.e., on the plinth, at the same width as the pelvis) and the knee should be flexed to 90°. If the hip is in neutral position, but the knee cannot be flexed, the rectus femoris is tight. If the hip is flexed, but lying in the plane of the body, the iliopsoas is tight. But if the hip remains flexed and abducted, the TFL is tight. Lack of flexibility of the TFL can be further confirmed in side lying by Ober's test. Thomas test needs to be performed on both legs, so a comparison between legs can be made. Hamstrings flexibility may be examined by a passive straight leg raise, once the lumbar spine is flattened on the plinth and the pelvis is stable. Normal length hamstrings should allow 80–85° of hip flexion, when the knee is extended and the lumbar spine is flattened.

Patellar Position

One of the most essential parts of patellofemoral evaluation in supine is assessing the orientation of the patella relative to the femur because the clinician is aiming to maximize the surface area of contact, so that for the same amount of force there is less pressure being distributed through the overloaded part of the joint. In order to maximize the area of contact of the patella with the femur, the patellar position should be optimal before the patella enters the trochlea. The clinician needs to consider the patellar position not with respect to the normal, but with respect to the optimal, because articular cartilage is nourished and maintained by evenly distributed, intermittent compression. An optimal patellar position is one where the patella is parallel to the femur in the frontal and the sagittal planes, and the patella is midway between the two condyles when the knee is flexed to 20°. The position of the patella is determined by examining four discrete components, glide, lateral tilt, anteroposterior tilt, and rotation, in a static and dynamic manner. An optimal position involves the patella being parallel to the femur in the sagittal plane.

Anteroposterior Tilt

A most common finding is a posterior displacement of the inferior pole of the patella (Fig. 3.2). This will result in fat pad irritation and often manifests itself as inferior patella

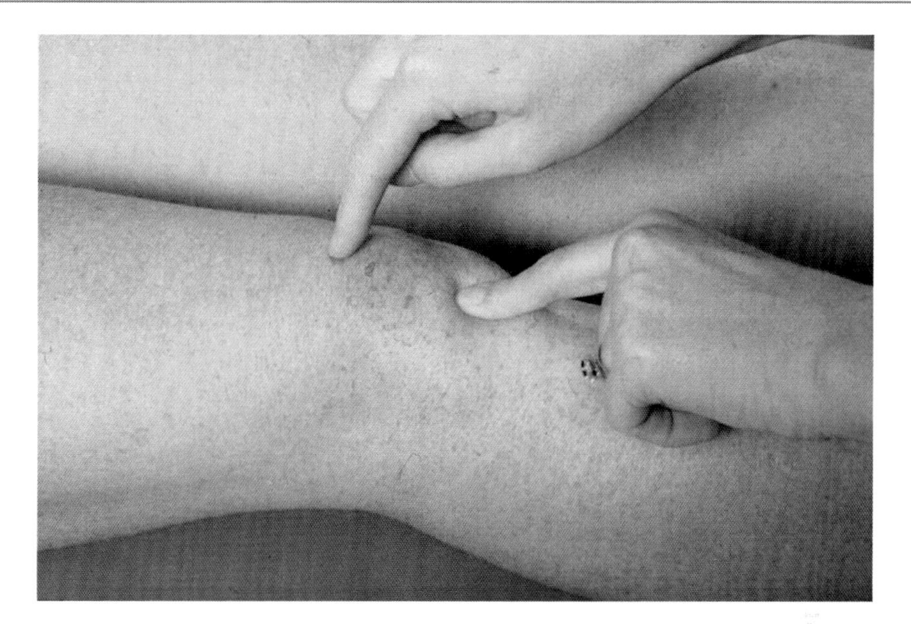

Fig. 3.2 Posterior tilt of the inferior pole of the patella. The inferior pole of the patella is embedded in the infrapatellar fat pad

pain, which is exacerbated by extension maneuvers of the knee. A dynamic posterior tilt problem can be determined during an active contraction of the quadriceps muscle as the inferior pole is pulled posteriorly, particularly in patients who hyperextend.

Glide

Determination of the glide component involves measuring the distance from the midpole of the patella to the medial and lateral femoral epicondyles. The patella should be sitting equidistant (±5 mm) from each epicondyle when the knee is flexed 20°. In some instances, the patella may sit equidistant to the condyles, but moves lateral, out of the line of the femur, when the quadriceps contracts, indicating a dynamic problem. The dynamic glide examines both the effect of the quadriceps contraction on patellar position as well as the timing of the activity of the different heads of quadriceps. The VMO and the VL should be activated simultaneously or slightly even earlier for the VMO.

Tilt

If the passive lateral structures are too tight, then the patella will tilt so that the medial border of the patella will be higher than the lateral border and the posterior edge of the lateral border will be difficult to palpate. This is a lateral tilt and if severe can lead to excessive lateral pressure syndrome. When the patella is moved in a medial direction, it should initially remain parallel to the femur. If the medial border rides anteriorly the patella has a dynamic tilt problem, which indicates that the deep lateral retinacular fibers are too tight, affecting the seating of the patella in the trochlea.

Rotation

To complete the ideal position, the long axis of the patella should be parallel to the long axis of the femur. In other words, if a line was drawn between the medial and lateral poles of the patella, this line should be perpendicular to the long axis of the femur. If the inferior pole is sitting lateral to the long axis of the femur, the patient has an externally rotated patella. If the inferior pole is sitting medial to the long axis of the femur, then the patient has an internally rotated patella. The presence of a rotation component indicates that a particular part of the retinaculum is tight.

Side Lying

In side lying the clinician assesses the flexibility of the lateral retinaculum—superficial and deep fibers, by gliding and tilting the patella medially. Any tightness of these structures can be addressed by soft tissue work as well as an injection of local anesthetic into the tight band to facilitate loosening of the structures.

Prone

Examination of some of the contributory factors to the patellofemoral problem is best performed in prone. In this position the clinician can examine foot position, anterior hip flexibility and, if necessary, palpate the lumbar spine and sacroiliac joints. The flexibility of the anterior hip structures can be examined with the patient in a figure-of-four position, where the bent leg is placed under the straight leg with the malleolus at the level of the tibial tubercle (Fig. 3.3). This position tests the available hip extension and external rotation, which is often limited because of chronic adaptive shortening of the anterior structures as a result of the underlying femoral anteversion. The distance of the ASIS from the plinth is measured, so the clinician has an objective measure of change.

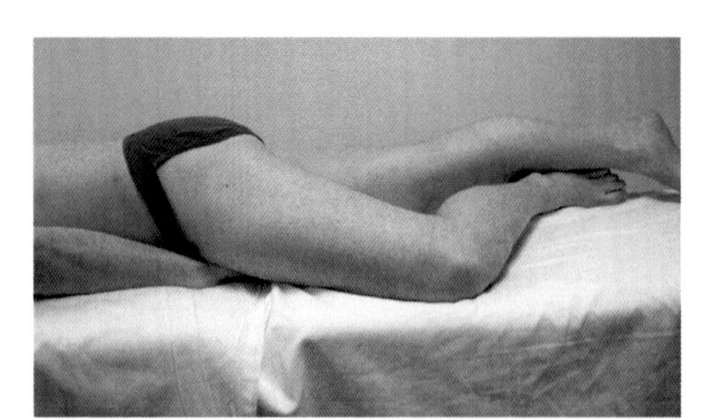

Fig. 3.3 Assessment of anterior structure hip tightness. This is done in prone figure 4 with the lateral malleolus of the bent leg at the level of the tibial tubercle. Ideally the patient's hip should be flat on the table

Treatment

Most patellofemoral conditions are successfully managed with nonoperative treatment. The aims of the treatment are twofold: first, to unload the painful structures around the PF joint by optimizing the patellar position and second, to improve the lower limb mechanics, which, if executed well, will significantly decrease the patient's symptoms.

Patellar Taping

Patellar taping is unique to each patient, as the component/s corrected, the order of correction and the tension of the tape is tailored for each individual based on the assessment of the patellar position. The worst component is always corrected first and the effect of each piece of tape on the patient's symptoms should be evaluated by reassessing the painful activity. It may be necessary to correct more than one component. After each piece of tape is applied, the symptom producing activity should be reassessed. The tape is kept on all day every day until the patient has learned how to activate his/her VMO at the right time, that is, the tape is like trainer wheels on a bicycle and is discontinued once the skill is established.

If a posterior tilt problem has been ascertained on assessment, it must be corrected first, as taping over the inferior pole of the patella will aggravate the fat pad and exacerbate the patient's pain. The posterior component is corrected together with a glide or a lateral tilt with the non-stretch tape being placed on the superior aspect of the patella, either on the lateral border to correct lateral glide or in the middle of the patella to correct lateral tilt. This positioning of the tape will lift the inferior pole out of the fat pad and prevent irritation of the fat pad.

Tape should immediately decrease the symptoms by at least 50 %. If the tape cannot change the patient's symptoms immediately or even worsens them, then one of the following must be considered:

1. The patient requires additional taping to further unload the inflamed IPFP.
2. The tape was poorly applied.
3. The assessment of patellar position was inadequate.
4. The patient has an intra-articular primary pathology which was inappropriate for taping.

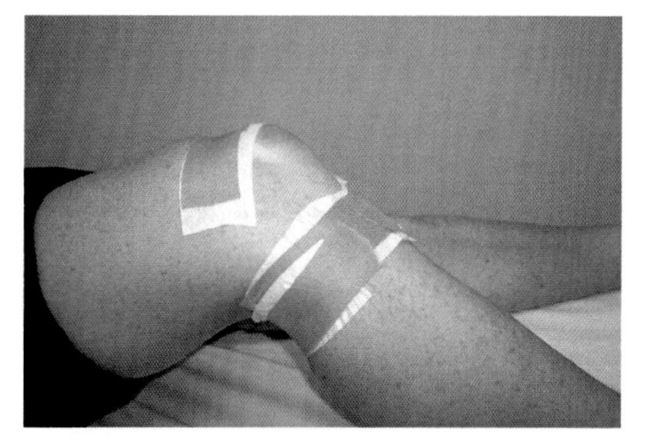

Fig. 3.4 Unloading the fat pad with tape. The patella is tipped out of the fat pad and then a muffin top is created with the soft tissues lifting them from the tibial tubercle up towards the patella. For the recalcitrant fat pad problem, a final piece of tape may be added. This commences posteriorly just below the popliteal fossa to pull the tibia forward and further unload the fat pad

Unloading

The principle of unloading is based on the premise that inflamed soft tissue does not respond well to stretch. For example, if a patient presents with a sprained medial collateral ligament, applying a valgus stress to the knee will aggravate the condition, whereas a varus stress will decrease the symptoms. The same principle applies for patients with an inflamed fat pad, an irritated iliotibial band, or a pes anserinus bursitis. The inflamed tissue needs to be shortened or unloaded. To unload an inflamed fat pad, for example, a "V" tape is placed below the fat pad, with the point of the "V" at the tibial tubercle coming wide to the medial and lateral joint lines. As the tape is being pulled towards the joint line, the skin is lifted towards the patella, thus shortening the fat pad. If this is not sufficient to decrease the patient's symptoms, a firm pull forward of the tibia just below the popliteal fossa is usually sufficient to decrease the pull on the fat pad created by the sag of the gastrocnemius (Fig. 3.4).

The patient should never train with or through pain or effusion, as it has been shown quite conclusively that effusion has an inhibitory effect on muscle activity [94, 95, 104]. If the patient experiences a return of the pain, then the patient should readjust the tape. If the activity is still painful, the patient must cease the activity immediately. The tape will loosen quickly if the lateral structures are extremely tight or the patient's job or sport requires extreme amounts of knee flexion.

Tape has been found to

1. Decrease pain [105–109]
2. Increase quadriceps muscle torque [108]
3. Increase loading knee flexion response [106]
4. Alter VMO timing [105, 107]
5. Alter joint position [110]

Other Taping to Enhance Muscle Activation

Frequently, the gluteal muscles are not firing well, so the patient exhibits adduction and internal rotation of the femur during weight-bearing activities, so taping the gluteal muscles can improve the stability of the pelvis. This tape is applied once a week for a couple of weeks, because improved gluteal activation occurs relatively quickly. Kilbreath and coworkers [111] demonstrated improved hip extension in a group of stroke patients following gluteal taping. The subjects who had experienced a stroke between 2 and 11 years ago walked at two different speeds (self-selected and fast) under three different conditions (control, therapeutic, and placebo tape). With the therapeutic tape in situ subjects went

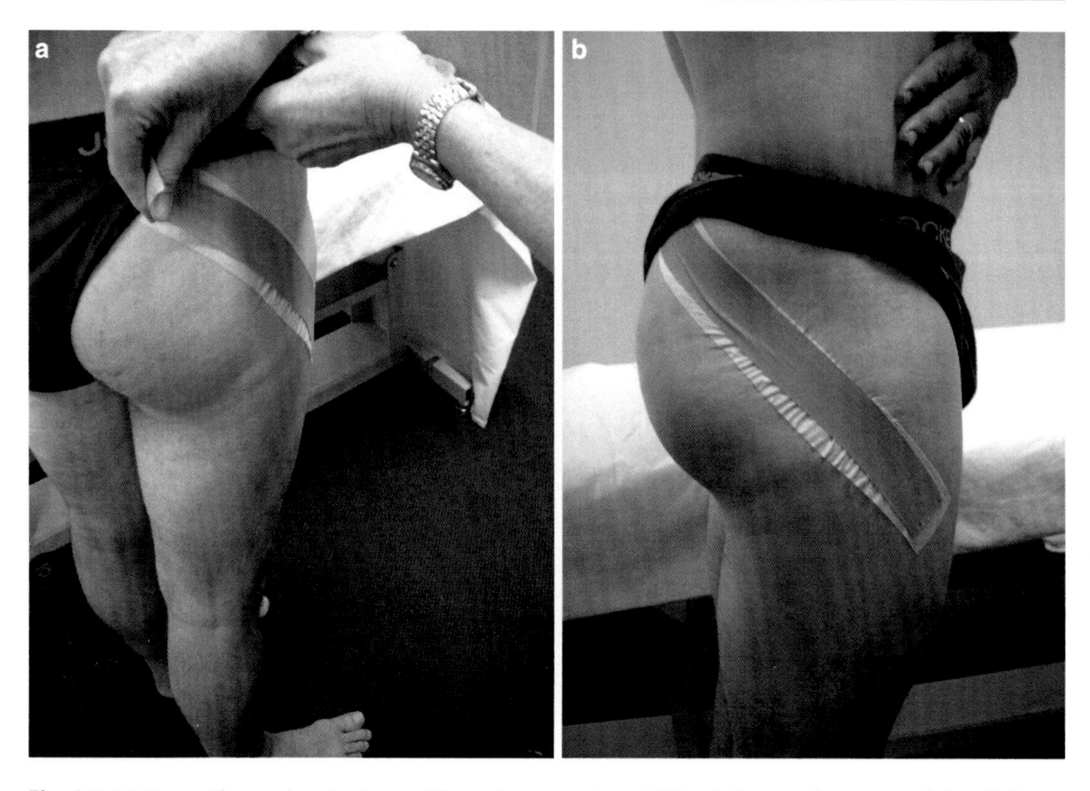

Fig. 3.5 (**a**) Externally rotating the femur. The patient keeps the feet anchored and turns the body away to create an external rotation of the femur (**b**). The tape commences on the *middle* of the anterior aspect of the thigh and finishes at the sacrum

from 3° of hip flexion in the control situation to 11° extension in self-selected walking speed and 8° in fast walking. No difference was found with placebo tape.

If the patient is unable to control the femoral position, tape may be used to externally rotate the femur giving a proprioceptive reminder to the patient, not to internally rotate (Fig. 3.5). Unfortunately, this tape is not as well tolerated because it causes a skin pull on the thigh and the sacrum during sitting. However, it usually only needs to be applied for a short period of time while the motor recruitment pattern changes.

If the patient is having difficulty recruiting the VMO or the VMO activity is less than the VL, the VL can be inhibited, by applying firm tapes from mid-thigh across the lateral aspect of the thigh. A recent within-subject placebo-controlled trial on asymptomatic individuals found that this inhibitory tape significantly reduced the EMG activity of VL compared with no tape or placebo tape in a stair descent task [112].

Stretching Tight Soft Tissue Structures

The deep lateral retinacular structures may require stretching. This can be done in side lying (as shown in Fig. 3.6). The anterior hip structures are usually tight as these individuals often have anteverted femurs. These structures may be stretched in a "figure-of-four" position in prone. The malleolus of the bent leg is placed under the straight leg at the level of the tibial tuberosity. The patient elongates the thigh towards the wall. The stretch is usually held for 5 s and repeated five times. If there is a pull anteriorly, the patient can hold the anterior soft tissues, lifting the adductors firmly towards the head to take the tension off these structures. The patient can also be given stretches for other soft tissues, such as hamstrings, gastrocnemius, rectus femoris, and TFL/ITB, which were found to be tight on the examination.

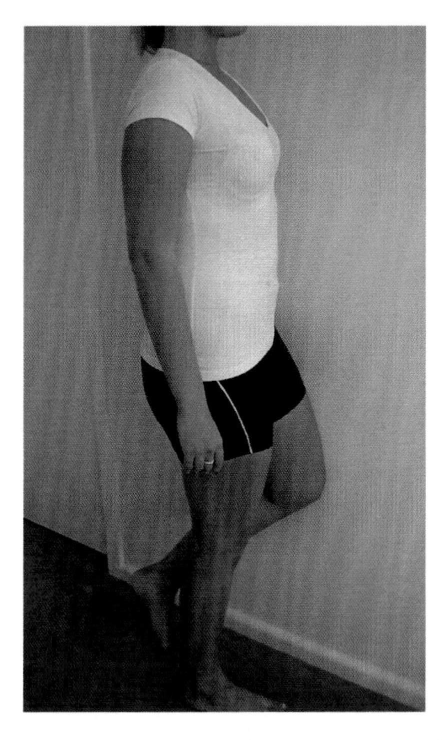

Fig. 3.6 Weight bearing gluteal exercise which simulates walking. The patient turns 45° into the wall, and puts the knee of the inside leg against the wall for balance. The knee of the standing leg is slightly flexed; the pelvis is tucked under and the weight is back through the heel. The patient turns the standing thigh out without moving the hip or the foot

Muscle Training

Individuals with patellofemoral pain need to up-train the VMO and the gluteal musculature to improve the dynamic stability of the patellofemoral joint. How is this achieved?

Before progressing further into exercise prescription, some discussion is required on the importance of training specificity. A recent study by Jensen and colleagues [113] comparing 4 weeks of strength training versus visuomotor skill training of the biceps brachii demonstrated statistically significant changes as measured by transcranial magnetic stimulation in corticospinal excitability in the skill training group but not in the strength training group. This study confirms what has been previously established in the literature about the importance of specific training to facilitate skill improvement [114–116]. It is possible to identify at least four aspects of strength training specificity:

1. Strength training effects are largely muscle specific [114].
2. The training effect is joint angle specific, that is, if a muscle is trained isometrically at one angle or dynamically through a limited range, then the increases in strength occur where the training has taken place with limited increases at other joint angles [116].
3. The training response is specific to the type of contraction and the velocity of the contraction [115].
4. Training is specific to limb position [114], that is, there is a postural specificity to training, so we are training synergistic muscle activation patterns.

For the patellofemoral joint, there is increasing evidence that weight-bearing or closed-chain training is more effective than open-chain exercises. Stensdotter and colleagues [117] found in asymptomatic subjects that closed-chain knee extension promoted a more simultaneous onset of EMG activity of the four different muscle portions of the quadriceps compared with open chain. In open chain, rectus femoris had the earliest EMG onset while the VMO was activated last with smaller amplitude than in closed chain. These authors concluded that closed kinetic chain exercise promotes a more balanced initial quadriceps activation than open kinetic chain exercise. This supports the previous finding of Escamilla and coworkers [118], who found that open kinetic chain exercises produced more rectus femoris activity with closed-chain exercises producing more vastii activity. Closed kinetic training allows simultaneous training not only of the vastii but also the gluteals and trunk muscles to control the limb position in weight bearing. A dual channel biofeedback with electrodes placed on the VMO and VL helps the patient to optimize the firing patterns of the VMO and VL, which significantly enhances the muscle training particularly in weight bearing.

Improving Local Control

Patients with patellofemoral pain usually have poor inner range quadriceps control, so small-range weight-bearing activities in front of a mirror are commenced early in the retraining program to ensure an optimal alignment of the lower limb. This must be performed in the pain-free range, in the first 30° of knee flexion, where the patellar position has been controlled by tape, and the patient can control the femoral position, by keeping the hip, knee, and foot aligned. The essential aspect of training in early stages of rehabilitation is that emphasis should be given to the timing and intensity of the VMO contraction relative to the VL. The patient starts with the feet positioned pelvis-width apart, facing forward, and with the weight distributed either equally on both feet or partially through the symptomatic limb. The patient is instructed to maintain the pelvis, hips, knees, and feet in a forward-facing alignment by squeezing the gluteals, while the knees are slowly flexed to 30° and then returned to full extension without locking the knees back.

VMO retraining can progress to small-range flexion and extension movements in the walk stance position, with the VMO constantly active. This position not only simulates the motion of the knee during the stance phase of walking, but it is also the position where VMO recruitment is poor and the seating of the patella in the trochlea is critical. Again, emphasis should be given to the timing and intensity of the contraction of VMO relative to VL.

Improving Proximal Control

Training the gluteal musculature to improve stance phase of gait is required to decrease the lack of femoral control in weight bearing and improve the stability of the lower extremity. The patient stands with the asymptomatic leg closest to the wall at a distance of a fist away from the wall. The patient's whole body is turned 30° into the wall and the weight is transferred to the outside (symptomatic) leg. The knee of the leg closest to the wall is flexed to 60° with the knee touching, not pushing the wall, for balance purposes. The foot is off the ground. The hips are kept in neutral position so the thighs are parallel. The patient's weight is directed through the heel of the weight-bearing leg, the pelvis is slightly posteriorly tilted, and the knee is slightly flexed. The patient externally rotates the standing leg without turning the foot, the pelvis, or the shoulders. The patient should sustain the contraction for 20 s, so a burning can be felt in the gluteus medius region. The patient can progress this by flexing the hip of the non-weight-bearing leg to 90°. Again, the knee just touches the wall for balance while the patient externally rotates the standing leg without moving the foot, pelvis, or shoulders (Fig. 3.7). These positions improve the patient's core control for the single-support phase of walking and the strike phase of running. The training may be progressed to standing on one leg where the pelvis is kept level and the lower abdominals and the glutei are worked together while the other leg is swinging back and forward, simulating the stance phase of gait. This is better performed in front of the mirror so the patient receives feedback about body alignment and limb position.

As these exercises require a degree of coordination, some patients may need to be more stable initially, so they can stand parallel to a wall, keeping both feet on the floor and isometrically abduct both legs, with the weight back through the heels and the knees slightly flexed. This triggers a less specific gluteal contraction, but it improves the patient's awareness of the gluteal musculature. Some patients also benefit from using an elasticized band/tubing around the ankles for resistance. The patient stands on the symptomatic leg while extending and abducting the asymptomatic leg to 45° without rotating or tilting the pelvis. The patient aims to do as many repetitions as he/she can without losing control of the pelvis. The number of repetitions and/or the thickness of the tubing can be increased as the patient improves.

If the patient has poor balance and is not be able to perform the weight-bearing exercises described above, a more stable position of side lying is preferable where the patient has the hips

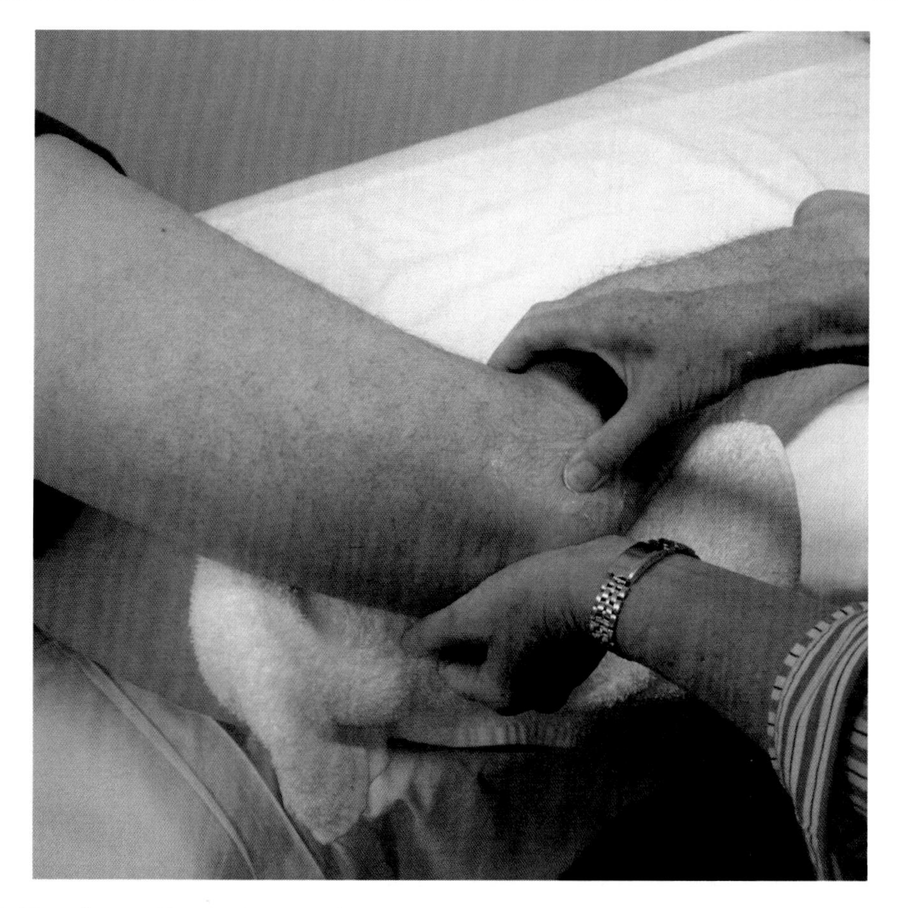

Fig. 3.7 Manually stretching the tight deep lateral retinacular tissue. Patient is in side lying with the knee flexed to 30°, the clinician pushes on the medial aspect of the patella to expose the lateral aspect and put the deep lateral retinacular tissues on stretch

and knees flexed to 90° and lifts the top knee away from the bottom knee while keeping the feet together (clam exercise). Once pelvic control has improved, step training can be implemented.

The patients need to practice stepping up and down, initially using a small step. This should be performed slowly, in front of a mirror, so that changes in limb alignment can be observed and deviations can be observed and corrected. Some patients may be able to do only a small number of repetitions with correct lower limb alignment. Since inappropriate practice can be detrimental to learning, a small number of exercises with correct alignment are sufficient. These exercises should be performed frequently throughout the day with the number of repetitions being increased as the skill level improves. For further progression, the patient can move to a larger step, initially decreasing the number of contractions and then slowly increasing the exercises again. As the patellofemoral pain improves, the patient can alter the speed of the stepping activity, the amount of range used and rate of the change of direction. Weights may be introduced in the hands or in a backpack. Initially, the number of repetitions and the speed of the movement should be decreased and slowly built back up again. The aim of retraining is to make the transition from functional exercises to functional activities. Training should be applicable to the patient's activities/sport, so that a jumping athlete, for example, should have jumping incorporated in the program. Figure-of-eight running, bounding, jumping off boxes, jumping and turning, and other plyometric routines are particularly appropriate for the high performance athlete. However, the patient's VMO needs to be monitored at all times for timing and level of contraction relative to the VL.

As the VMO plays an important stabilizing role for the patellofemoral joint, endurance training is the ultimate goal. The number of repetitions performed by the patient at a training session will depend upon the onset of muscle fatigue. Initially, it is important to emphasize quality and not quantity, progressing to increase the number of repetitions before the onset of fatigue. Patients should be taught to recognize muscle fatigue or quivering, so that they do not train through the fatigue and risk exacerbating their symptoms.

Improving Distal Control

It may be necessary to control the foot position with an orthotic. Both rigid and soft orthotics have been found to be equally effective for controlling patellofemoral symptoms [119]. Compliance is the biggest issue with orthotics but comfort of the orthotic will improve the compliance. If the athlete is involved in change of direction sport, they are better off in a soft orthotic as there will be fewer issues with blisters.

Additionally the clinician can help the patient train the supinators of the foot, specifically tibialis posterior, particularly if the patient demonstrates prolonged pronation during the mid-stance in gait. With the foot supinated, the base of the first metatarsal is higher than the cuboid, which will allow the peroneus longus to work more efficiently to increase the stability of the first metatarsal complex for push-off. The therapist can train this action to improve the efficiency of push-off. The position of training is in mid-stance; the patient is instructed to lift the arch while keeping the first metatarsal head on the floor and then pushing the first metatarsal and great toe into the floor. If the patient is unable to keep the first metatarsophalangeal joint on the ground when the arch is lifted, then the foot deformity is too large to correct with training alone and orthotics will be necessary to control the excessive pronation. If the patient has a stiff subtalar joint, the therapist can increase the mobility of the subtalar joint by mobilizing the calcaneum to increase eversion. The mobilization position should simulate the position of heel strike. This can be achieved by having the patient in side lying with the talocrural joint in a close-packed position and the tibia stabilized. The clinician then glides the calcaneum laterally. Tape can be used to help maintain any gains in range.

Daily Strategies

Patellofemoral pain is not cured but is managed by ensuring that the exercise regime is incorporated into the patient's daily routine. The exercises should only take 5 min otherwise the patient is unlikely to continue with the exercises. The patient needs to realize that to keep the knee in "good health," these exercises are like cleaning their teeth—essential part of body maintenance. No more than four, but preferably three exercises should be given and should consist of weight-bearing gluteal training, small squats, and anterior hip stretches, where no equipment is needed so the patient can do the exercises at any time and place. Patients need advice on how to stand and how to get out of a chair. The patient should stand with the heel of front foot positioned into the instep of the back foot, so the legs are slightly externally rotated, the knees should be soft, and some part of one leg should touch the other leg (like third position in ballet—Fig. 3.8). This position enhances slight gluteal and abdominal activation, improving femoral control. When getting out of a chair, the patient's tibia should remain directly underneath the femur to decrease the valgus loading on the knee.

Evidence

It has been found that 6 weeks of 1 session per week of physical therapy treatment changes the onset timing of VMO relative to VL during stair-stepping

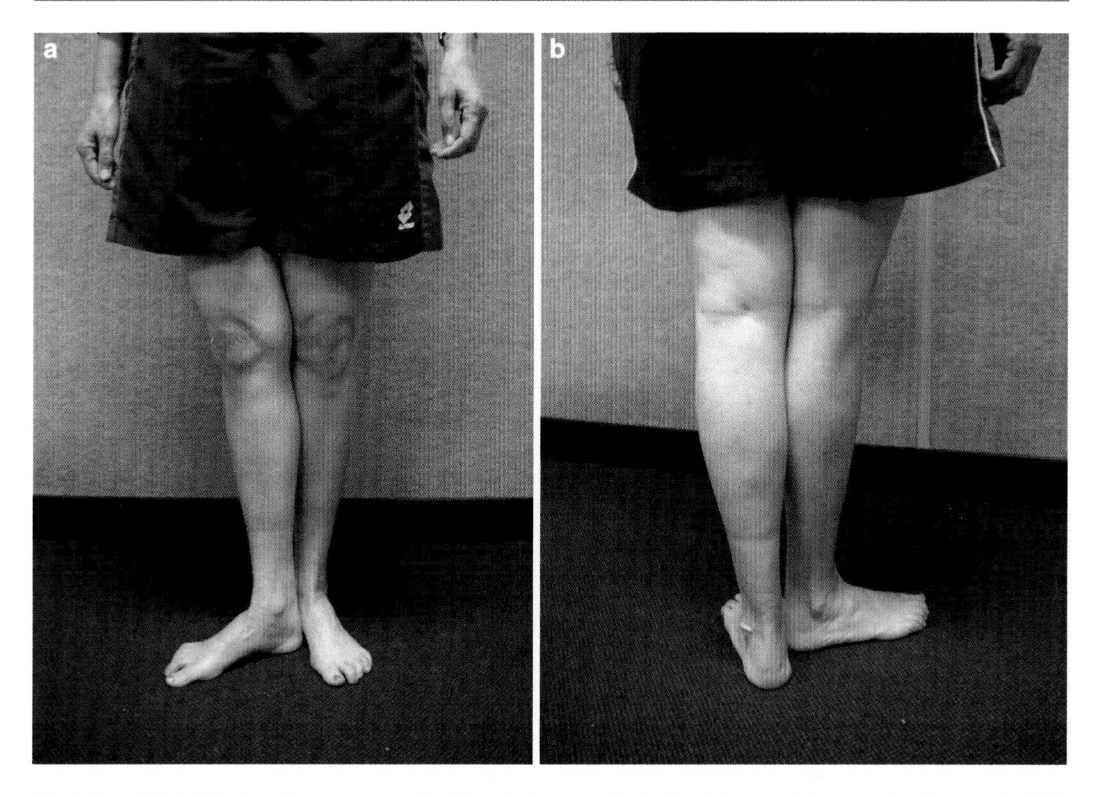

Fig. 3.8 (**a**) Ballet third position—an easy standing strategy to activate the gluteals and decrease the stress on the ITB. The knees should be soft, not be locked back (**b**) Ballet third position from behind

and postural perturbation tasks. At baseline in both the placebo and treatment groups, the VMO came on significantly later than the VL. Following treatment, there was no change in muscle onset timing of the placebo group, but in the physiotherapy group, the onset of VMO and VL occurred simultaneously during concentric activity, and VMO preceded VL during eccentric activity [120].

A recent six treatment randomized, double-blind, placebo-controlled trial which included specific weight-bearing gluteal and VMO training, as well as anterior hip structure stretches, showed that the physical therapy group demonstrated a significantly better response to treatment and greater improvements in pain and functional activities than the placebo group [121]. Hence, physical therapy is effective in improving pain and function in patellofemoral pain patients as well as altering VMO onset relative to VL.

Surgical Intervention

In most circumstances, surgical intervention is not warranted for patellofemoral pain, and if the patient has a surgical procedure to improve pain the symptoms often worsen. However, there are some recalcitrant problems where surgery may be helpful but only after comprehensive nonoperative management has been tried.

1. Lateral release is indicated if the patient has extremely tight lateral retinaculum, particularly the deep fibers.
2. Chondroplasty ± osteoplasty is indicated if the patient is experiencing recurrent effusions and locking of the knee. Minimal intervention is required here.
3. MPFL reconstruction is indicated for a patient with recurrent patellofemoral subluxation.

4. In extremely rare cases, for recurrent patellofemoral dislocation a realignment procedure may be helpful, but the outcome of these procedures is extremely variable.

Conclusion

Management of patellofemoral pain is no longer be difficult if the clinician can determine the underlying causative factors and address those factors in treatment. It is imperative that the patient's symptoms are significantly reduced. This is often achieved by taping the patella, which not only decreases the pain but also promotes an earlier activation of the VMO and increases quadriceps torque. Management will need to include specific VMO training, gluteal control work, stretching tight lateral structures, and appropriate advice regarding the foot, be it orthotics, training, or taping.

References

1. Baquie P, Brukner P. Injuries presenting to an Australian sports medicine centre: a 12 month study. Clin J Sport Med. 1997;7:28–31.
2. Clement DB, Taunton JE, Smart GW, et al. A survey of overuse injuries. Phys Sportsmed. 1981;9:47–58.
3. DeHaven KE, Lintner DM. Athletic injuries: comparison by age, sport and gender. Am J Sports Med. 1986;14:218–24.
4. Devereaux M, Lachmann S. Patellofemoral arthralgia in athletes attending a sports injury clinic. Br J Sports Med. 1984;18:18–21.
5. James SL, Bates BT, Osternig LR. Injuries to runners. Am J Sports Med. 1978;6(2):40–50.
6. Kannus P, Aho H, Järvinen M, et al. Computerised recording of visits to an outpatient sports clinic. Am J Sports Med. 1987;15(1):79–85.
7. Macintyre JG, Taunton JE, Clement DB, et al. Running injuries: a clinical study of 4,173 cases. Clin J Sport Med. 1991;1:81–7.
8. Pagliano JW, Jackson DW. A clinical study of 3,000 long distance runners. Ann Sports Med. 1987;3(2): 88–91.
9. Fulkerson J, Hungerford D. Disorders of the patellofemoral joint. Baltimore MD: Williams and Wilkins; 1997.
10. Grelsamer RP, Klein JR. The biomechanics of the patellofemoral joint. J Orthop Sports Phys Ther. 1998;28(5):286–98.
11. Gresalmer R, McConnell J. The patella – a team approach. Gaithersburg, MD: Aspen Publications; 1998.
12. Fucentese SF, von Roll A, Koch PP, et al. The patella morphology in trochlear dysplasia–a comparative MRI study. Knee. 2006;13(2):145–50.
13. Grelsamer RP, Tedder JL. The lateral trochlear sign. Femoral trochlear dysplasia as seen on a lateral view roentgenograph. Clin Orthop Relat Res. 1992;281: 159–62.
14. Pfirrmann CW, Zanetti M, Romero J, et al. Femoral trochlear dysplasia: MR findings. Radiology. 2000; 216(3):858–64.
15. Labelle H, Roussouly P, Berthonnaud E, et al. Spondylolisthesis, pelvic incidence, and spinopelvic balance: a correlation study. Spine. 2004;29(18): 2049–54.
16. Wenger DE, Kendell KR, Miner MR, et al. Acetabular labral tears rarely occur in the absence of bony abnormalities. Clin Orthop Relat Res. 2004; 426:145–50.
17. Eckhoff DG, Montgomery WK, Kilcoyne RF, et al. Femoral morphometry and anterior knee pain. Clin Orthop Relat Res. 1994;302:64–8.
18. Amed A, Shi S, Hyder A et al. The effect of quadriceps tension characteristics on the patellar tracking pattern. In Transactions of the 34th Orthopaedic Research Society, Atlanta, 1988, p. 280.
19. Heegard J, Leyvraz P, van Kampen A, et al. Influence of soft structures on patellar three dimensional tracking. Clin Orthop Relat Res. 1994;299:235–43.
20. van Kampen A, Huiskes R. The three-dimensional tracking pattern of the human patella. J Orthop Res. 1990;8:372–82.
21. Dye S, Vaupel G, Dye C. Conscious neurosensory mapping of the internal structures of the human knee without intra-articular anaesthesia. Am J Sports Med. 1998;26(6):773–7.
22. Bennell K, Hodges P, Mellor R, et al. The nature of anterior knee pain following injection of hypertonic saline into the infrapatellar fat pad. J Orthop Res. 2004;22(1):116–21.
23. Fujikawa K, Seedhom B, Wright V. Biomechanics of the patellofemoral joint. Part 1&II study of the patellofemoral compartment and movement of the patella. Eng Med. 1983;12(1):3–21.
24. Wiberg G. Studies of the femoropatellar joint. Acta Orthop Scand. 1941;12:319–410.
25. Baumgartl F. Das kniegelenk. Berlin: Springer; 1964.
26. Grana WA, Kriegshauser LA. Scientific basis of extensor mechanism disorders. Clin Sports Med. 1985;4(2):247–57.
27. Insall J. Chondromalacia patellae:patellar malalignment syndrome. Orthop Clin North Am. 1979;10: 117–25.
28. Reider B, Marshall J, Koslin B, et al. The anterior aspect of the knee. J Bone Joint Surg. 1981;63A(3): 351–6.
29. Senavongse W, Amis AA. The effects of articular, retinacular, or muscular deficiencies on patello-

femoral joint stability. J Bone Joint Surg Br. 2005;87(4):577–82.
30. Micheli L, Slater J, Woods E, et al. Patella alta and the adolescent growth spurt. Clin Orthop Relat Res. 1986;213:159–62.
31. Fulkerson JP, Shea KP. Current concepts review: disorder of patellofemoral alignment. J Bone Joint Surg Am. 1990;72A:1424–9.
32. Conlan T, Garth WP, Lemons JE. Evaluation of the medial soft-tissue restraints of the extensor mechanism of the knee. J Bone Joint Surg Am. 1993;75A:682–93.
33. Desio SM, Burks RT, Bachus KN. Soft tissue restraints to lateral patellar translation in the human knee. Am J Sports Med. 1998;26(1):59–65.
34. Hautamaa PV, Fithian DC, Kaufman K, et al. Medial soft tissue restraints in lateral patellar instability and repair. Clin Orthop Relat Res. 1998;349:174–82.
35. Amis AA, Firer P, Mountney J, Senavongse W, Thomas NP. Anatomy and biomechanics of the medial patellofemoral ligament. Knee. 2003;10(3): 215–20.
36. Lieb FJ, Perry J. Quadriceps function. An anatomical and mechanical study. J Bone Joint Surg Am. 1968;50A(8):1535–48.
37. Bose K, Kanagasuntheram R, Osman MBH. Vastus medialis obliquus; an anatomic and physiologic study. Orthopedics. 1980;3:883–0.
38. Raimondo RA, Ahmad CS, Blankevoort L, et al. Patellar stabilization: a quantitative evaluation of the vastus medialis obliquus muscle. Orthopaedics. 1998;21(7):791–5.
39. Scharf W, Weinstable R, Othrner E. Anatomical separation and clinical importance of two different parts of the vastus medialis muscle. Acta Anat (Basel). 1985;123:108–11.
40. Thiranagama R. Nerve supply of the human vastus medialis muscle. J Anat. 1990;170:193–8.
41. Goh JC, Lee PY, Bose K. A cadaver study of the function of the oblique part of vastus medialis. J Bone Joint Surg Br. 1995;77B(2):225–31.
42. Hallisey M, Doughty N, Bennett W, Fulkerson J. Anatomy of the junction of the vastus lateralis tendon and the patella. J Bone Joint Surg. 1987;69A(4):545.
43. Bull AMJ, Senavongse WW, Taylor AR, et al. The effect of the oblique portions of the vastus medialis and lateralis on patellar tracking. In Proceedings of the 11th Conference of the ESB, Toulouse, France; 1998.
44. Cowan SM, Bennell KL, Hodges PW, et al. Delayed onset of electromyographic activity of vastus medialis obliquus relative to vastus lateralis in subjects with patellofemoral pain syndrome. Arch Phys Med Rehabil. 2001;82(2):183–9.
45. Karst GM, Willet GM. Onset timing of electromyographic activity in the vastus medialis oblique and vastus lateralis muscles in subjects with and without patellofemoral pain syndrome. Phys Ther. 1995; 75(9):813–23.
46. Lange GW, Hintermeister RA, Schlegel T, et al. Electromyographic and kinematic analysis of graded treadmill walking and the implications for knee rehabilitation. J Orthop Sports Phys Ther. 1996; 23(5):294–301.
47. Morrish GM, Woledge RC. A comparison of the activation of muscles moving the patella in normal subjects and in patients with chronic patellofemoral problems. Scand J Rehabil Med. 1997;29(1):43–8.
48. Powers CM, Landel RF, Perry J. Timing and intensity of vastus muscle activity during functional activities in subjects with and without patellofemoral pain. Phys Ther. 1996;76:946–55.
49. Reynolds L, Levin T, Medeiros J, et al. EMG activity of vastus medialis obliquus and vastus lateralis and their role in patella alignment. Am J Phys Med. 1983;62:61.
50. Ahmed AM, Burke DL, Hyder A. Force analysis of the patellar mechanism. J Orthop Res. 1987;5:69–85.
51. Brindle TJ, Mattacola C, McCrory J. Electromyographic changes in the gluteus medius during stair ascent and descent in subjects with anterior knee pain. Knee Surg Sports Traumatol Arthrosc. 2003;11(4):244–51.
52. Ireland ML, Willson JD, Ballantyne BT, et al. Hip strength in females with and without patellofemoral pain. J Orthop Sports Phys Ther. 2003;33(11): 671–6.
53. Reilly D, Martens M. Experimental analyses of the quadriceps muscle force and patellofemoral joint reaction force for various activities. Acta Orthop Scand. 1972;43:126–37.
54. van Eijden TMG, Kouwenhoven E, Verburg J, Weijs WA. A mathematical model of the patellofemoral joint. J Biomech. 1986;19(3):219–29.
55. Huberti HH, Hayes WC, Stone JL, Shybut GT. Force ratios in the quadriceps tendon and ligamentum patellae. J Orthop Res. 1984;2(1):49–54.
56. Carson W, James S, Larson R, Singer K, Winternitz W. Patello-femoral disorders - parts I and II. Clin Orthop Relat Res. 1984;185:165–74.
57. Burgess R. Patellofemoral joint transverse displacement and tibial rotation. Unpublished Project Report Graduate Diploma Manipulative Therapy, SAIT, Adelaide; 1985.
58. Goodfellow J, Hungerford D, Zindel M. Patellofemoral joint mechanics & pathology, 1 & 2. J Bone Joint Surg Br. 1976;58B(3):287–99.
59. Bandi W. Chondromalacia patellae und femoropatellare arthrose. Helv Chir Acta. 1972;1(supp): 3–70.
60. Dye S. The knee as a biologic transmission with an envelope of function : a theory. Clin Orthop. 1996;325:10–8.
61. Torres L, Dunlop DD, Peterfy C, Guermazi A, Prasad P, Hayes KW, Song J, Cahue S, Chang A, Marshall M, Sharma L. The relationship between specific tissue lesions and pain severity in persons with knee osteoarthritis. Osteoarthr Cartil. 2006;14: 1033–40.
62. Hill CL, Hunter DJ, Niu J, Clancy M, Guermazi A, Genant H, Gale D, Grainger A, Conaghan P, Felson

DT. Synovitis detected on magnetic resonance imaging and its relation to pain and cartilage loss in knee osteoarthritis. Ann Rheum Dis. 2007;66:1599–603.
63. Sengupta M, Zhang YQ, Niu JB, Guermazi A, Grigorian M, Gale D, Felson DT, Hunter DJ. High signal in knee osteophytes is not associated with knee pain. Osteoarthritis Cartilage. 2006;14:413–7.
64. Bierdert R, Stauffer E, Niklaus NF. Occurence of free nerve endings in the soft tissue of the knee joint. A histologic investigation. Am J Sport Med. 1992; 20:430–3.
65. Fulkerson JP, Tennant R, Jaivin JS, et al. Histological evidence of retinacular nerve injury associated with patellofemoral malalignment. Clin Orthop Relat Res. 1985;197:196–205.
66. Sanchis-Alfonso V, Rosello-Sastre E. Immunohistochemical analysis for neural markers of the lateral retinaculum in patients with isolated symptomatic patellofemoral malalignment. Am J Sport Med. 2000;28:725–31.
67. Dye SF, Chew MH. The use of scintigraphy to detect increased osseous metabolic activity about the knee. J Bone Joint Surg Am. 1993;75A:1388–406.
68. Hoffa A. The influence of the adipose tissue with regard to the pathology of the knee joint. JAMA. 1904;43:795–6.
69. Dragoo JL, Johnson C, McConnell J. Evaluation and treatment of disorders of the infrapatellar fat pad. Sports Med. 2012;42:51–67.
70. Clements KM, Ball AD, Jones HB, Brinckmann S, Read SJ, Murray F. Cellullar and histopathological changes in the infrapatellar fat pad. Osteoarthritis Cartilage. 2009;17:805–12.
71. Witonski D, Wagrowska-Danielewicz M. Distribution of substance-P nerve fibers in the knee joint of patients with anterior knee pain. A preliminary report. Knee Surg Sports Traumatol Arthrosc. 1999;7:177–83.
72. Bohnsack M, Meier F, Walter GF, Hurschler C, Schmolke S, Wirth CJ, Rühmann O. Distribution of substance-P nerves inside the infrapatellar fat pad and the adjacent synovial tissue: a neurohistological approach to anterior knee pain syndrome. Arch Orthop Trauma Surg. 2005;125(9):592–7.
73. Bohnsack M, Hurschler C, Demirtas T, Rühmann O, Stukenborg-Colsman C, Wirth CJ. Infrapatellar fat pad pressure and volume changes of the anterior compartment during knee motion: possible clinical consequences to the anterior knee pain syndrome. Knee Surg Sports Traumatol Arthrosc. 2005;13(2):135–41.
74. Tang G, Niitsu M, Ikeda K, Endo H, Itai Y. Fibrous scar in the infrapatellar fat pad after arthroscopy: MR imaging. Radiat Med. 2000;18(1):1–5.
75. Apostolaki E, Cassar-Pullicino VN, Tyrrell PN, McCall IW. MRI appearances of the infrapatellar fat pad in occult traumatic patellar dislocation. Clin Radiol. 1999;54(11):743–7.
76. Hodges PW, Mellor R, Crossley K, Bennell K. Pain induced by injection of hypertonic saline into the infrapatellar fat pad and effect on coordination of the quadriceps muscles. Arthritis Rheum. 2009;61: 70–7.
77. Juhn SK, Li W, Kim JY, Javel E, Levine S, Odland RM. Effect of stress-related hormones on inner ear fluid homeostasis and function. Am J Otol. 1999;20:800–6.
78. Van de Kar LD, Blair ML. Forebrain pathways mediating stress-induced hormone secretion. Front Neuroendocrinol. 1999;20:1–48.
79. Powers CM. The influence of altered lower-extremity kinematics on patellofemoral joint dysfunction: a theoretical perspective. J Orthop Sports Phys Ther. 2003;33(11):639–46.
80. McConnell J. The physical therapist's approach to patellofemoral disorders. In: Fithian D, editor. Injuries to the extensor mechanism of the knee. Clin Sports Med. 2002;21(3):363–87.
81. Buchbinder R, Naparo N, Bizzo E. The relationship of abnormal pronation to chondromalacia patellae in distance runners. J Am Podiatry Assoc. 1979;69(2): 159–61.
82. Tiberio D. The effect of excessive subtalar joint pronation on patellofemoral mechanics; a theoretical model. J Orthop Sports Phys Ther. 1987;9(4):160–5.
83. Powers CM, Maffucci R, Hampton S. Rearfoot posture in subjects with patellofemoral pain. J Orthop Sports Phys Ther. 1995;22(4):155–60.
84. Powers CM, Chen PY, Reischl SF, Perry J. Comparison of foot pronation and lower extremity rotation in persons with and without patellofemoral pain. Foot Ankle Int. 2002;23(7):634–40.
85. Mellor R, Hodges P. Motor unit synchronization between medial and lateral vasti muscles. Clin Neurophysiol. 2005;116(7):1585–95.
86. Wickiewicz TL, Roy RR, Powell PL, et al. Muscle architecture of the human lower limb. Clin Orthop Relat Res. 1983;179:275–83.
87. Voight M, Weider D. Comparative reflex response times of the vastus medialis and the vastus lateralis in normal subjects with extensor mechanism dysfunction. Am J Sports Med. 1991;19(2):131–7.
88. Souza DR, Gross M. Comparison of vastus medialis obliquus: vastus lateralis muscle integrated electromyographic ratios between healthy subjects and patients with patellofemoral pain. Phys Ther. 1991;71(4):310–20.
89. Grabiner MD, Koh TJ, Draganich LF. Neuromechanics of the patellofemoral joint. Med Sci Sports Exerc. 1994;26(1):10–21.
90. Witvrouw E, Lysens R, Bellemans J, et al. Intrinsic risk factors for the development of anterior knee pain in an athletic population. A two year prospective study. Am J Sports Med. 2000;28(4):480–9.
91. Cowan SM, Hodges PW, Bennell KL, et al. Altered vastii recruitment when people with patellofemoral pain syndrome complete a postural task. Arch Phys Med Rehabil. 2002;83(7):989–95.
92. Cowan S, Bennell K, Hodges P, et al. Simultaneous feedforward recruitment of the vasti in untrained

postural tasks can be restored by physical therapy. J Orthop Res. 2003;21(3):553–8.
93. Abernathy PJ, Townsend P, Rose R, Radin E. Is chondromalacia a separate clinical entity? J Bone Joint Surg Br. 1978;60(B(2)):205–10.
94. Spencer J, Hayes K, Alexander I. Knee joint effusion and quadriceps reflex inhibition in man. Arch Phys Med. 1984;65:171–7.
95. Stokes M, Young A. Investigations of quadriceps inhibition: implications for clinical practice. Physiotherapy. 1984;70:425–8.
96. Maitland GD. Vertebral manipulation. London: Butterworths; 1986.
97. McConnell J. Promoting effective segmental alignment. In: Crosbie J, McConnell J, editors. Key issues in musculoskeletal physiotherapy. Oxford: Butterworth–Heinemann; 1993.
98. McConnell J. Rehabilitation and nonoperative treatment of patellar instability. Sports Med Arthrosc. 2007;15(2):95–104.
99. Broom MJ, Fulkerson JP. The plica syndrome: a new perspective. Orthop Clin North Am. 1986;17(2): 279–81.
100. Patel D. Plica as a cause of anterior knee pain. Orthop Clin North Am. 1986;17(2):273.
101. Jackson R, Marshall D, Fujisawa Y. The pathological medial shelf. Orthop Clin North Am. 1982; 13(2):307.
102. O'Neill D, Micheli L. Overuse injuries in the young athlete. Clin Sports Med. 1989;7(3):591–610.
103. Perry J. Gait analysis. Thorofare, NJ: Slack; 1992.
104. Henriksen M, Rosager S, Aaboe J, Graven-Nielsen T, Bliddal H. Experimental knee pain reduces muscle strength. J Pain. 2011;12(4):460–7.
105. Gilleard W, McConnell J, Parsons D. The effect of patellar taping on the onset of vastus medialis obliquus and vastus lateralis muscle activity in persons with patellofemoral pain. Phys Ther. 1998; 78(1):25–32.
106. Powers C, Landel R, Sosnick T, et al. The effects of patellar taping on stride characteristics and joint motion in subjects with patellofemoral pain. J Orthop Sports Phys Ther. 1997;26(6):286–91.
107. Cowan S, Bennell K, Hodges P. Therapeutic patellar taping changes the timing of vasti muscle activation in people with patellofemoral pain syndrome. Clin J Sport Med. 2002;12(6):339–47.
108. Conway A, Malone T, Conway P. Patellar alignment/tracking alteration: effect on force output and perceived pain. Isokinet Exerc Sci. 1992;2:9–17.
109. Handfield T, Kramer J. Effect of McConnell taping on perceived pain and knee extensor torques during isokinetic exercise performed by patients with patellofemoral pain syndrome. Physiotherapy Canada; 2000, pp. 39–44.
110. Derasari A, Brindle TJ, Alter KE, Sheehan FT. McConnell taping shifts the patella inferiorly in patients with patellofemoral pain: a dynamic magnetic resonance imaging study. Phys Ther. 2010; 90(3):411–9.
111. Kilbreath SL, Perkins S, Crosbie J. McConnell J Gluteal taping improves hip extension during stance phase of walking following stroke. Aust J Physiother. 2006;52(1):53–6.
112. Tobin S, Robinson G. The effect of McConnell's vastus lateralis inhibition taping technique on vastus lateralis and vastus medialis obliquus activity. Physiotherapy. 2000;26(4):173–83.
113. Jensen JL, Marstrand PC, Nielsen JB. Motor skill training and strength training are associated with different plastic changes in the central nervous system. J Appl Physiol. 2005;99(4):1558–68.
114. Sale D, MacDougall D. Specificity of strength training: a review for coach and athlete. Can J Appl Sport Sci. 1981;6(2):87–92.
115. Sale D. Influence of exercise and training on motor unit activation. Exerc Sport Sci Rev. 1987;5:95–151.
116. Kitai T, Sale D. Specificity of joint angle in isometric training. Eur J Appl Physiol. 1989;64:1500.
117. Stensdotter AK, Hodges PW, Mellor R, Sundelin G, Hager-Ross C. Quadriceps activation in closed and in open kinetic chain exercise. Med Sci Sports Exerc. 2003;35(12):2043–7.
118. Escamilla RF, Fleisig GS, Zheng N, et al. Biomechanics of the knee during closed kinetic chain and open kinetic chain exercises. Med Sci Sports Exerc. 1998;30(4):556–69.
119. Collins N, Crossley K, Beller E, Darnell R, McPoil T, Vicenzino B. Foot orthoses and physiotherapy in the treatment of patellofemoral pain syndrome: randomised clinical trial. Br J Sports Med. 2009; 43(3):169–71.
120. Cowan SM, Bennell KL, Crossley K, et al. Physical therapy alters recruitment of the vasti in patellofemoral pain syndrome. Med Sci Sports Exerc. 2002;34(12):1879–85.
121. Crossley K, Bennell K, Green S, et al. Physical therapy for patellofemoral pain: a randomized, double-blinded, placebo-controlled trial. Am J Sports Med. 2002;30(6):857–65.

4 Surgical Treatment of Patellar Instability in Skeletally Immature Athletes

J. Lee Pace, William L. Hennrikus, and Mininder S. Kocher

Introduction

Management of patellofemoral instability in the skeletally immature patient has a unique set of challenges. These patients are commonly the most active group of patients seen in a sports practice with several years of participation in organized sport ahead of them. On a social level, organized athletics creates a peer network and it often becomes an "identity meaning" activity for the young athlete. Strong peer, coach, and family pressure coupled with a strong desire to participate may reduce compliance with therapy and activity restrictions. In addition, children with collagen disorders such as Ehlers–Danlos syndrome, Marfan's disease, and Down syndrome commonly present with patellar instability. These patients require unique management in contrast to the majority of patients where anatomic restoration may be sacrificed in the name of stability [1].

From a surgical perspective, the presence of open growth plates limits some reconstructive options, namely, tibial tubercle osteotomies. In addition, the physes can be damaged during soft tissue reconstruction and lead to growth disturbances with associated disability that may require more invasive corrective procedures. Conversely, future growth potential leaves open the possibility of correction of patellar instability due to certain anatomic malalignments via guided growth principles. Surgical treatment of the unstable patellofemoral joint in the skeletally immature patient follows the same mechanical principles as adult treatment: to realign and rebalance the extensor mechanism and provide smooth, stable patellofemoral motion. Like adults, children may need proximal, distal, or combined realignment.

Epidemiology

Adolescents represent the highest risk group for acute traumatic patellar dislocation [2, 3]. Reports vary somewhat on incidence. Waterman et al. used the National Electronic Injury Surveillance System (NEISS) to estimate an incidence rate of approximately 11.19/100,000 person-years in the 15–19 age group that presented to an emergency room [3]. The incidence in the 10–14 age group was close to 7/100,000 person-years [3]. The authors acknowledged that

J.L. Pace, M.D.
Surgery Department, Orthopaedic Surgery, Children's Hospital Los Angeles, Los Angeles, CA, USA

Orthopaedic Surgery Department, Keck School of Medicine, University of Southern California, Los Angeles, CA, USA

W.L. Hennrikus, M.D.
Orthopaedics Department, Penn State College of Medicine, Hershey, PA, USA

M.S. Kocher, M.D., M.P.H. (✉)
Orthopaedic Surgery, Sports Medicine, Children's Hospital Boston, Harvard Medical School, 300 Longwood Avenue, Hunnewell 2, Boston, MA 02115, USA
e-mail: mininder.kocher@childrens.harvard.edu

R.V. West and A.C. Colvin (eds.), *The Patellofemoral Joint in the Athlete*,
DOI 10.1007/978-1-4614-4157-1_4, © Springer Science+Business Media New York 2014

these numbers might be an underestimation due to sampling bias of patients exclusively from emergency rooms. Fithian found the incidence in patients aged 10–17 to be 29/100,000 (95 % CI 21–37) in the Kaiser Permanente system in San Diego [2]. Nietosvaara et al. reported an incidence of 43/100,000 for the entire pediatric population and 107/100,000 for the age range of 9–15 years in Helsinki. The average age for a first-time dislocation in Nietosvaara's group was 13.3 years (range 9.2–15.9) [4]. Some have reported that the most "at-risk" age for an acute patella dislocation is 15 [4, 5]. While several studies have found females to have a higher rate of patellar instability [2, 4, 6–8], Waterman found no difference in gender [3]. Fithian reported the incidence of patellar instability to be 33/100,000 (95 % CI 22–44) in females compared to 25/100,000 (95 % CI 16–34) in males in the 10–17-year age group [2]. The incidence of an associated osteochondral fracture in the pediatric and adolescent age group is thought to be higher than adults, and studies have reported rates anywhere from 25 to 75 % [9].

Anatomy

The medial patellofemoral ligament (MPFL) is the main checkrein to lateral translation of the patella from 0 to 30° of knee flexion [10–12]. An elegant cadaver study in adult patients by Baldwin has shown the femoral origin of the MPFL is in a groove between the medial epicondyle and the adductor tubercle and is immediately superior to the origin of the superficial MCL from which the MPFL receives an oblique decussation of fibers [11]. The MPFL joins with the inferior portion of the vastus medialis obliquus (VMO) tendon to insert on the upper two-thirds of the medial patella [11].

The distal femoral physis has a characteristic undulating structure with relatively proximal medial and lateral borders (Fig. 4.1) [13–15]. Within this macroscopic appearance are smaller undulations which increase the surface area of the physis [13]. It is the largest and fastest growing physis in the body [16, 17]. It contributes

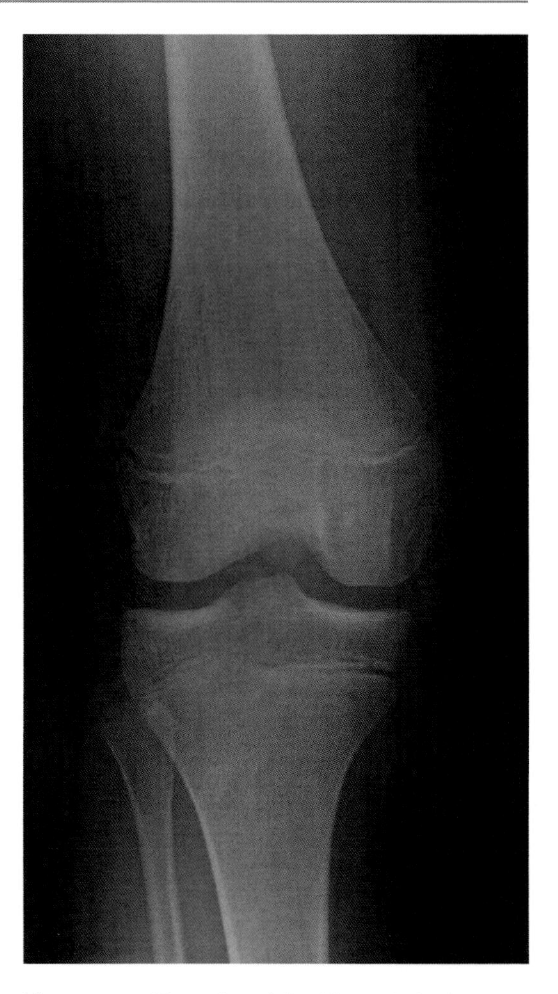

Fig. 4.1 Any illustration of distal femoral physis

approximately 70 % of the length of the femur and 37 % of the length of the entire limb. On average, this physis contributes 1 cm of growth per year and from age 7 to skeletal maturity, it contributes 1.3 cm of growth per year except the last 2 years when it contributes 6 mm each year [16, 17]. This growth plate fuses with the metaphysis between 14 and 16 years in females and 16 and 18 years in males [16, 17].

The proximal tibial physis has a much more flat macroscopic appearance. 3D modeling shows it to have a slight proximally directed biconcave structure with a pit located central and posterior that corresponds to the epiphyseal attachment of the PCL [13, 14]. This physis contributes approximately 55 % of the length of the tibia and 25 % of the length of the entire limb. On average it contributes 0.65 cm of growth per year and from age 7 to skeletal maturity, it contributes 9 mm of growth per year except the last 2 years when it contributes 4–5 mm. This physis fuses with the metaphysis between 13 and 15 years in females and 15 and 19 years in males [16, 17].

The tibial tubercle apophysis develops as an extension of the proximal tibial physis around 13 weeks gestation and typically develops a secondary ossification center around 8 years of age [16, 17]. This center starts distally and progresses proximally towards the proximal tibial epiphysis with an average age of fusion of 17 years. The apophysis fuses with the underlying metaphysis between 13 and 15 years in females and 15 and 19 years in males [16, 17]. The tibial tubercle apophysis is unique from the proximal tibial physis in that the apophyseal cartilage is fibrocartilage as opposed to columnar, which is seen in the epiphysis [13, 18].

The patella is completely cartilaginous at birth and begins to ossify between 2 and 4 years of age. There are multiple ossification centers that coalesce over time. Ossification is typically complete in late adolescence [16, 19].

The articular cartilage-subchondral bone transition zone is unique in adolescents. In the juvenile patient, long interdigitating fingers of uncalcified cartilage project into the subchondral bone. As the child matures, these projections are gradually replaced with calcified matrix to form the eventual cement line. Both the cement line in the adult and the interdigitating uncalcified cartilage fingers in the juvenile provide adequate toughness to the osteochondral region. In the adolescent, as these cartilage fingers are replaced, this zone becomes relatively weak and more susceptible to shear forces thus increasing the risk of an osteochondral fracture during a patella dislocation or in isolation [9, 20, 21].

Management

Primary Dislocation

There are few studies looking specifically at the management of pediatric and adolescent athletes with patellar instability. Thus, while there are general recommendations from the adult literature, these may not be directly applicable in the skeletally immature population. Most practitioners recommend conservative treatment of a primary traumatic patella dislocation in the absence of cartilaginous damage warranting immediate surgical intervention [8, 22]. Treatment focuses on activity restriction, swelling reduction, lower extremity flexibility with focus on the quadriceps, hamstrings, and iliotibial band, and a strengthening program focused on the VMO/quadriceps, gluteals, and core [23, 24]. Return to sports is usually permitted after 3 months given appropriate progress in therapy. Even with compliant patients, the redislocation rate in adolescent patients is high with percentages ranging from 16 to 70 % [8, 25]. Approximately half of patients with recurrent instability will have an event in the first 2 years after the initial dislocation [8]. Recurrent subluxation, which is hard to quantitate, is also high in this age group with rates ranging from 33 to 91 % [8, 25].

The few studies that have looked exclusively at initial treatment in the pediatric and adolescent age group seem to conclude that surgical stabilization for first-time dislocations does not reduce the dislocation rate in this age group compared to nonoperative treatment [8, 22]. Palmu et al. conducted the largest study to date examining exclusively a pediatric and adolescent age group. They carried out a prospective, randomized study designed to evaluate nonoperative vs. operative treatment of acute, traumatic patella dislocations in 62 patients (64 knees) under 16 years of age with 14-year follow-up. Operative repair involved medial tissue repair directed at the specific site of injury (i.e., medial patellotibial ligament, midsubstance vs. femoral or patellar MPFL insertion tears) and lateral release in 25 knees. Four knees had medial repair only and seven knees had lateral release only due to an inability to dislocate the patella laterally during an exam under anesthesia. The dislocation rates were similar amongst the two groups: 71 % for the operative group and 67 % for the nonoperative group [8]. Fifty-two percent of patients experienced a recurrent dislocation within 2 years after their index dislocation. Furthermore, the authors reported the only statistically significant predictive factor found for recurrent dislocation in this age group was a positive family history. This held true for patients treated operatively or nonoperatively. Factors such as trochlear dysplasia, age, gender, and patellar height were not shown to increase risk in either group [8]. It should be noted that in the patients treated operatively that the authors performed repair "at the site of injury without aponeurotic or tendinous augmentation." We are unsure if this statement means that the damaged and elongated tissue was not imbricated at the time of repair. Other studies have found similar results in this age group. Apostolovic et al. conducted a smaller prospective randomized study in 37 adolescents. Patients were randomized to initial stabilization if they had a significant loose body found on initial imaging studies. With a mean follow-up of 6.1 years, the authors noted no significant differences in functional outcomes, subjective outcomes, or episodes of recurrent instability [22]. Nikku et al. conducted a prospective study comparing initial nonoperative vs. operative treatment in patient group consisting of 60 % adolescents. While they found no differences between the two groups regarding subjective outcomes or recurrent instability, they did not separate patients by age group for the reader to make a firm conclusion regarding outcomes for the skeletally immature population [26].

In the event of an associated osteochondral fracture, immediate surgical intervention aimed at removal or repair of the fragment is indicated [9]. The decision to perform a concomitant stabilization procedure can be made between patient, family, and treating surgeon. Generally, if a small loose body is removed arthroscopically, stabilization is less likely performed. In the case of a sizeable fragment requiring arthrotomy, a stabilization procedure can be performed. There are no firm recommendations guiding treatment for pediatric and adolescent patients in this situation.

Recurrent Dislocation

If a patient sustains a second patellar dislocation, surgery is more seriously considered. Continued nonoperative care can be instituted if that is the wish of the patient and family. This decision should be reached after appropriate counseling regarding risk of further damage to articular cartilage with subsequent dislocations and the potential need for long-term brace use and/or activity modification. The decision to proceed with surgery should be made between the patient, family, and physician after risks, benefits, and alternatives are discussed. The type of surgery performed should be individualized and take each patient's anatomy into consideration. Physical exam findings such as genu valgum, *Q*-angle, femoral anteversion, external tibial torsion, and generalized ligamentous laxity should be noted [21, 27–30]. Radiographs should be evaluated for patella alta, patellar tilt, lateral patellar overhang, open physes, and loose bodies [7, 31, 32]. Sulcus and congruence angles are noted but they rarely affect surgical planning in this age group [33]. If magnetic resonance imaging (MRI) is obtained, the tibial tubercle to trochlear groove distance (TT–TG) is recorded and any other injuries are noted as well [34]. Trochlear dysplasia, usually better seen on MRI, is noted mainly for counseling purposes [33].

In patients who have growth remaining and patellar instability that has failed conservative measures, surgical planning must take the physes into consideration. Patients who are candidates for distal realignment cannot undergo a tibial tubercle osteotomy, as the proximal tibial physis and tibial tubercle apophysis will be violated and result in a recurvatum deformity or possible distal migration of the apophysis [35, 36]. Soft tissue realignment procedures must be considered. Surgical options include the Galeazzi and Roux–Goldthwait procedures [37–41]. Proximal realignment risks damage to the distal femoral physis. This is particularly pertinent when considering certain methods of MPFL reconstruction. Primary MPFL/medial retinacular plication and MPFL reconstruction techniques not requiring femoral bone tunnels are viable options [21, 42–45]. If MPFL reconstruction with a femoral bone tunnel is considered, fluoroscopic assistance is mandatory to avoid physeal disturbance in addition to determining appropriate tunnel placement [46–48].

Surgical Options

Proximal Realignment

Senior Author's Preferred Technique: Open Medial Plication

It is standard practice for the senior author (MSK) to perform proximal realignment with an open medial plication with or without lateral release as first-line treatment, unless there is compelling evidence to add a distal procedure. The procedure closely resembles that of Nam and Karzel [49]. Diagnostic arthroscopy is performed in standard fashion. Any internal derangement is repaired as indicated. Patellar tracking is visualized and the need for a lateral release is determined. If performed, the lateral release is accomplished with curved Mayo scissors through the lateral portal. The soft tissue overlying the lateral retinaculum is bluntly dissected off with the scissors in the closed position prior to performing the release. Any cut branches of the lateral geniculate artery or other vessels are cauterized with an Oratec probe (Oratec Interventions, Inc, Menlo Park, CA). The release is usually carried proximally to the level of the vastus lateralis muscle. A partial release stopping short of this level can be performed if adequate release is deemed to be achieved as evidenced by eversion of the patella beyond neutral. Alternately, the lateral release can be performed with an underwater electrocautery device. After completion of arthroscopy and possible lateral release, a 4-cm medial parapatellar incision is made and sharp dissection is carried down to the level of the medial retinacular structures. Soft tissue flaps are created laterally over the anterior aspect of the patella and medially near the adductor tubercle and medial epicondyle. A longitudinal incision 1.5 cm medial to the patella is made through the retinacular structures down to synovium. This incision is typically the length of the patella with proximal extension into the inferior fibers of the VMO if advancement is planned. In cases of acute traumatic patellar dislocation with an intra-articular loose body that requires immediate surgical intervention, the site of the MPFL tear should be addressed directly (i.e., repair at the site of the MPFL tear: patella, mid-substance, femur). In the recurrent dislocator who is having elective surgery, the MPFL is typically healed, albeit in an elongated fashion, so the standard incision 1.5 cm medial to the patella can be made. Heavy, nonabsorbable suture such as #2 Fiberwire (Arthrex, Naples, FL) is used and is typically placed in vertical mattress fashion (Fig. 4.2). The other senior author (WLH) typically uses a large Ethibond (Ethicon, Somerville, NJ). While the exact amount of plication can be different, in general, about 1 cm of tissue on either side of the incision is taken up with the suture. Sutures are passed, cut, and tagged and the adequacy of the plication is determined prior to definitive suture tying. Data exist showing MPFL repair to be less strong than several reconstruction techniques in cadaver models [50]. Thus, sometimes the repair will overcorrect patellar alignment but not to the point of causing medial subluxation. This decision can be made on a case-by-case basis and depends on patient factors such as constitutional

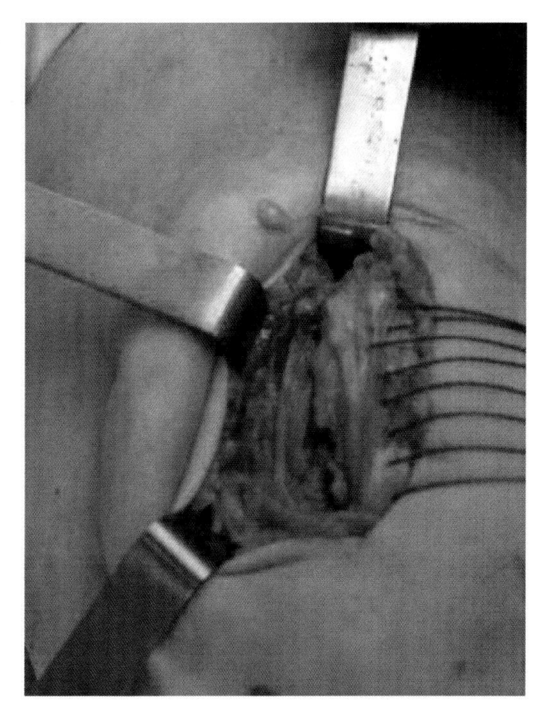

Fig. 4.2 Intraop photo of open medial plication

flexibility, shallow trochlear groove, and patella alta. Postoperatively, the patient is placed in a flexible brace aimed at medializing the patella. Full weight bearing and motion are encouraged immediately. Depending on the patient, full weight bearing may be best accomplished in full extension as this help minimize risks of flexion contracture and quad atrophy. Early motion helps the patella settle in the trochlear groove and attain a new level of tensioning taking advantage of the fact that MPFL repairs sometimes "stretch out" postoperatively. Isometric quadriceps exercises and straight leg raises are started 1 week after surgery and progressed to resistive exercises after 6 weeks. This procedure differs from Nam and Karzel's technique in that they incised the retinacular structures off the medial border of the patella and advanced them onto the anterior patellar surface [49].

MPFL Reconstruction with Quadriceps Tendon Autograft

If MPFL reconstruction is deemed appropriate, there are a few techniques that do not require femoral bone tunnels and, thus, minimize risk to the distal femoral physis. Noyes and Albright have described a technique using quadriceps tendon autograft [43]. The technique begins with standard arthroscopic examination of the knee with lateral release as needed and addressing any other internal derangement. A 5–6-cm longitudinal medial parapatellar incision is made centered on the widest aspect of the patella. Skin flaps are raised to allow visualization from the medial epicondyle and intermuscular septum to the medial half of the patella and distal quadriceps tendon and VMO. An 8 × 70-mm-full-thickness graft is harvested from the medial quadriceps tendon, leaving its attachment secure on the patella. Two to three millimeters of medial tendon adjacent to the VMO is left intact for later closure. If more length is needed, the tendon can be carefully dissected subperiosteally off the patella an additional 1 cm before turning it medially. A suture anchor can be placed here to reinforce the transition. Medial dissection along the length of the patella between the medial retinaculum and capsule is performed to the medial epicondyle, and a soft tissue hole is made at this level for graft passage. The graft is passed through the hole deep to the medial retinaculum. With the knee in 30–45° of flexion, the medial retinaculum is imbricated and the tendon harvest site is closed. Appropriate imbrication is determined if the patella can be laterally translated approximately 25 % of its width and the knee flexed easily to at least 90°. With this amount of tension, the tendon graft is sewn to the medial intermuscular septum at the level of the medial epicondyle and adductor tubercle to recreate the MPFL. Suturing the graft to adjacent patellar periosteum and overlying imbricated retinaculum also reinforces its attachment on the patella. The procedure is displayed in Fig. 4.3 [43].

Steensen et al. also reported a similar procedure using quadriceps tendon autograft [42]. While the technique differs only slightly, they used a K-wire in the femur to determine graft isometry and also secured the graft by passing suture through femoral bone tunnels. As already discussed, these bone tunnels place the distal femoral physis at risk for damage.

It must be noted that while the senior authors (MSK, WLH) has used this procedure with good effect, there are no published studies beyond the above case reports examining outcomes in a series of patients.

MPFL Reconstruction with Semitendinosus Autograft

Deie et al. described a technique using the semitendinosus to reconstruct the MPFL without bone tunnels in four skeletally immature patients (six knees) with an average age of 8.5 years (6–10) [45]. The tendon is harvested through an incision on the anteromedial tibia using an open tendon stripper leaving it attached to the tibia. A second 2-cm incision is made over the origin of the MCL on the femur, and a 1-cm slit is created in the posterior 1/3 of the MCL origin. A third incision is created on the medial patella and a tunnel is created between the medial retinaculum and the knee capsule. The tendon is brought under the posterior 1/3 of the MCL origin and through the retinacular tunnel to the attachment site of the MPFL on the medial patella. With the knee at 30°

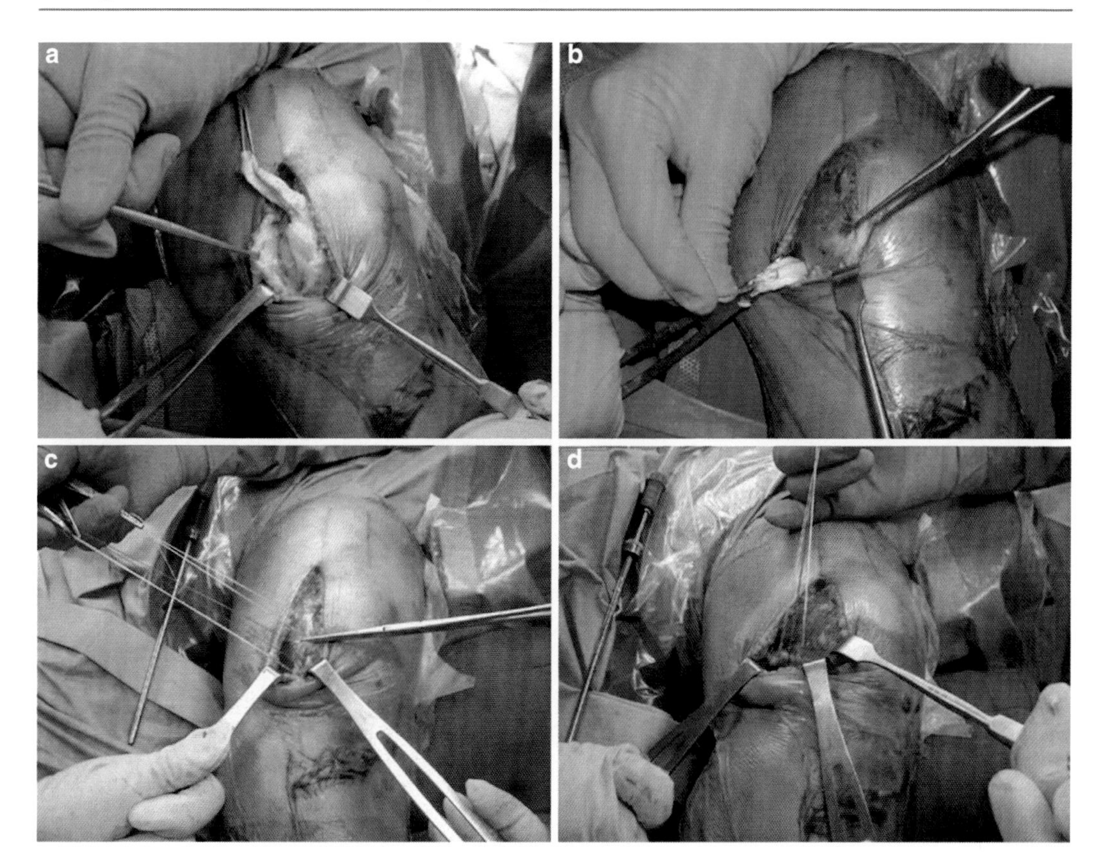

Fig. 4.3 (**a**) Subcutaneous dissection deep to the medial retinaculum posteriorly to the medial epicondyle and the medial intermuscular septum; (**b**) puncture of the medial retinaculum distal to the VMO, anterior to the intermuscular septum, and superficial to the medial epicondyle. Setting of tension on the medial side with (**c**) imbrication of the medial retinaculum and (**d**) tensioning and securing of the graft to the medial retinaculum. From Noyes FR, Albright JC. Reconstruction of the medial patellofemoral ligament with autologous quadriceps tendon. Arthroscopy. Aug 2006;22(8):904 e901–907. Reprinted with permission from Elsevier Limited

of flexion, the graft is sutured to the anterior patella after appropriate tensioning has been determined (Fig. 4.4). At an average of 7.4 years of follow-up, the authors reported no recurrent instability and a mean Kujala score of 96.3 [45].

MPFL Reconstruction with Adductor Magnus Tendon Autograft

Recently, Sillanpää et al. [44] described a modification of an earlier technique described by Avikainen et al. [51] to reconstruct the MPFL with adductor magnus tendon autograft. After diagnostic arthroscopy, a single 3–4-cm longitudinal incision is made midway between the medial patellar border and the adductor tubercle. Flaps are raised medially and laterally exposing the adductor magnus tendon, adductor tubercle, and medial patella. A tendon stripper is used to harvest the medial 2/3 of the adductor magnus tendon for a length of 12–14 cm, leaving it attached distally. The graft is tunneled between the retinaculum and capsule and fixed to the patella with suture anchors. Appropriate tensioning is done with the knee in approximately 30° of flexion. The authors have no experience with this technique, and it is unclear why 12–14 cm of tendon is harvested other than it is the approximate length of available tendon. A study evaluating outcomes in a series of patients undergoing this procedure has yet to be published.

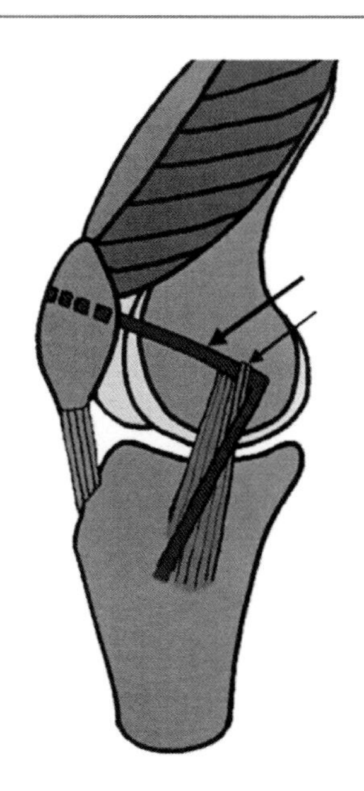

Fig. 4.4 Reconstruction of the MPFL. The semitendinosus is transferred to the patella by passing it under the posterior one-third of the proximal aspect of the superficial MCL and then anchoring on the patella

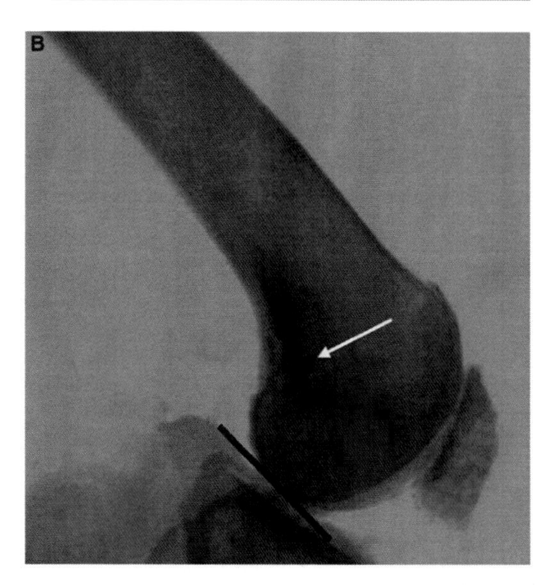

Fig. 4.5 Two perpendiculars to line 1 are drawn, intersecting the contact point of the medial condyle and the posterior cortex (point 1, line 2) and intersecting the most posterior point of the Blumensaat line (point 2, line 3). For determination of the vertical position, the distance between line 2 and the lead ball center is measured as well as the distance between line 2 and line 3. From Schottle PB, Schmeling A, Rosenstiel N, Weiler A. Radiographic landmarks for femoral tunnel placement in medial patellofemoral ligament reconstruction. Am J Sports Med 2007;35:801–4. Reprinted with permission from SAGE Publications

MPFL Reconstruction Using Femoral Bone Tunnels

Various methods for MPFL reconstruction using femoral bone tunnels are discussed elsewhere in this book. In children, MPFL reconstruction using a femoral bone tunnel risks distal femoral physeal damage. In adult patients, the MPFL femoral origin has been determined in a cadaver study and correlated to radiographic landmarks on a lateral X-ray by Schöttle et al. [46] (Fig. 4.5). The femoral insertion of the MPFL is near the distal femoral physis, and there is disagreement as to whether the insertion is proximal or distal to the physis. Shea et al. determined the femoral MPFL insertion to be, on average, 2–5 mm proximal to the physis by finding Schöttle's point on lateral radiographs of skeletally immature patients [52]. This finding has been disputed. In a similar study by Nelitz et al., Schöttle's point was determined on a lateral radiograph and then cross-referenced to the corresponding location on the AP view [47]. This indirect determination placed the MPFL origin, on average, 6.4 mm (range 4.1–12) distal to the medial physis. The authors posited that the portion(s) of the physis seen on the lateral radiograph is(are) the central portion(s) and the undulating structure of the physis produces a more proximal medial location (Fig. 4.6). Others have also questioned the relation of the MPFL origin to the distal femoral physis. Ladd et al. conducted an MRI study using the origin of the MCL, an easily identifiable landmark, as a surrogate for the MPFL origin. They found the MCL origin to be, on average, 1.33 cm distal to the physis [53]. Kepler et al. also conducted an MRI study looking at the MPFL insertion directly. They found 86 % of patients had an insertion distal to the physis, while 7 % had an insertion directly on the physis and the other 7 % inserting proximal to the physis. Relative to the physis, the average insertion site was 5 mm distal to the physis (range 7.5 mm proximal to 16 mm distal) [54]. Despite the differing results, all of these studies suggest that the MPFL insertion is very close to the physis and at risk during MPFL

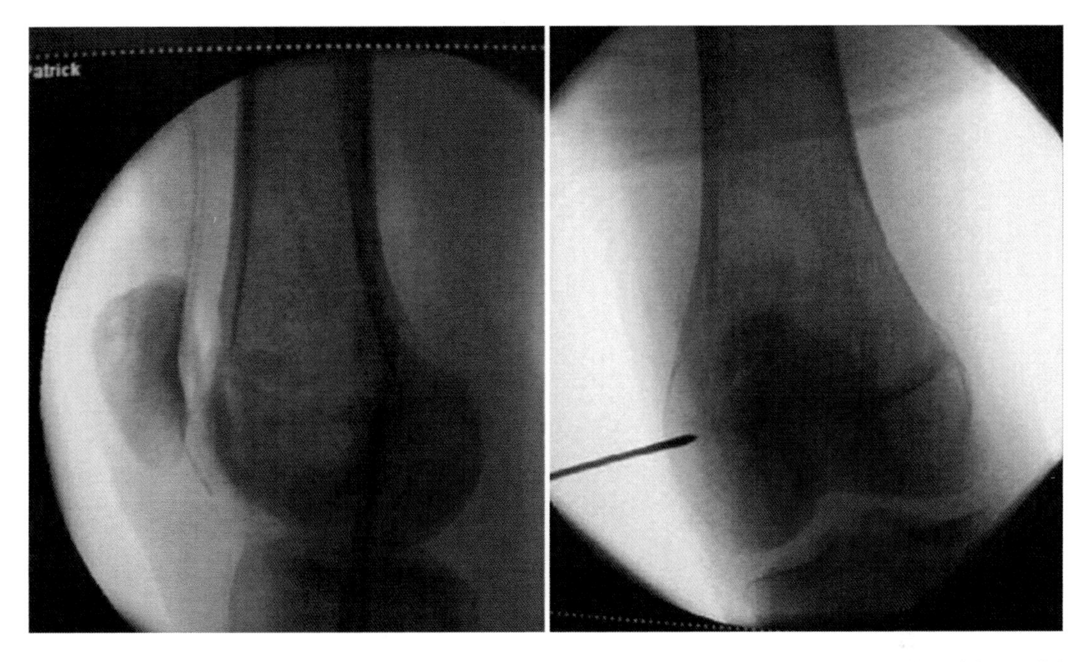

Fig. 4.6 Intraoperative cross-reference of the physis on the lateral view onto an AP view reveals the distance between the medial most part of the physis and the central part of the physis as seen on the lateral view. From Nelitz M, Dornacher D, Dreyhaupt J, Reichel H, Lippacher S. The relation of the distal femoral physis and the medial patellofemoral ligament. Knee Surg Sports Traumatol Arthrosc 2011;19:2067–71. Reprinted with permission from Springer

reconstruction. From a mechano-developmental standpoint, it seems most logical for the MPFL origin to be epiphyseal. An epiphyseal origin maintains a constant patellofemoral relationship during skeletal growth. If the origin were metaphyseal, it seems possible for the MPFL origin to always be migrating proximal during growth. At the time of this writing, no cadaver study in skeletally immature patients has been conducted to verify the relation of the MPFL to the distal femoral physis.

Distal Realignment

Modified Roux–Goldthwait Procedure

Roux [55] and Goldthwait [56] first described a medial transfer of the lateral half of the patellar tendon for patellar instability in the late nineteenth century. This procedure has changed little since its inception. Marsh et al. reported on a modification in which a lateral release is added in 20 skeletally immature patients (30 knees) [39]. Fondren et al. also reported on the procedure but their patient population was a mix of children and adult patients and the procedure was decidedly more invasive [38]. While no firm recommendations exist, this procedure is typically indicated for skeletally immature patients with patellar instability and an associated increased *Q*-angle or TT–TG distance [34, 39, 57]. The procedure begins with diagnostic arthroscopy in which the lateral release is performed and any other internal derangement is repaired. It is common to include a proximal procedure with this. Both proximal and distal procedures can be performed through a single incision or through separate incisions, at the discretion of the treating surgeon. For an isolated lateral tendon transfer, a longitudinal incision is made on the medial border of the patellar tendon. Blunt dissection deep to the subcutaneous fat proceeds laterally over the patellar tendon and medially to the sartorius insertion. The tendon is incised longitudinally at its midpoint and the lateral half is detached distally at its insertion on the tibial tubercle. The free end is reinforced

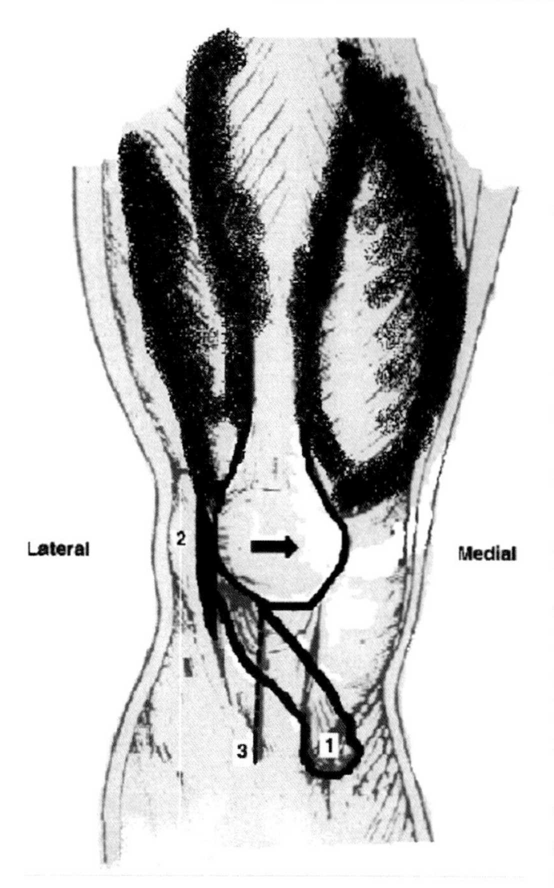

Fig. 4.7 Modified Roux–Goldthwait technique: patellar tendon split and transferred medially onto the tibial insertion of the sartorius muscle (1); modification of the classical Roux–Goldthwait operation by adding a lateral release (2); and medial half of patellar tendon (3). From Marsh JS, Daigneault JP, Sethi P, Polzhofer GK. Treatment of recurrent patellar instability with a modification of the Roux–Goldthwait technique. Journal of pediatric orthopedics. Jul-Aug 2006;26(4):461–465. Reprinted with permission from Wolters Kluwer Health

with heavy suture and brought underneath the intact, medial tendon. With little to no distalization, the tendon is translated medially to the insertion of the sartorius where it is sutured in place (Fig. 4.7). Appropriate tension can be judged by the presence of any slack in the intact, medial portion of the tendon. If slack is present, too much distalization of the graft has occurred. Care is taken to avoid suturing the tendon to the underlying gracilis and semitendinosus. The authors immobilized their patients in full extension for 4 weeks with subsequent progressive motion. They did not comment on weight bearing. In Marsh's study, the average age was 14.2 years (3–18) with an average follow-up of 6.2 years (3–18). Of the 20 patients, 10 carried a diagnosis of ligamentous laxity, 8 with Nail-Patella syndrome, and 1 with Down syndrome. Ten patients had unilateral instability and the other 10 had bilateral instability that underwent surgical intervention. The authors' main outcome measures were radiographic and physical examination criteria as opposed to subjective outcomes or episodes of recurrent instability. Nevertheless, they noted that 26 knees had an excellent result as determined by a *Q*-angle of 14° or less. They also noted significant improvements in congruence angle, lateral patellar deviation, and lateral patellar angle [39]. While they did not state a redislocation rate, the authors noted that the patient with Down syndrome had recurrent instability requiring reoperation and one patient with extreme ligamentous laxity had only fair radiographic improvement [39].

While this procedure may decrease the dislocation rate, it may increase the risk of early arthritis in the patellofemoral joint. Sillanpää et al. retrospectively reviewed a group of patients who underwent either a MPFL reconstruction with adductor magnus autograft or a modified Roux–Goldthwait procedure for recurrent patellar instability [1]. Fifteen patients with an average age at the time of surgery of 20 (range 19–22) were reviewed at a median follow-up of 10.1 years (8–13) in the MPFL reconstruction group. Twenty-one patients with an average age at the time of surgery of 20.2 (19–22) were reviewed at a medial follow-up of 7 years (5–11). All patients were male conscripts in the Finnish military and had comparable baseline characteristics with regard to baseline health, number of prior patellar dislocations, and status of articular cartilage at the time of surgery [1]. At the time of follow-up, the redislocation rate was similar between both groups (6.7 % in MPFL group, 14.3 % in Roux–Goldthwait group, $p=0.52$) as were Kujala and Tegner scores (88 and 4 in MPFL group, 86 and 5 in Roux–Goldthwait group). Follow-up MRIs showed an equal number of International Cartilage Repair Society grade II–IV lesions [58] in both groups. Follow-up radiographs at final follow-up revealed at least Ahlbäck grade I arthritic changes [59] in the patellofemoral joint of 5 patients in the Roux–Goldthwait group compared with no patients in the MPFL group ($p=0.04$). No patients in either group had radiographic signs of arthritis in either tibiofemoral compartment at final follow-up or any signs of arthritis in any knee compartment prior to index surgery [1]. The authors did not postulate a mechanism for this observation, and they also noted that the functional scores were similar in both groups so the implication of this finding on overall outcome is not totally clear. With that said, it may be reasonable to reserve this procedure for lower demand patients (Down syndrome, Nail-Patella syndrome, Ehler's Danlos, etc.) and more of a salvage option in an otherwise normal young athlete.

Galeazzi Procedure

This procedure involves transferring the semitendinosus tendon to the patella. It was first described by Galeazzi in 1922 [60] and there have been several reports on it use subsequently [37, 40, 57, 61]. The technique has become less invasive over time. Similar to the Roux–Goldthwait procedure, no firm recommendations exist for patient selection. However, skeletally immature patients without an increased *Q*-angle and/or TT–TG distance and possibly with patella alta are considered appropriate candidates [57]. The most recent description of this technique by Moyad and Blakemore utilizes two 3–4-cm incisions for the entirety of the reconstruction [40]. The first incision is longitudinal and made directly over the patella with extra-periosteal exposure of the entire bone. If needed, a lateral release and medial plication are performed through this incision. A second longitudinal incision is made over the insertion of the pes tendons on the anteromedial tibia. The semitendinosus tendon is isolated under the sartorius fascia and freed from surrounding adhesions. Using an open tendon stripper from a standard anterior cruciate ligament (ACL) hamstring harvest set, the tendon is detached from its proximal muscle belly and reinforced with heavy suture. Its distal insertion on the tibia is left undisturbed. A bone tunnel directed inferomedial to superolateral is drilled in the patella. The semitendinosus tendon is tunneled deep to the subcutaneous fat, passed through the patellar bone tunnel, and excess tendon is secured to the anterior patella with heavy absorbable suture (Fig. 4.8). Prior to definitive fixation, the reconstruction is tensioned to ensure appropriate tracking and excursion of the patella. A few studies have reported results on this procedure. Baker et al. reported on 42 patients with an average age of 12 years (5–17) and average follow-up of 5 years (0.5–12). They defined an excellent outcome as having no pain, stiffness, crepitus, or loss of function. A good outcome was defined as having only minimal pain or stiffness and limitation only in strenuous sports.

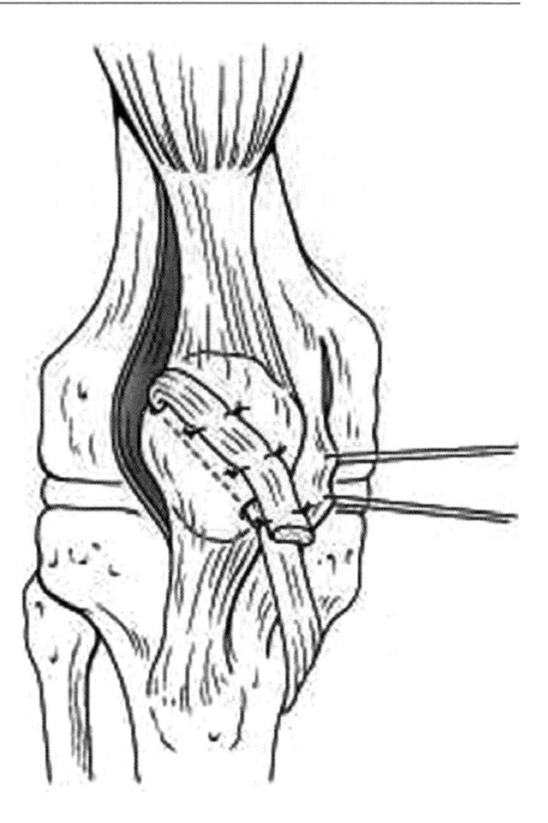

Fig. 4.8 The patella drill hole is oriented from inferomedially to superolaterally. After passage of the tendon, the remaining semitendinosus is sutured over the anterior patella in line with the bone tunnel. From Moyad TF, Blakemore L. Modified Galeazzi technique for recurrent patellar dislocation in children. Orthopedics. Apr 2006;29(4):302–304. Reprinted with permission from Laurel C. Blakemore, MD

Eighty-one percent achieved either an "excellent" or "good" outcome and there were two known recurrent dislocations (5 %). 30 % (patients with an "excellent" rating) were able to return to unlimited strenuous sports and had an otherwise asymptomatic knee [37]. Letts et al. reported on 26 knees in 22 patients who underwent this procedure [57]. The average age was 14 (9–18) and average follow-up was 3 years (2–7). In addition to objective findings, they utilized the Lysholm [62] questionnaire, portions of the Zarins-Rowe [63] questionnaire, and subjective patient assessments of instability and return to activities to quantify outcomes. Similar to Baker, an excellent outcome was an asymptomatic knee with full function, no pain, no instability, and complete return to sports and activities. A good outcome allowed for minimal pain during exertional activities and infrequent subluxation episodes without dislocation. Their results mirrored those of Baker [37] with 27 % obtaining an excellent outcome and 55 % with a good outcome. There was one recurrent lateral dislocation that required tightening of the semitendinosus tenodesis and one with medial subluxation that required loosening of the tenodesis. Both patients had relief of symptoms after the second procedure [57]. Hall et al. have also reported on this procedure but their results are difficult to interpret in this setting as 73 % of patients underwent a concomitant tibial tubercle transfer [61].

Complete Patellar Tendon Transfer

Recently, Luhmann et al. described a technique of complete patellar tendon transfer for skeletally immature patients with patellar instability and a *Q*-angle greater than 15° [64]. Simply put, the tendon is sharply incised off its insertion on the tibial tubercle apophysis and translated medially 50 % of its width where it is sutured in place. Luhmann et al. reported performing this procedure on two patients as part of larger study in which other operations were performed on a mixed group of skeletally immature and mature adolescents. The objective and subjective outcomes of these two specific patients were not reported separately in their study. This procedure sounds technically simple and seems to preserve anatomy and is thus a new, attractive option. Additional study is required to determine its utility and safety before recommending it on a more outright basis.

Combined Proximal and Distal Realignment

Distal realignment procedures are often accompanied by a concomitant proximal procedure such as MPFL repair or reconstruction. Joo et al. reported on six knees in five patients who underwent a "four-in-one" procedure of proximal tube realignment [65], lateral release, semitendinosus tenodesis, and Roux–Goldthwait. All patients were female, two had Down syndrome and one had William's syndrome. All patients had significant ligamentous laxity and trochlear aplasia observed intraoperatively. The mean age was 6.1 years (4.6–6.9) and mean follow-up was 54.5 months (31–66) [41]. No redislocations occurred and Kujala scores averaged 95.3 (88–98). While this procedure was quite effective in their patient population, it may be too invasive for the more typical active older child/adolescent population.

Brown and Ahmad described a technique of combined medial patellotibial and MPFL reconstruction with autogenous semitendinosus tendon [66]. The authors note the utility of medial patellotibial ligament (MPTL) reconstruction as it may play a role as a secondary stabilizer of the patella as evidenced by a previous biomechanical study [67]. The procedure is performed through a 10-cm midline incision. The semitendinosus graft is harvested proximally with an open tendon stripper and left attached distally. A docking hole, typically 5 mm in diameter is drilled in the medial patella at the site of the native MPFL insertion. Two divergent drill holes are made at the base of the docking tunnel, and a 2.4-mm pin with an eyelet is used to shuttle both ends of a passing suture leaving a loop of suture on the medial patella to draw the graft into the docking tunnel. The graft is tensioned at 60° of knee flexion and the free end of the graft is sutured to the origin of the MCL. The distal limb of the reconstruction recreates the medial patellotibial

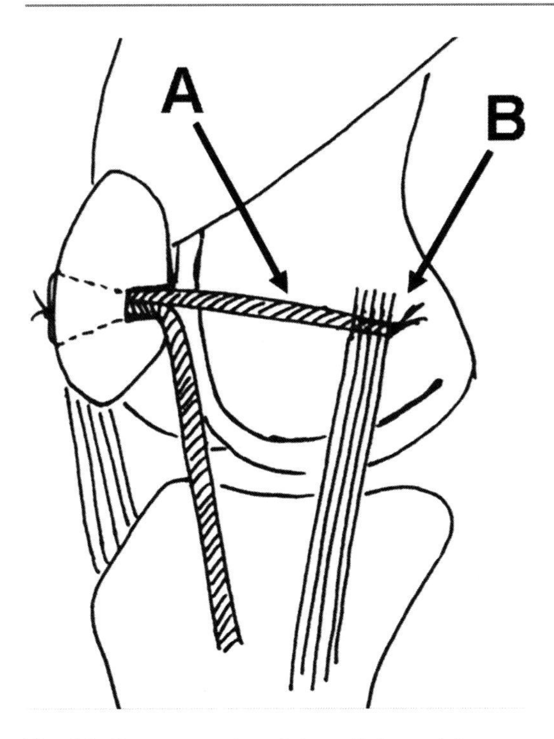

Fig. 4.9 Reconstructed medial patellofemoral ligament (a). Semitendinosus graft sutured to the proximal medial collateral ligament (b). From Brown GD, Ahmad CS. Combined medial patellofemoral ligament and medial patellotibial ligament reconstruction in skeletally immature patients. The journal of knee surgery. Oct 2008;21(4):328–332. Reprinted with permission from Thieme Publishing Group

ligament, and the proximal limb recreates the MPFL (Fig. 4.9). A medial retinacular imbrication and VMO advancement are included in the procedure [66]. In additional to potential biomechanical advantage, the authors note that addition of the MPTL reconstruction adds no morbidity to the procedure. They reported favorable results in two case reports utilizing this procedure [66].

Guided Growth

There are several known anatomic risk factors for patellar maltracking and instability including femoral anteversion, external tibial torsion, patella alta, increased *Q*-angle, genu valgum, and lateral femoral condyle hypoplasia [28, 30, 31, 33, 68, 69]. Of these conditions, genu valgum in the skeletally immature patient has the potential to be corrected by guided growth principles [70, 71] and thus avoid more invasive procedures such as osteotomies. Genu valgum in excess of 10° has been associated with patellofemoral pain and instability [29, 72, 73]. Recent reports describe the success of guided growth techniques utilizing a tension band on the medial physis to correct this angular deformity [70, 72, 73]. Kearney and Mosca reported their results utilizing guided growth to treat patellar instability with associated genu valgum [74]. They reviewed 28 knees in 16 patients. The average age was 12 years (9–15) and average follow-up was 31.5 months. All patients underwent hemiepiphysiodesis at the medial distal femoral physis, and 2 patients had additional hemiepiphysiodesis at the proximal medial tibial physis. Staples were used prior to the advent of the plate and screw construct [70]. The average lateral distal femoral angle improved from 78° preoperatively to 83° postoperatively. 82 % of patients noted complete resolution of symptoms and the remaining 18 % note a significant reduction. All competitive athletes returned to full sports participation. 19 knees (66 %) underwent hardware removal at an average of 9.6 months postoperatively. One patient required reinsertion of a loose staple [74].

General guidelines for guided growth include extra-periosteal plate application [70], application after 8 years of age due to risk of spontaneous rebound [72, 73], application with at least 1 year of growth remaining, and careful monitoring to prevent overcorrection [70, 73]. If there is growth remaining, hardware is removed to prevent overcorrection. In the case of rebound deformity, hardware can be safely reapplied [72]. While the speed of correction slows as the child approaches skeletal maturity, one can expect 0.7° per month of correction in the distal femur and 0.3° per month of correction in the tibia [71–73].

Outcomes

Reports on long-term functional outcomes from nonoperative treatment of patellar instability and surgical patellar realignment for recurrent dislocators in this age group are rare [7, 64]. In addition to studies mentioned previously in this chapter [8, 22, 26], Atkin et al. conducted a prospective study of Kaiser Permanente patients in the San Diego area who were treated conservatively after a first-time traumatic patellar dislocation [7]. There were 74 patients in the group and 51 (69 %) were in the 10–19-year age group. There were 37 men and 37 women. They found a significant reduction in the amount of hours per week spent playing sports in all age groups. Specifically in the 10–19-year age group, the average reduction in sports participation decreased from an average of 6.9 to 2.6 h/week 24 weeks after injury [7]. The authors commented this likely represents a gradual return to sports. No longer-term studies regarding functional outcomes for nonoperative treatment of acute patellar dislocation in this age group have been reported.

Luhmann et al. reported a retrospective review on functional outcomes after surgery for patellar instability in children and adolescents [64]. They collected IKDC [75], Lysholm [62], and Tegner [75] scores on 27 knees in 23 patients. The average age was 14 years (range 8.8–18.3) with 22 knees belonging to female patients and 5 knees belonging to male patients. There were four patients with significant associated diagnoses: Down syndrome, Charcot–Marie–Tooth disease, juvenile rheumatoid arthritis, and Ehlers–Danlos syndrome. Mean follow-up was 5 years (3.2–7.4). Twenty-one patients had proximal and distal realignment. Proximal realignment consisted of lateral release and MPFL repair. Distal realignment was tibial tubercle osteotomy for skeletally mature patients (19 patients) and complete patellar tendon transfer for skeletally immature patients (2 patients). The mean IKDC score was 65.6 (31–100), the mean Lysholm score was 69.3 (38–100), and the mean Tegner activity level was 5.4 (1–9). In the group of four patients with associated disease, the mean scores were 57.5, 60.5, and 3.5, respectively [64]. Given the retrospective nature of the study, there were no baseline pre-injury or pre-surgery scores for comparison. Further analysis revealed that patients with a Lysholm and IKDC score ≥70 were significantly younger (13.1 vs. 14.9), were all patellar dislocators (vs. 66 % in the <70 group), and had a significantly shorter length of symptoms prior to surgery (13 vs. 24 months). Also, the Tegner scores were significantly higher in the ≥70 group (6.8 vs. 4.3) [64]. No other factors such as sex, anatomic alignment, and presence of preoperative crepitus had a significant correlation to functional outcome. It may have been hard to determine the effect of gender given the large majority of females in this study.

Conclusions

Patellar instability is common in the adolescent age group and this group represents the highest risk group for first-time and recurrent dislocation. Nonoperative management is advocated for first-time dislocators except in cases of loose bodies requiring timely surgical intervention. Surgical options for skeletally immature patients can be different from adults, especially when considering distal realignment or MPFL reconstruction with bone tunnels to minimize risk of physeal damage. While several unique options are available, quality data with adequate power are lacking to document safety and efficacy. Patients with associated conditions such as Down syndrome and Ehlers–Danlos require unique management that may compromise anatomic restoration in order to maximize stability. Functional outcome reports are rare in both conservatively and surgically treated patients and thus represent exciting research opportunities going forward.

References

1. Sillanpaa P, Mattila VM, Visuri T, Maenpaa H, Pihlajamaki H. Ligament reconstruction versus distal realignment for patellar dislocation. Clin Orthop Relat Res. 2008;466(6):1475–84.
2. Fithian DC, Paxton EW, Stone ML, et al. Epidemiology and natural history of acute patellar dislocation. Am J Sports Med. 2004;32(5):1114–21.
3. Waterman BR, Belmont Jr PJ, Owens BD. Patellar dislocation in the United States: role of sex, age, race, and athletic participation. J Knee Surg. 2012; 25(1):51–7.

4. Nietosvaara Y, Aalto K, Kallio PE. Acute patellar dislocation in children: incidence and associated osteochondral fractures. J Pediatr Orthop. 1994;14(4):513–5.
5. Cash JD, Hughston JC. Treatment of acute patellar dislocation. Am J Sports Med. 1988;16(3):244–9.
6. Nikku R, Nietosvaara Y, Aalto K, Kallio PE. Operative treatment of primary patellar dislocation does not improve medium-term outcome: a 7-year follow-up report and risk analysis of 127 randomized patients. Acta Orthop. 2005;76(5):699–704.
7. Atkin DM, Fithian DC, Marangi KS, Stone ML, Dobson BE, Mendelsohn C. Characteristics of patients with primary acute lateral patellar dislocation and their recovery within the first 6 months of injury. Am J Sports Med. 2000;28(4):472–9.
8. Palmu S, Kallio PE, Donell ST, Helenius I, Nietosvaara Y. Acute patellar dislocation in children and adolescents: a randomized clinical trial. J Bone Joint Surg Am. 2008;90(3):463–70.
9. Kramer DE, Pace JL. Acute traumatic and sports-related osteochondral injury of the pediatric knee. Orthop Clin North Am. 2012;43(2):227–36. vi.
10. Bicos J, Fulkerson JP, Amis A. Current concepts review: the medial patellofemoral ligament. Am J Sports Med. 2007;35(3):484–92.
11. Baldwin JL. The anatomy of the medial patellofemoral ligament. Am J Sports Med. 2009;37(12):2355–61.
12. Philippot R, Chouteau J, Wegrzyn J, Testa R, Fessy MH, Moyen B. Medial patellofemoral ligament anatomy: implications for its surgical reconstruction. Knee Surg Sports Traumatol Arthrosc. 2009;17(5):475–9.
13. Craig JG, Cody DD, Van Holsbeeck M. The distal femoral and proximal tibial growth plates: MR imaging, three-dimensional modeling and estimation of area and volume. Skeletal Radiol. 2004;33(6):337–44.
14. Harcke HT, Synder M, Caro PA, Bowen JR. Growth plate of the normal knee: evaluation with MR imaging. Radiology. 1992;183(1):119–23.
15. Roberts JM. Operative treatment of fractures about the knee. Orthop Clin North Am. 1990;21(2):365–79.
16. Beaty JH, Kumar A. Fractures about the knee in children. J Bone Joint Surg Am. 1994;76(12):1870–80.
17. Pritchett JW. Longitudinal growth and growth-plate activity in the lower extremity. Clin Orthop Relat Res. 1992;275:274–9.
18. Rockwood CA, Beaty JH, Kasser JR. Rockwood and Wilkins' fractures in children. 7th ed. Philadelphia, PA: Wolters Kluwer/Lippincott, Williams & Wilkins; 2010.
19. Green NE, Swiontkowski MF. Skeletal trauma in children. 4th ed. Philadelphia, PA: Saunders/Elsevier; 2009.
20. Flachsmann R, Broom ND, Hardy AE, Moltschaniwskyj G. Why is the adolescent joint particularly susceptible to osteochondral shear fracture? Clin Orthop Relat Res. 2000;381:212–21.
21. Micheli LJ, Kocher MS. The pediatric and adolescent knee. 1st ed. Philadelphia, PA: Saunders/Elsevier; 2006.
22. Apostolovic M, Vukomanovic B, Slavkovic N, et al. Acute patellar dislocation in adolescents: operative versus nonoperative treatment. Int Orthop. 2011;35(10):1483–7.
23. Powers CM. Rehabilitation of patellofemoral joint disorders: a critical review. J Orthop Sports Phys Ther. 1998;28(5):345–54.
24. Beasley LS, Vidal AF. Traumatic patellar dislocation in children and adolescents: treatment update and literature review. Curr Opin Pediatr. 2004;16(1):29–36.
25. McManus F, Rang M, Heslin DJ. Acute dislocation of the patella in children. The natural history. Clin Orthop Relat Res. 1979;139:88–91.
26. Nikku R, Nietosvaara Y, Kallio PE, Aalto K, Michelsson JE. Operative versus closed treatment of primary dislocation of the patella. Similar 2-year results in 125 randomized patients. Acta Orthop Scand. 1997;68(5):419–23.
27. Smith TO, Hunt NJ, Donell ST. The reliability and validity of the Q-angle: a systematic review. Knee Surg Sports Traumatol Arthrosc. 2008;16(12):1068–79.
28. Colvin AC, West RV. Patellar instability. J Bone Joint Surg Am. 2008;90(12):2751–62.
29. Fabry G, MacEwen GD, Shands Jr AR. Torsion of the femur. A follow-up study in normal and abnormal conditions. J Bone Joint Surg Am. 1973;55(8):1726–38.
30. Reider B, Marshall JL, Warren RF. Clinical characteristics of patellar disorders in young athletes. Am J Sports Med. 1981;9(4):270–4.
31. Dejour H, Walch G, Nove-Josserand L, Guier C. Factors of patellar instability: an anatomic radiographic study. Knee Surg Sports Traumatol Arthrosc. 1994;2(1):19–26.
32. Walker P, Harris I, Leicester A. Patellar tendon-to-patella ratio in children. J Pediatr Orthop. 1998;18(1):129–31.
33. Bollier M, Fulkerson JP. The role of trochlear dysplasia in patellofemoral instability. J Am Acad Orthop Surg. 2011;19(1):8–16.
34. Balcarek P, Jung K, Frosch KH, Sturmer KM. Value of the tibial tuberosity-trochlear groove distance in patellar instability in the young athlete. Am J Sports Med. 2011;39(8):1756–61.
35. Macnab I. Recurrent dislocation of the patella. J Bone Joint Surg Am. 1952;34(A(4)):957–67. passim.
36. Harrison MH. The results of a realignment operation for recurrent dislocation of the patella. J Bone Joint Surg Br. 1955;37-B(4):559–67.
37. Baker RH, Carroll N, Dewar FP, Hall JE. The semitendinosus tenodesis for recurrent dislocation of the patella. J Bone Joint Surg Br. 1972;54(1):103–9.
38. Fondren FB, Goldner JL, Bassett 3rd FH. Recurrent dislocation of the patella treated by the modified Roux-Goldthwait procedure. A prospective study of

forty-seven knees. J Bone Joint Surg Am. 1985;67(7): 993–1005.
39. Marsh JS, Daigneault JP, Sethi P, Polzhofer GK. Treatment of recurrent patellar instability with a modification of the Roux-Goldthwait technique. J Pediatr Orthop. 2006;26(4):461–5.
40. Moyad TF, Blakemore L. Modified Galeazzi technique for recurrent patellar dislocation in children. Orthopedics. 2006;29(4):302–4.
41. Joo SY, Park KB, Kim BR, Park HW, Kim HW. The 'four-in-one' procedure for habitual dislocation of the patella in children: early results in patients with severe generalised ligamentous laxity and aplasia of the trochlear groove. J Bone Joint Surg Br. 2007;89(12): 1645–9.
42. Steensen RN, Dopirak RM, Maurus PB. A simple technique for reconstruction of the medial patellofemoral ligament using a quadriceps tendon graft. Arthroscopy. 2005;21(3):365–70.
43. Noyes FR, Albright JC. Reconstruction of the medial patellofemoral ligament with autologous quadriceps tendon. Arthroscopy. 2006;22(8):904 e1–7.
44. Sillanpaa PJ, Maenpaa HM, Mattila VM, Visuri T, Pihlajamaki H. A mini-invasive adductor magnus tendon transfer technique for medial patellofemoral ligament reconstruction: a technical note. Knee Surg Sports Traumatol Arthrosc. 2009;17(5):508–12.
45. Deie M, Ochi M, Sumen Y, Yasumoto M, Kobayashi K, Kimura H. Reconstruction of the medial patellofemoral ligament for the treatment of habitual or recurrent dislocation of the patella in children. J Bone Joint Surg Br. 2003;85(6):887–90.
46. Schottle PB, Schmeling A, Rosenstiel N, Weiler A. Radiographic landmarks for femoral tunnel placement in medial patellofemoral ligament reconstruction. Am J Sports Med. 2007;35(5):801–4.
47. Nelitz M, Dornacher D, Dreyhaupt J, Reichel H, Lippacher S. The relation of the distal femoral physis and the medial patellofemoral ligament. Knee Surg Sports Traumatol Arthrosc. 2011;19(12):2067–71.
48. Farr J, Schepsis AA. Reconstruction of the medial patellofemoral ligament for recurrent patellar instability. J Knee Surg. 2006;19(4):307–16.
49. Nam EK, Karzel RP. Mini-open medial reefing and arthroscopic lateral release for the treatment of recurrent patellar dislocation: a medium-term follow-up. Am J Sports Med. 2005;33(2):220–30.
50. Mountney J, Senavongse W, Amis AA, Thomas NP. Tensile strength of the medial patellofemoral ligament before and after repair or reconstruction. J Bone Joint Surg Br. 2005;87(1):36–40.
51. Avikainen VJ, Nikku RK, Seppanen-Lehmonen TK. Adductor magnus tenodesis for patellar dislocation. Technique and preliminary results. Clin Orthop Relat Res. 1993;297:12–6.
52. Shea KG, Grimm NL, Belzer J, Burks RT, Pfeiffer R. The relation of the femoral physis and the medial patellofemoral ligament. Arthroscopy. 2010;26(8):1083–7.
53. Ladd PE, Laor T, Emery KH, Salisbury SR, Parikh SN. Medial collateral ligament of the knee on magnetic resonance imaging: does the site of the femoral origin change at different patient ages in children and young adults? J Pediatr Orthop. 2010;30(3):224–30.
54. Kepler CK, Bogner EA, Hammoud S, Malcolmson G, Potter HG, Green DW. Zone of injury of the medial patellofemoral ligament after acute patellar dislocation in children and adolescents. Am J Sports Med. 2011;39(7):1444–9.
55. Roux C. The classic. Recurrent dislocation of the patella: operative treatment. Clin Orthop Relat Res. 1979;144:4–8.
56. Goldthwait JE. Dislocation of the patella. Trans Am Orthop Assoc. 1895;8:237.
57. Letts RM, Davidson D, Beaule P. Semitendinosus tenodesis for repair of recurrent dislocation of the patella in children. J Pediatr Orthop. 1999;19(6):742–7.
58. Brittberg M, Winalski CS. Evaluation of cartilage injuries and repair. J Bone Joint Surg Am. 2003;85-A Suppl 2:58–69.
59. Ahlback S. Osteoarthrosis of the knee. A radiographic investigation. Acta Radiol Diagn (Stockh). 1968;Suppl 277:277–72.
60. Galeazzi R. New tendonous and muscular transplant applications [in Italian]. Arch Ortop. 1922;38:315–25.
61. Hall JE, Micheli LJ, McManama Jr GB. Semitendinosus tenodesis for recurrent subluxation or dislocation of the patella. Clin Orthop Relat Res. 1979;144:31–5.
62. Tegner Y, Lysholm J. Rating systems in the evaluation of knee ligament injuries. Clin Orthop Relat Res. 1985;198:43–9.
63. Zarins B, Rowe CR. Combined anterior cruciate-ligament reconstruction using semitendinosus tendon and iliotibial tract. J Bone Joint Surg Am. 1986; 68(2):160–77.
64. Luhmann SJ, O'Donnell JC, Fuhrhop S. Outcomes after patellar realignment surgery for recurrent patellar instability dislocations: a minimum 3-year follow-up study of children and adolescents. J Pediatr Orthop. 2011;31(1):65–71.
65. Insall J, Bullough PG, Burstein AH. Proximal "tube" realignment of the patella for chondromalacia patellae. Clin Orthop Relat Res. 1979;144:63–9.
66. Brown GD, Ahmad CS. Combined medial patellofemoral ligament and medial patellotibial ligament reconstruction in skeletally immature patients. J Knee Surg. 2008;21(4):328–32.
67. Hautamaa PV, Fithian DC, Kaufman KR, Daniel DM, Pohlmeyer AM. Medial soft tissue restraints in lateral patellar instability and repair. Clin Orthop Relat Res. 1998;349:174–82.
68. Redziniak DE, Diduch DR, Mihalko WM, et al. Patellar instability. J Bone Joint Surg Am. 2009;91(9): 2264–75.
69. Monk AP, Doll HA, Gibbons CL, et al. The pathoanatomy of patellofemoral subluxation. J Bone Joint Surg Br. 2011;93(10):1341–7.
70. Stevens PM. Guided growth for angular correction: a preliminary series using a tension band plate. J Pediatr Orthop. 2007;27(3):253–9.

71. Ballal MS, Bruce CE, Nayagam S. Correcting genu varum and genu valgum in children by guided growth: temporary hemiepiphysiodesis using tension band plates. J Bone Joint Surg Br. 2010;92(2):273–6.
72. Boero S, Michelis MB, Riganti S. Use of the eight-Plate for angular correction of knee deformities due to idiopathic and pathologic physis: initiating treatment according to etiology. J Child Orthop. 2011;5(3):209–16.
73. Guzman H, Yaszay B, Scott VP, Bastrom TP, Mubarak SJ. Early experience with medial femoral tension band plating in idiopathic genu valgum. J Child Orthop. 2011;5(1):11–7.
74. Kearney SP, Mosca VS. Selective hemiepiphysiodesis for patellar instability with associated genu valgum. Paper presented at: Pediatric Orthopaedic Society of North America 2011 (Annual Meeting 2011); Montreal, Quebec, Canada.
75. Wright RW. Knee injury outcomes measures. J Am Acad Orthop Surg. 2009;17(1):31–9.

Cartilage Restoration in the Patellofemoral Joint

5

Nicolas Brown, Geoffrey S. Van Thiel, and Brian J. Cole

Epidemiology

The exact incidence of patellofemoral chondral lesions is unknown as these lesions may present with a wide range of symptom severity, and it is unclear what percentage of patients with these defects are ever evaluated by a healthcare provider. The incidence of patellofemoral pain, however, is relatively high. A study of 1,525 military recruits from the United States Naval Academy demonstrated that 15 % of females and 12 % of males at the time of study enrollment had patellofemoral pain syndrome as evidenced by pain with stairs, hopping/jogging, prolonged sitting, kneeling, squatting, and absence of examination findings to suggest alternate pathology. Many of these cases of patellofemoral pain were undoubtedly not due to chondral lesions; however, there is a high prevalence of these lesions in the general population as demonstrated by other studies. Widuchowski et al. [1] studied 25,124 patients who received arthroscopy for knee pain of any etiology and found a 60 % incidence of chondral lesions, with the patellar articular surface accounting for 36 % of these lesions. A similar study by Curl et al. examined 31,516 knee arthroscopies and found a similar incidence of articular cartilage lesions, with chondral lesions visualized in 63 % of patients. This study does not state the exact percentage, but found Outerbridge grade III lesions of the patella to be the most common [2].

The prevalence of patellofemoral cartilage defects in athletes is thought to be even greater than the general population given the stresses placed on the knee by athletic activity. However, the athletic population may also have lower average BMI than nonathletes, which may mitigate this effect to some degree. There are a number of studies that specifically investigate the athletic population with regard to prevalence and location of chondral defects. Walczak et al. studied 28 asymptomatic NBA players with MRI and found that 12 of 28 (44 %) showed patellar cartilage changes and 7 of 28 (26 %) had trochlear changes [3]. The relatively high incidence of patellar defects suggests the possibility of sport-specific defects. It is theorized that basketball, which requires frequent jumping, places a larger amount of stress on the patellofemoral joint than other sports. In contrast, Mithofer and colleagues [4] reported that in high-level soccer players, 48 % of cartilage defects occurred on the medial femoral condyle, 23 % occurred on the lateral femoral condyle, and only 29 % occurred in the patellofemoral joint. Biomechanical studies such as one performed by Eckstein and colleagues [5]

N. Brown, M.D. • B.J. Cole, M.D., M.B.A.
Rush University Medical Center, Chicago, IL, USA

G.S. Van Thiel, M.D., M.B.A. (✉)
Sports Medicine Division, Department of Orthopedics, Rush University Medical Center, Chicago, IL, USA

Rockford Orthopedic Associates, 324 Roxburg Road, Rockford, IL 61107, USA
e-mail: gvanthiel@rockfordortho.com

R.V. West and A.C. Colvin (eds.), *The Patellofemoral Joint in the Athlete*,
DOI 10.1007/978-1-4614-4157-1_5, © Springer Science+Business Media New York 2014

reinforce this idea of varying stresses on the patellofemoral joint with different activities. They studied knee movement and demonstrated using MRI and three-dimensional digital image analysis that certain activities lead to different amounts of patellar cartilage deformation as measured by volume before and after activity. Patellar cartilage deformation was 5.9 % after knee bends, 4.7 % after squatting, 2.8 % after normal walking, 5.0 % after running, and 4.5 % after cycling. Patellar cartilage was the most affected knee area except when the activity was high-impact loading, in which case the tibial plateau was most affected. Interestingly, there was no difference in athletes vs. nonathletes indicating that cartilage is not "trained" to resist stresses in the athletes. However, there are studies that have demonstrated relative lower rates of symptomatic osteoarthritis in long-distance runners, indicating that athletic activity might have a protective effect on knee articular cartilage [6, 7]. These studies often show an increased rate of radiographic arthritis, but lower rates of symptoms. However, opposing studies have shown that long-distance running increases rates of symptomatic osteoarthritis [8] arguing against a protective effect. Overall, one of the most comprehensive studies of full-thickness chondral defects specifically in the knees of athletes was performed by Flanigan et al., which included 931 subjects and 40 % professional athletes. The prevalence of full-thickness defects was 36 %, with the most common being patellofemoral (37 %). Interestingly, 14 % of athletes with these defects were asymptomatic [9].

Natural History

The natural history of chondral defects of the knee is mostly unknown. Articular cartilage is known at a basic science level to have limited ability to heal or regenerate. It is generally believed that large chondral defects may expand in size and lead to degenerative arthritis. However, there is limited published evidence to support this statement. While this contention seems logical given what is known about the basic science of cartilage, there is no proof. It is difficult to perform these studies as asymptomatic lesions are difficult to follow, and symptomatic lesions have a wide range of available treatment options. Many of the studies are performed on ACL-reconstructed patients as cartilage lesions are often noted at the time of surgery, but not corrected because they are asymptomatic. A study of 125 patients with Outerbridge grade III or IV lesions that were discovered but not addressed at the time of ACL reconstruction noted a statistically significant, but not necessarily clinically significant, decrease in knee scores at reevaluation (medial compartment defect, 94.0 vs. 95.2, and lateral compartment, 92.8 vs. 95.9) [10]. A similar study by Widuchowski et al. [11] studied 42 patients at 10-year follow-up and 36 patients at 15-year follow-up and found that untreated deep cartilage lesions incidentally found during ACL repair do not affect clinical outcome. However, the lesions in these studies are asymptomatic and the findings are not necessarily generalizable to all chondral lesions, especially patellofemoral lesions. Progression may depend upon size, location, depth, condition of surrounding cartilage, age, concomitant pathology, joint alignment and stability, and body mass index. Progression of lesions may lead to asymptomatic radiographic changes that are essentially clinically insignificant. Also, patients with prior chondral lesions may experience symptoms of knee pain, but these symptoms cannot always be attributed to the defect, just because one exists. Finally there are no level one studies that examine the natural history of the lesions by comparing a treatment group to a control group. Many of the studies are level IV studies, which, historically, overstate the benefit of the treatment under consideration. This lack of evidence leads to a clinical dilemma. There is no strong evidence supporting the treatment of these lesions, but the alternative would be nonsurgical, conservative treatment in a painful, marginally functional knee. On the other end of the spectrum is arthroplasty, which may be a far too extreme procedure in a young patient and is not an option in a competitive athlete. Therefore, while the natural history is mostly unknown, it is generally accepted that full-thickness Outerbridge grade III or IV lesions are suitable for treatment. This statement is particularly true when concerning a high-level athlete who desires a treatment that will allow for return to play.

Historical Perspective

The Scottish anatomist and physician William Hunter famously noted in his eighteenth-century treatise entitled "On the Structure and Diseases of Articulating Cartilages" that [12] "If we consult the standard chirurgical writers from Hippocrates down to the present age, we shall find, that an ulcerated cartilage is universally allowed to be a very troublesome disease; that it admits of a cure with more difficulty than carious bone; and that, when destroyed, it is not recovered." Over 100 years later, Paget stated, "There are, I believe, no instances in which a lost portion of cartilage has been restored, or a wounded portion repaired with new and well-formed permanent cartilage, in the human subject." As evidenced from these quotes, the difficulty of treating cartilage lesions has been known at least as far back as 1742, but it was over 150 years from this declaration that real attempts were made to treat these lesions. In the early 1900s, orthopedic surgeons first tried using allograft tissue to repair joint lesions, with the first reported cartilage transfer being performed in 1908 by Judet when he transplanted posttraumatic fragments into their defects and obtained pain relief. In the 1940s, open treatments were used to removed damaged cartilage or any other knee structures that could be causing pain [13]. These were essentially debridement techniques and there was no repair of damaged tissues. The earliest attempts at repair were microfracture techniques used in dogs, which date back to the 1930s [14]. However, use in humans really began in the last 1950s with the priddie drilling technique [15] which involved drilling into subchondral bone to allow for fibrocartilage to fill the resultant defect. Arthroscopic techniques began with limited use in the 1930s, but arthroscopic cartilage restoration was not widely utilized until abrasion arthroplasty became more popular in the 1980s. However, many of the techniques we use today, which are described in this chapter, are relatively new and were developed in the 1990s. This includes modern microfracture technique, osteochondral autograft/allograft transplantation, and autologous chondrocyte implantation.

Basic Science

While bone has the ability to completely heal itself and remodel in response to the specific stresses placed on it, cartilage does not possess this inherent characteristic as it is avascular, aneural, and alymphatic with only sparsely distributed chondrocytes within an extracellular matrix. These chondrocytes rarely undergo mitosis and are dependent upon diffusion for their nutrition. This combination of factors clearly does not lend itself towards regeneration.

Articular cartilage is histologically divided into four discrete levels, which include the superficial, transitional, deep radial, and calcified layers. The superficial layer functions to secrete lubrication for the joint and has low permeability to fluids, and its collagen fibrils are arranged parallel to the underlying tissue. The orientation of these fibers renders this layer to be particular adept at resisting shear stress. The deep layer, on the other hand, contains collagen arranged perpendicular to the surface and allows this layer to resist compression and distribute load. A transition zone is present between the superficial and deep layers and is aptly named as it retains physical properties intermediate between the two due to its mix of collagen fibril orientation. The deepest layer is the calcified layer, which is important because progenitor cells and nutrients are contained beneath this layer and breach of this level is necessary for "natural repair." Therefore, both intentional and unintentional violations of this layer may provide opportunity for healing through the formation of a fibrin clot, vascular proliferation, and migration of pluripotent marrow cells. The biological restorative potential of these released cells and molecular factors is the molecular basis of the microfracture technique.

Unfortunately, the resulting tissue that fills the defect is fibrocartilage, which lacks the durability and functionality of native hyaline cartilage and is a major limitation to this technique. While violation of the calcified layer is an absolute necessity with the microfracture technique, it is imperative to preserve this layer when performing autologous chondrocyte implantation. Autologous chondrocyte implantation is performed with the intent of restoring hyaline cartilage, and thus, the fibrocartilage inducing milieu that occurs with subchondral bone violation can theoretically undermine this goal.

Etiology and Pathophysiology

As noted in the prior sections, cartilage is avascular, alymphatic, and aneural, which means that pain cannot be generated directly from a cartilage lesion. Consequently, it is unknown why some chondral lesions cause pain and others are asymptomatic. It is logical that exposed bone and its associated nerves would generate a pain response when there is a full-thickness defect of this tissue. However, this does not address why some partial-thickness lesions are symptomatic. It is theorized that bone senses increased force transmission through weakened cartilage. Other theories suggest that pain from partial lesions is not due to the defect, but rather from irritated surrounding synovial tissue or other damaged structures. This question is yet unresolved, which is unsatisfying as these lesions can cause considerable pain and dysfunction but are lacking in a definitive pathophysiologic explanation.

Patellofemoral joint chondral injuries can arise from an acute event, such as direct trauma, a torn ligament, and patellar dislocation, or can result from a more indolent chronic process that leads to repetitive microtrauma and subsequent cartilage incongruity. There are a number of predisposing factors to both acute and chronic injuries, which include bone and soft tissue variances that lead to lateral maltracking/instability. Those factors related to anatomical bone variations include valgus knee alignment, a large *Q* angle, increased tibial tubercle–trochlear groove distance on superimposed CT imaging, and dysplasia of the trochlea. Influences related to soft tissue include lateral retinacular tightness, medial retinacular laxity, and medial patellofemoral ligament laxity. These aforementioned factors combined with muscular imbalances, decreased core strength, and variants of foot anatomy can all predispose the patella to increased contact stresses or instability. The forces on the patellofemoral joint are enormous and range from 3× body weight with stair climbing to up to 20× body weight with athletic activities. Therefore, proper biomechanics are essential as patellar maltracking can concentrate these immense forces on a smaller area and lead to acute or chronic damage. Lateral maltracking at its extreme can lead to dislocation, which has been shown in the literature to be associated with a 95 % incidence of chondral lesions [16]. Predisposition to lateral maltracking and its resultant effect on the underlying cartilage are the basis of the anteromedialization techniques that are used to correct maltracking of the patella to relieve these stresses. Performing an anteromedialization procedure simultaneously with cartilage restoration can aid in the survival of restored cartilage and help produce successful outcomes following these procedures.

On a histologic level, cartilage injuries can be viewed as partial-thickness, full-thickness, or osteochondral injuries. Partial-thickness tears involve only the superficial zone of cartilage and lead to decreased proteoglycan content, increased hydration, and resultant stiffness. These changes predispose the cartilage to further injury as well as increase the forces on subchondral bone, as the damaged cartilage has decreased ability to absorb energy. Full-thickness defects involve destruction of the entire cartilage thickness with sparing of the subchondral bone and often result in visible flaps or splits in the tissue. While some minor healing due to chondrocyte proliferation and increased extracellular matrix production may occur, substantive regeneration is not possible because this layer has no access to underlying pluripotent cells or vasculature. Osteochondral injuries involve damage to both cartilage and subchondral bones. These injuries are more common in adolescents and can be due to acute injury or chronic microfracture as is seen with osteochondritis dissecans. As described previously in this chapter, damage to this layer yields an inflammatory response that leads to the formation of fibrocartilage filling the defect.

Classification of Chondral Injuries

Chondral injuries are most commonly classified using either the Outerbridge or international cartilage repair classification system.

Diagnosis

History

The diagnosis of patellofemoral cartilage injury begins with a comprehensive history. These injuries have a highly variable presentation, which ranges from being completely asymptomatic to causing debilitating pain, swelling, and limited function. The majority of patients who present with a lesion that requires treatment will complain of anterior knee pain, but more posteriorly located distribution of pain is also possible. Condylar or tibial plateau defects, in comparison, will typically present with pain along the joint line. Any activity which increases patellar contact stress can exacerbate this pain and includes many facets of athletic competition including running, jumping, and squatting as well as non-athletic activities such as kneeling or stair climbing. Other non-pain-related, however nonspecific, symptoms that patients may experience include crepitus, locking, giving way, and catching. A history of traumatic knee injuries, especially dislocation, is very important to elicit as these have been correlated with a high rate of chondral injury [16]. A thorough history of all prior treatment modalities both surgical and nonsurgical is imperative as current treatment decisions are nearly always influenced by those of the past. Finally, it is necessary to explore patient expectations, goals, and level of athletic competition as these factors are important in the decision-making process.

Physical Exam

The physical exam findings at the patellofemoral joint are useful in suggesting the presence of lateral patellar tracking, which can lead to increased patellar contact stresses. Positive findings are present in a wide-spectrum disease severity ranging from isolated pain due to patellofemoral syndrome, chronic microtrauma from increased stress, and lateral subluxation/dislocation with acute chondral injury. Therefore, physical exam findings often help predict a predisposition to disease rather than being sensitive/specific diagnostic tests for cartilage injury. The physical exam includes evaluation of gait, which can demonstrate foot pronation, abductor weakness, knee subluxation, patellar tracking, and overall antalgia. Other anatomic observations during physical exam that may predispose to patellar maltracking include intoeing, valgus knee alignment, and femoral anteversion. Abductor weakness can be tested with patient standing on one foot. A compensatory shift in weight to the contralateral side reflects a phenomenon that occurs during gait and predisposes the affected side to increased lateral stresses. A tight IT band (Ober's test), muscular imbalance (VMO wasting), excess patellar mobility, patellar tilt, apprehension with lateral patellar force at 30° of knee flexion, and patellar J sign (lateral dislocation during knee extension) all suggest underlying factors which predispose an athlete to altered contact stress or subluxation/dislocation which can ultimately cause chondral injury.

Imaging

Radiographs should include anteroposterior, lateral, Rosenberg (PA with knee in 45° of flexion), long leg alignment, and Merchant views of the knee. While osteochondral lesions are typically not visualized using this modality, bony anatomy can suggest a predisposition to disease (trochlear dysplasia, patellar tilt, *Q* angle, and tibiofemoral alignment) as well as rule out other causes of pain (osteoarthritis, rheumatoid arthritis, loose bodies). Of note, the *Q* angle, which has often been cited as a key measurement in patellofemoral disorders, can be associated with significant interobserver variation [17]. Additionally, it is important to recognize that osteoarthritis and joint space narrowing can be visualized with the Merchant view (45° of flexion), but patellar maltracking and condylar dysplasia are better visualized at 30° of flexion [17].

CT and/or MRI is often more useful than roentgenograms for evaluating cartilage disease. These modalities may transition from helpful to necessary in obese patients as physical examination may yield limited information. A CT scan can more precisely define patellar and trochlear osseous anatomy than can a Merchant view because the entire trochlea can be assessed. CT also allows for determination of tibial tubercle to trochlear groove distance (TT–TG), where an increased distance (>20 mm) suggests patellar maltracking. This value is determined by measuring the distance between the deepest portion of the trochlear groove and the tibial tubercle when superimposed on axial cuts. More than 50 % of patients with patellar maltracking have a TT–TG distance of greater than 20 mm, whereas this is true in less than 5 % of asymptomatic knees [18].

MRI can also be used to calculate the TT–TG distance with accuracy equivalent to that of CT [19]. Also, MRI can be very useful for directly detecting cartilage lesions. However, it is important to separate correlation from causation as the presence of an osteochondral or chondral defect visualized on MRI is not always the source of a patient's symptoms.

Arthroscopy

Arthroscopy is clearly the most invasive of the diagnostic tests, but is also the most definitive at it allows direct visualization of the cartilage surfaces. It allows for a definitive diagnosis, determination of the extent of pathology (size, depth, degree of containment), identification of associated pathologies, and inspection of opposing cartilage surfaces and is an opportunity for debridement and lavage or biopsy for an autologous chondrocyte implantation procedure. In fact, cells from such a biopsy can be cryopreserved for up to 2 years. Finally, if a patient has had previous surgery, arthroscopy can be necessary to evaluate the surrounding cartilage and supporting knee structures. Further, prior arthroscopic surgery does not necessarily negate the need for diagnostic arthroscopy as the lesion in question or condition of the surrounding cartilage may have changed since the original evaluation and visualization.

Differential Diagnosis

The differential diagnosis for anterior knee pain is broad and includes maltracking, patellar articular cartilage defects, trochlear articular cartilage defects, meniscal tears, ligamentous injury, patellar tendinitis, plicae, prepatellar bursitis, fractures, referred pain from hip pathology, infectious, neoplastic, vascular, and psychiatric disease.

Treatment Options Overview

The treatment goals for patellofemoral cartilage defects in the athlete are aimed at decreasing pain, increasing function, and returning the athlete to his or her sport. These objectives are achieved through a variety of operative and nonoperative means. Nonoperative treatment aims to either correct patellar maltracking or simply reduce pain. Correction of patellar maltracking can decrease the likelihood of subluxation, reduce patellofemoral contact stress, and unload diseased cartilage. Pain reduction can be achieved through correction of patellar maltracking as well as a myriad of other treatment modalities. Physical therapy includes stretching and strengthening knee musculature with emphasis on vastus medialis obliquus (VMO), hip abductors, and core musculature. There is debate as to whether this is best achieved with closed- versus open-chain exercises [20]. Additional options to be used alone or in conjunction with physical therapy include weight loss, taping, bracing, cooling, NSAIDs, glucosamine supplements, and intra-articular injections with corticosteroids or viscosupplements. Nonoperative modalities are typically implemented for a minimum of

6 months with demonstration of improvement in VMO, core musculature, and hip abductor strength before surgical intervention will be considered. However, in the high-level athlete with economic incentives to hasten return to play, there is a lower threshold to initiate operative intervention. Surgical treatments are divided between those that correct alignment and unload the abnormal stresses and those that directly address the cartilage lesion. Unloading can be accomplished with proximal realignment of the quad tendon, VMO advancement, MPFL (medial patellofemoral ligament) reconstruction, medial retinacular plication, lateral retinacular release, and tibial tubercle osteotomy. Tibial tubercle osteotomy most commonly involves anteromedialization and may be done in conjunction with a procedure that directly addresses the lesion. These defect-specific treatments include primary repair, debridement, microfracture, osteochondral autografting, osteochondral allografting, and autologous chondrocyte implantation, which is the most common procedure to combine with tibial tubercle osteotomy. If the aforementioned treatments fail and the patient is left with debilitating pain or minimal function, total knee arthroplasty is an option. TKA has demonstrated successful results with regard to patient satisfaction and implant longevity. Clearly this is not a valid option in an athlete looking to return to high-level competition. However, patients with TKA can satisfactorily participate in lower impact sports such as golf and swimming. Also, while TKA is more often being performed in younger patients, this population may also benefit from an isolated patellofemoral resurfacing operation.

Debridement and Lavage

Debridement and lavage is an older technique that involves direct arthroscopic visualization of the lesion, debridement of loose cartilage or subchondral bone, and lavage, which may remove additional debris and, in theory, eliminate inflammatory cytokines and proteases. This treatment is typically reserved for low-demand, older patients with limited symptoms and small (<2 cm) lesions. Therefore, this technique is of limited use unless a quite liberal definition of the term "athlete" is assumed. This treatment is rarely definitive, typically used for more generalized osteoarthritis, but can provide temporary alleviation of symptoms while allowing direct arthroscopic visualization of the cartilage defects and surrounding tissues. This treatment is also a useful adjunct in patients whom the primary source of pain is not a cartilage lesion. The recovery time is short, patients may bear weight as tolerated, and early rehabilitation is acceptable. Fond et al. [21] published a cohort study which followed 36 patients with mean age of 64.5 who received debridement of meniscal lesions, stabilization of chondral defects, removal of impinging osteophytes, and notchplasty. He demonstrated successful outcomes using arthroscopic debridement in 88 % of patients at 2 years and 69 % of patients at 5 years. This treatment was most successful in patients with preoperative flexion contractures less than 10° and preoperative HSS scores greater than 22. This study did not specifically comment on what percentage of these patients had patellofemoral lesions.

Microfracture

Overview

Microfracture, or marrow stimulation, is a cartilage restorative technique in which a surgical awl is used to penetrate subchondral bone. The resultant violation of subchondral bone that allows bleeding and the formation of a "superclot" where pluripotent cells and other molecular factors, which are normally contained under the calcified layer of hyaline cartilage, have access to the chondral defect. These cells along with their necessary growth factors differentiate and fill the defect with fibrocartilage. The fact that the resultant fibrocartilage cells come from underlying mesenchymal cells as opposed to migration of surrounding cells was demonstrated in a study that used radiolabeled cells and observed their migration [22]. Unfortunately, fibrocartilage does

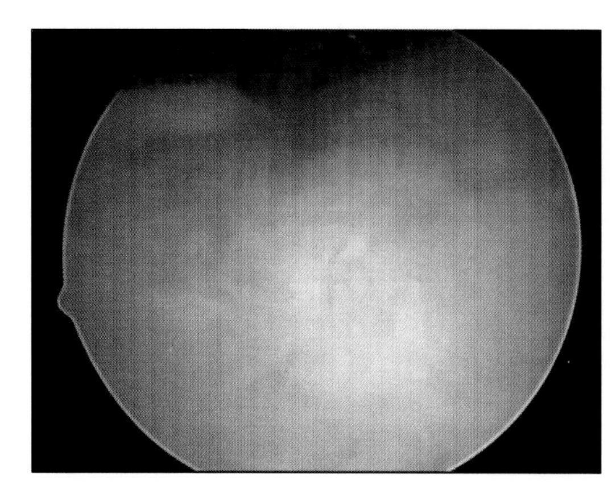

Fig. 5.1 Defect in the trochlea prior to microfracture

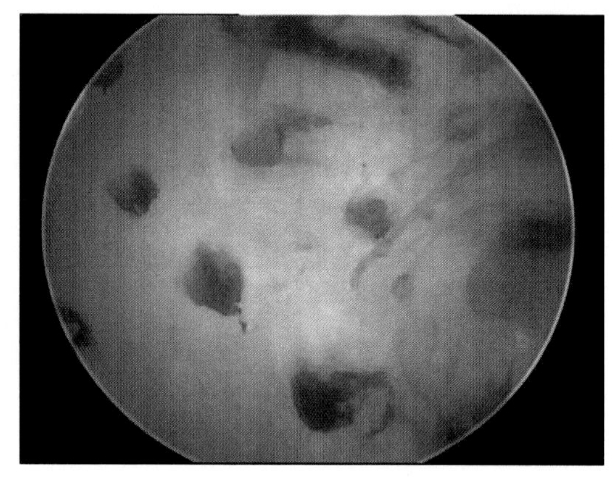

Fig. 5.2 Post-microfracture of the trochlea

not have the same durability and mechanical properties as native hyaline cartilage. Therefore, this technique is more often used as a first-line treatment for low-demand patients with small lesions (<2 cm), and its use is less applicable in the athletic population. Further, the decreased wear resistance of fibrocartilage makes microfracture less suitable for the patellofemoral joint and its associated high contact pressures.

Technique

Standard arthroscopic evaluation is performed for the purpose of identifying the lesion, characterizing it, and ruling out or treating other pathology prior to the microfracture (Fig. 5.1). A curette and mechanical shaver is used to expose subchondral bone and create a "well-shouldered" lesion. A ring curette can be useful when preparing a lesion in the patellofemoral joint. Utilize an assistant to provide counterpressure and stabilize the patella during preparation of the patellar underside while removing the calcified cartilage layer.

Following lesion preparation, a microfracture awl is used to produce holes perpendicular to the surface 3–4 mm apart and 2–4 mm deep. These are created from outside in to maximize the number that can be placed. Fat globules originating in the marrow should be visualized (Fig. 5.2). The fluid pressure is then decreased to allow blood flow to the microfracture sites, the scope is removed, and the wounds are closed using standard technique.

Continuous passive motion (CPM) is started on the day of surgery, 6–8 h daily, for a length of 4–6 weeks. In the patellofemoral joint, immediate weight bearing is allowed while in a hinged knee brace allowing 30–45° of flexion. After 8 weeks, patients begin active range-of-motion exercises and progress to full flexion. Cutting, twisting, and jumping sports are prohibited for a minimum of 6 months.

Results

Studies of the microfracture technique have demonstrated that it results in decreased pain and increased function in the majority of patients. A review of this literature also revealed some prognostics indicators of a successful result. The main difficulty with interpreting the literature on this subject is that most of it pertains to the general population as opposed to just the athletic population and the knee as a whole rather than just the patellofemoral articulation. For example, Mithoefer et al. [23] performed microfracture in 48 patients with isolated full-thickness defects of the femur, but only 23 % of which were at the trochlea, and these lesions were not independently analyzed. However, at average follow-up of 41 months, 32 patients (67 %) reported good or excellent subjective results, 12 (25 %) had fair knee function, and only 4 (8 %) reported poor function, suggesting relative success. The best results were seen in patient with low body mass index and a short duration of preoperative symptoms. Kreuz et al. [24] independently evaluated knee lesions in different knee compartments and demonstrated similarly successful results. These results are more useful despite small numbers, because they provide data specific to the patellofemoral joint. There were 16 patients with average age of 41.6 years with grade III–IV trochlear defects and 11 patients with average age of 38.5 years with grade III–IV patellar defects. Both groups had improved function at 36 months compared to pre-op using Cincinnati knee and ICRS scores. Interestingly, there was improvement from pre-op to 6 months, continued improvement from 6 to 18 months, but significant decrease between 18 and 36 months. This was present in all knee compartments except in the femoral condyles, where they continued to show increased scores. Overall, however, there was still an increase in scores at 36 months compared to preoperative values. They concluded that the best prognostic factors were young patients with femoral condyle defects. Both of those studies demonstrated successful short-term results. Steadman et al. [25] have a comprehensive study of 72 patients with full-thickness defects, age less than 45, without associated meniscus or ligamentous injury with a longer, average 11-year follow-up after microfracture technique. Thirty-nine of these patients had lesions that involved the patellofemoral joint. Significant improvement was demonstrated in average Lysholm scores (59–89) and Tegner scores (3–6), and most importantly, 80 % of the patients rated themselves as "improved."

Osteochondral Autograft

Overview

Osteochondral autografting is a procedure where one or more cylindrical autografts are harvested from non-weight-bearing areas of the femur and are inserted into the cartilage defect to recreate a cartilage-covered surface. If more than one plug is transplanted, it is referred to as a mosaicplasty. This technique is limited by the amount of donor tissue available as well as morbidity at the donor site. The complex geometry of the patellofemoral articulation results in relative decreased utilization of the technique at this site.

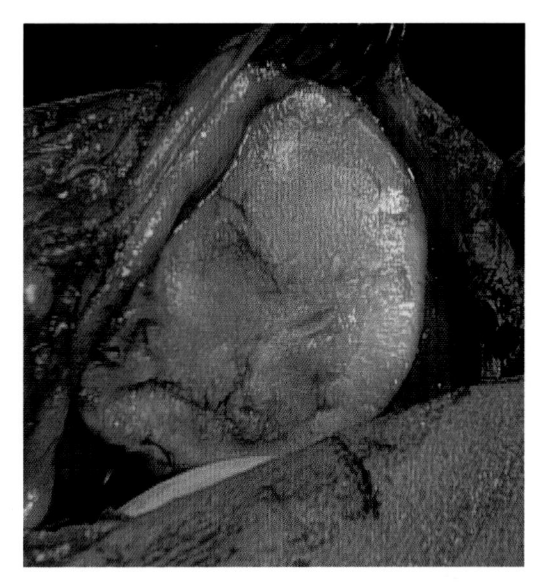

Fig. 5.3 Defect in the patella prior to osteochondral autografting

Technique

Place the patient supine, and begin the exposure utilizing a midline approach with either a medial or lateral arthrotomy. The majority of autologous bone grafts are removed from the lateral femoral condyle above the sulcus terminalis, the superolateral aspect of the intercondylar notch, or the peripheral aspect of the medial femoral condyle. Harvest the plugs using a T-handle device, which is inserted perpendicular to the surface at a depth of 1.5 cm and rotated to harvest the tissue (Fig. 5.3).

Prepare the recipient site by sizing the lesion and choose a reamer with a diameter similar to the size of the harvested grafts. Ream the recipient holes 1–2 mm apart and with 1–2 mm of excess depth beyond that measured from the size

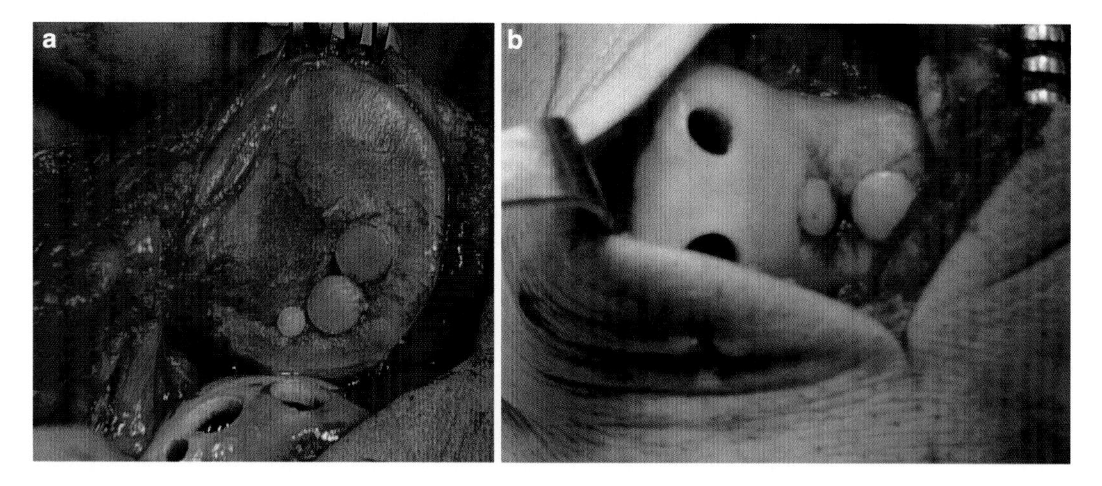

Fig. 5.4 Osteochondral autografting to the patella (**a**) and the trochlea (**b**)

of the harvested plugs. Further expand the holes as needed.

With the graft in a delivery tube, place it perpendicular to the recipient hole and drive it in using mallet strikes. Excessive force can lead to cell death, and therefore, caution should be taken with this step. Remove the delivery tube once the graft is close to flush with the surface and gently finish the impaction (Fig. 5.4).

Results

As with microfracture, reports of autografting demonstrate positive short-term clinical results at the patellofemoral joint, with better results in other knee compartments. Hangody et al. [26] evaluated 1,097 autografting procedures with grade III, grade IV, or osteochondral lesions, 147 of which were implemented at the patellofemoral joint. Eighty-one percent had a simultaneous procedure, including ACL reconstruction, realignment osteotomy, meniscus surgery, or patellofemoral realignment. Fortunately, there was independent evaluation of results in each anatomic zone of the knee. Seventy-four percent of patients with patellar and/or trochlear pain had good to excellent results, which was lower than the 92 % of patients with femoral condylar implantations and 87 % with tibial resurfacings that experienced good to excellent results. This study also contained an evaluation of 93 professional athletes who underwent autologous osteochondral mosaicplasties. There were 26 soccer players, 16 handball players, 10 track and field athletes, 8 water polo players, 7 wrestlers, 6 gymnasts, and 19 from other sports. The average age of the patients was 26 (14–39) and only ten included the patellofemoral joint. Sixty-four percent of the patients returned to the same level of sports activity (five of the patients participated in the Olympic Games in 1996, 2000, and 2004); 19 % were able to return a lower level of sports activity and 17 % were unable to continue athletic activities.

A study with longer term follow-up was performed by Bentley et al. [27] who randomized 100 patients to receive either ACI or mosaicplasty. The mean age of the patients at the time of surgery was 31.3 years and the mean duration of symptoms preoperatively was 7.2 years. Twenty-eight of these lesions were at the patellofemoral articulation but these were not independently analyzed. The number of patients whose repair had failed at 10 years was 10 of 58 (17 %) in the ACI group and 23 of 42 (55 %) in the mosaicplasty group ($P<0.001$). However, a closer analysis reveals that most of the mosaicplasty lesions did very well for about 2 years and then afterward went on to failure, indicating very successful short-term, but not long-term, results.

Osteochondral Allograft

Overview

Osteochondral allografting is typically used for larger lesions or those with substantial bone loss and is often a second-line procedure. However, it may be used as first-line treatment in athletes or high-demand patients. It has the advantage of filling defects with hyaline cartilage and provides the ability to restore lost bone. Tissue matching is not necessary as cartilage is avascular, aneural, and alymphatic, the chondrocytes are relatively isolated, and the implanted tissue is not exposed to the host immune system. Fresh or frozen allograft tissue can be transplanted. While frozen tissue can last many years, fresh tissue is typically stored at 4 °C and is used within 28 days of harvest.

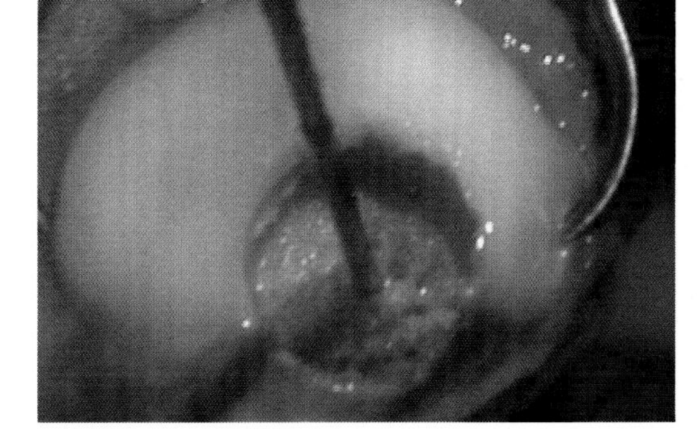

Fig. 5.5 Sizing the patellar defect for an osteochondral allograft

Technique

Place the patient supine, and begin the exposure utilizing a midline approach with either a medial or lateral arthrotomy. Next, size the recipient site, place a guide pin, and use a cannulated reamer to a depth of 6–8 mm (Fig. 5.5). Trim the sidewalls with a 15 blade and irrigate the site. Once this is complete, the depth of the cylindrical socket is measured at the 12, 3, 6, and 9 o'clock positions, and this is recorded. A more intricate freehand construct may be necessary at the patellofemoral joint due to the more complex architecture.

The donor tissue is fixed in a jig and a harvesting device is used to remove the plug. The goal is to match the curvature and architecture of the plug to that of the recipient site (Fig. 5.6). This is clearly a difficult task at the patellofemoral articulation. The graft is then extracted and remeasured according to the recipient site measurements, and necessary adjustments to the donor plug are made in order to allow for an optimal fit.

Dilate the recipient hole of an additional 0.5 mm and press fit the graft using minimal force as chondrocyte injury or death may occur if excess energy is used. The donor tissue is shaped

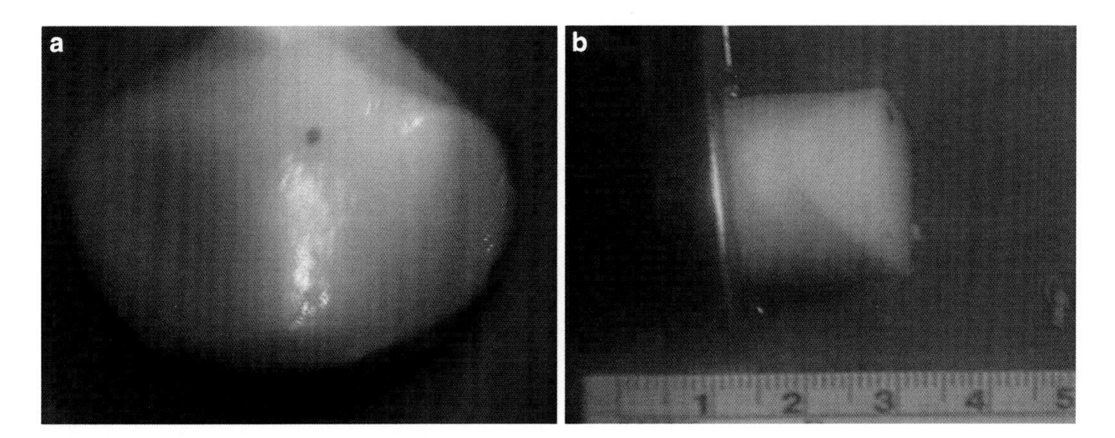

Fig. 5.6 Patella allograft (**a**) with cylindrical graft removed from the patellar allograft (**b**)

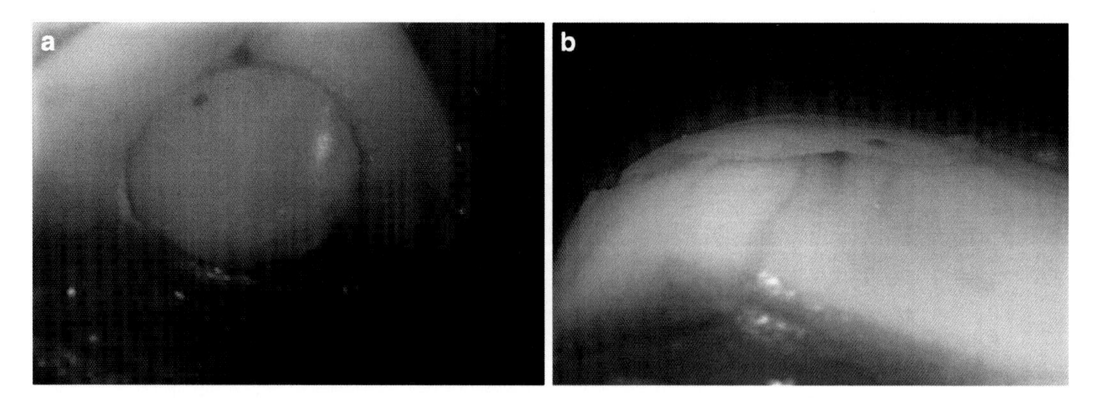

Fig. 5.7 (**a** and **b**) Patellar allograft placed into the patellar defect

to have minimal bone (usually composite thickness of 5–8 mm) with the goal of establishing a physiologic composite thickness (Fig. 5.7). Headless, variable pitch, and bioabsorbable screws may be used to fix the shell allografts or to augment the fixation of allograft plugs.

Early weight bearing and range of motion are allowed and encouraged. With a multiple plug technique, full range of motion and protected weight bearing are advised for the first 4 weeks and full weight bearing after that point. Sporting activities are typically allowed at around 4–6 months postoperatively.

Results

Osteochondral allografting has shown relatively successful clinical results at the knee joint [28–30]. While most of these studies are not specific for the patellofemoral joint, there are some more recent studies that specifically evaluate osteochondral allografting in this area. Unfortunately, these studies are not specific to the athletic population. Torga Spak and Teitge [31] evaluated 14 allografts implanted into the knees of 11 patients younger than 55 years all with advanced secondary osteoarthritis. Eight grafts had survived at an average follow-up of 10 years. Of the six that failed, three were in place for over 10 years. Average knee society scores improved from 46 to 82 points. This study presents effective results of allografting at the patellofemoral joint. A similar study by Jamali et al. [32] evaluated 20 knees in 18 patients with average age of 42 years who were treated with osteochondral allografting at the patellofemoral joint. Kaplan–Meier survivorship analysis demonstrated a 67 % survival rate at 10 years with improved clinical knee scores in the remaining patients. A recent study by Krych et al. [33] specifically evaluated return to athletic activity after osteochondral allograft transplantation in the knee and demonstrated that at 2.5 years follow-up, 38 of 43 athletes returned to sport at some level and 34 of 43 returned to pre-injury level. However, the majority of the treated lesions were not on the patellofemoral joint.

Autologous Chondrocyte Implantation

Overview

Autologous chondrocyte implantation is a technique wherein the patient's own chondrocytes are biopsied, cultured outside of the body, and replaced within the defect to stimulate healing with hyaline cartilage. This technique is best suited for symptomatic, well-contained lesions in patients who are high demand, have large lesions, or have failed alternative surgical measures. This technique is also particularly well suited for repairing lesions at the patellofemoral joint due to the complex topography of the area. Therefore, this procedure is often used in athletes with patellofemoral defects. However, if used at the patella or central/lateral trochlea, it is typically combined with a realignment procedure of the tibial tubercle. This is typically done to decrease the TG–TT distance and thereby causes the patella to track more medially, which will reduce patellar contact pressures and ultimately decrease stress on the graft. However, care must be taken not to overly medialize the tubercle as this also can lead to abnormal mechanics with increased medial wear. Contraindications to this procedure include inflammatory arthritis, loss of subchondral bone, disease in the tibiofemoral joint, probable noncompliance, and bipolar lesions. The success of this procedure and complication rates are improving as surgical technique and materials are optimized. Formerly, a common complication was hypertrophy of the periosteal patch that is used as coverage of the implanted cells. However, complications rates have decreased substantially since implementation of synthetic collagen patch in place of the periosteum [34].

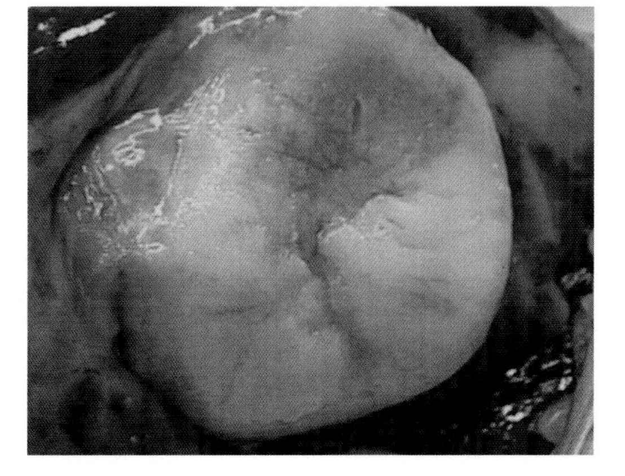

Fig. 5.8 Patellar defect prior to autologous chondrocyte implantation

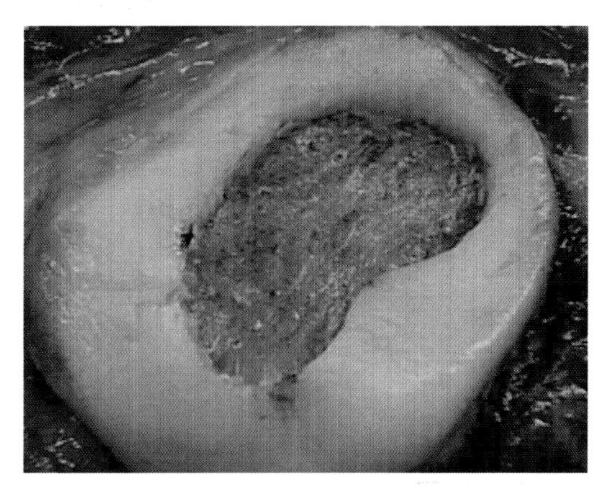

Fig. 5.9 Preparation of the patellar defect

Technique

An arthroscopic evaluation of the lesion must be performed to evaluate the lesions and to assess possibility of ACI. Cartilage is biopsied at this time and cultured to allow adequate cellular growth.

A midline utility incision that extends to the tibial tubercle gives adequate exposure if only ACI is being performed. If an anteromedialization procedure is also planned, the incision should extend 8 cm distal to the tibial tubercle. A lateral arthrotomy which extends from the vastus lateralis to the anterior capsule allows adequate exposure and is less morbid than a medial arthrotomy as it spares the vastus medialis. It is helpful to release the fat pad and to dissect the anterior horn of the meniscus from the capsule to increase exposure. The patella is subluxated or everted medially with varying amounts of knee flexion to maximize the view of the trochlea.

To prepare the recipient site (Fig. 5.8), create vertical walls at the periphery of the chondral lesion using a 15 blade and then debride the defect using a ring curette. Remove all cartilage in the defect with the exception of the calcified cartilage layer and create a "well-shouldered" recipient site without penetrating the underlying bone as this will cause bleeding (Fig. 5.9). Following lesion preparation, a template is pressed into the defect and is sized to cover the defect. Release the tourniquet and achieve hemostasis. This step is critical as bleeding may lead to a result more similar to microfracture with the repaired cartilage composition having increased fibrocartilage rather than hyaline cartilage. Thrombin-soaked Gelfoam can assist in this step. Control persistent bleeding with the application of fibrin glue to the base of the recipient site and hold pressure for 5 min. Ensure that there is adequate surrounding cartilage available to pass suture through in order to provide secure fixation of the patch.

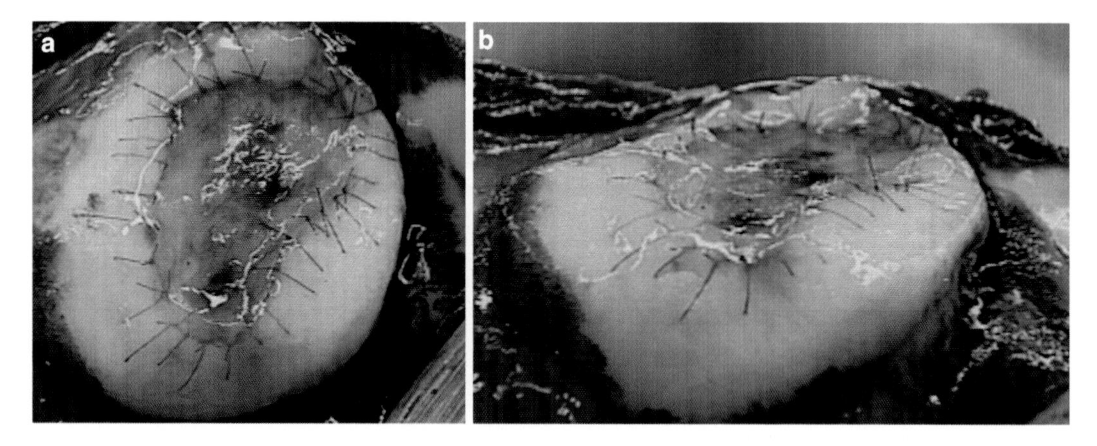

Fig. 5.10 Autologous chondrocyte implantation with a fibrous cover placed over the chondrocytes

Cut the patch to fit the defect and suture it in place using 6-0 Vicryl interrupted sutures achieving a water tight seal with a small opening into which the ACI cell mixture can be injected. Applying mineral oil to the suture can aid in passage through the cartilage. Tie the sutures on the patch side at the intersection of the patch and surrounding tissues. Suture anchors can be placed to provide additional fixation if necessary (Fig. 5.10). Alternatively, a collagen patch may be used rather than cartilage. The same technique is utilized; however, some of the cells may be seeded on a collagen patch prior to suturing it into place. Use fibrin glue to reinforce the seal and test it with saline. However, skip this step if there are cells embedded on the patch.

Postoperatively, a hinged knee brace locked in extension is applied with range of motion advanced by 15° weekly. Continuous passive motion is initiated on the first postoperative day for 6–8 h per day. The objective is to obtain 90° of flexion by weeks 6–8, but not generally sooner than 4 weeks. Return to full activity is not permitted until 8 months postoperatively to protect the lesion until the cartilage has sufficiently matured.

Results

A number of studies have demonstrated both successful short-term and longer term results of autologous chondrocyte implantation at the patellofemoral joint [27, 35–37]. Pascual-Garrido et al. [38] studied a cohort that included 62 patients (63 knees) who underwent autologous chondrocyte implantation of the PF joint with mean defect size of 4.2 cm^2, average age of 31.8 years (range, 15.8–49.4), and mean follow-up of 4 years (range, 2–7). Thirty-five patients had concomitant procedures performed, including AMZ (28), lateral release (4), lateral meniscal transplant (2), and osteochondral autograft (1). This study demonstrated statistically and clinically significant improvement in a variety of knee scores including Lysholm (37–63, $P<0.001$), International Knee Documentation Committee (31–57, $P<0.001$), KOOS Pain (48–71, $P<0.001$), KOOS Symptoms (51–70, $P<0.001$), KOOS Activities of Daily Living (60–80, $P<0.001$), KOOS Sport (25–42, $P<0.001$), KOOS Quality of Life (24–49, $P<0.001$), Short Form-12 Physical (38–41, $P<0.05$), Cincinnati (43–63, $P<0.005$), and Tegner (4–6, $P<0.05$). Also, having a prior failed cartilage restorative procedure did not significantly affect the outcome. This finding further emphasizes that the role of ACI can play following a prior failed cartilage restoration. Additionally, they found that the patients who had concomitant anteromedialization showed a trend towards better outcomes. Unfortunately, a relatively high percentage (44 %) of patients required a subsequent procedure. However, these further procedures were not necessarily "failures" of the ACI procedure specifically as they were most commonly due to graft hypertrophy, painful hardware, or new cartilage lesions. There were four true clinical failures (7.7 %), which were defined as progression to arthroplasty or conversion to osteochondral allograft transplantation. Most importantly, 72 % of patients stated that they would be willing to have the surgery again.

Farr et al. [39] demonstrated similar improvements in knee scores, reoperation rates, incidence of concomitant procedures, and treatment failures over a comparable time course. He evaluated 38 patients (39 knees, average age 31.2 years) with unipolar or bipolar patellofemoral lesions treated with ACI and simultaneous biomechanical correction procedure, the majority anteromedialization (74 %) at mean 3.1 years follow-up. There was a statistically significant improvement in Cincinnati knee, Lysholm, and VAS pain scores. At mean 1.2 years, there was a median 11 of 12 score on ICRS cartilage repair assessment. As with the previously discussed study, there was a high rate of reoperation (26 knees in 25 patients had 32 subsequent operations); however, only 3 (7.8 %) were technically considered treatment failures (2 required microfracture and one had septic knee with patch removal of implant). Perhaps most importantly, 80 % of patients rated their function as good, very good, or excellent at the latest follow-up.

Minas and Bryant [36] prospectively studied 45 patients with average age of 37.5 years at minimum 2-year follow-up after treatment involving ACI at the patellofemoral articulation. They demonstrated a postoperative improvement as measured by the Short Form-36, Western Ontario and McMaster University Score, Knee Society Score, modified Cincinnati Score, and a patient satisfaction survey. There was a higher rate of failure in this study (eight patients, 18 %). However, the procedure was still relatively successful as 71 % of patients rated their outcomes as good or excellent, 22 % rated outcome as fair, and 7 % rated outcome as poor.

The previously discussed studies demonstrate successful short-term results. However, there are a few studies that evaluate the longer term results of ACI. Peterson et al. [40] performed a study of ACI and independently evaluated 17 patients who were treated at the patellofemoral joint. At mean 7.4-year follow-up, he demonstrated that 13 of these 17 patients rated their overall clinical score as good or excellent. Another of the longer term studies was discussed earlier in this chapter. The report by Bentley et al. [27] in which he randomized 100 patients to ACI versus mosaicplasty showed only a 17 % failure rate at average 10 years of follow-up.

DeNovo

Overview

The use of particulated juvenile cartilage allograft (DeNovo Natural Tissue [NT]; ISTO, St. Louis, MO) for the treatment of articular cartilage lesions has been reported in the literature. This repair strategy uses bioactive cells to drive a biological process in a matrix scaffold that provides architectural support and facilitates the integration of the repaired tissue with the contiguous tissue. Until recently, allograft treatment options have been limited to osteochondral grafts, as graft incorporation to host tissue was only possible at the bone level. The concept that cartilage could be transplanted without its underlying bony component is a new concept. However, the potential safety and efficacy of DeNovo NT are changing the paradigm.

While the phenomenon of hyaline cartilage repair using particulated articular cartilage is relatively new to the English-speaking literature, a thorough literature review reveals a published report by Albrecht et al. in the German literature dating back to 1983 [41]. Their work showed that cartilage autograft implantation without bone can lead to cartilage defect healing if the cartilage is cut into small pieces. Dr. Jian Q. Yao noted these early preclinical reports and decided to evaluate similar studies using particulated juvenile cartilage allograft (DeNovo NT; distributed by Zimmer, Warsaw, IN) in place of autograft. This alternative approach was based on two factors (1) allograft allows conceptually no limit to the amount of harvested tissue and (2) juvenile cartilage has the potential of more robust cellular

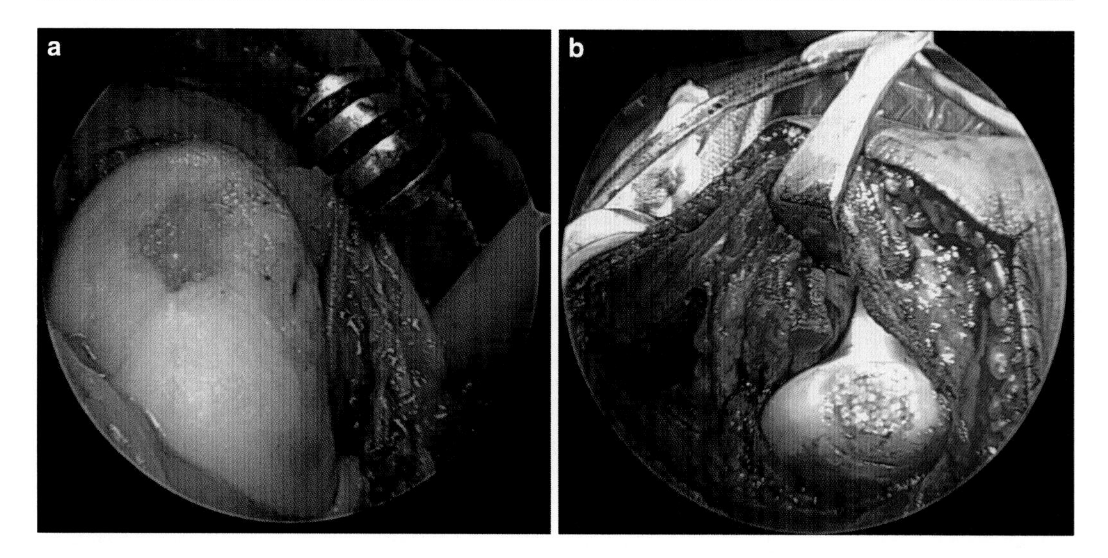

Fig. 5.11 (**a**) Femoral condyle prior to implementation of DeNovo, demonstrating the cartilage defect. (**b**) After the implant of DeNovo

activity than older cartilage tissue. DeNovo is currently available for use in clinical applications without an IDE (investigational device exemption) study, and to date, over 2,200 patients have received this product.

DeNovo represents an excellent option in the patellofemoral compartment for two main reasons. One, it is an "off-the-shelf" treatment that does not require staging of multiple procedures. Two, it allows conformity in the patellofemoral articulation. DeNovo can be placed into any defect and will conform to the shape of the defect. This is essential in the patellofemoral joint.

Technique

After confirmatory arthroscopy, a limited medial or lateral arthrotomy is performed to fully visualize the lesion (Fig. 5.11). The defect is outlined with a scalpel to create a shoulder (vertical peripheral wall) of normal or nearly normal host articular cartilage. The cartilage within the outlined area is removed carefully with a curette to the vertical wall of the host cartilage shoulder and the base of the defect. The base is cleared of all cartilage tissue including the calcified layer without entering into the subchondral bone. No marrow stimulation procedure is performed. Hemostasis, without a tourniquet, is achieved with epinephrine-soaked Cottonoids and fibrin glue. After measuring the defect dimensions and recording the visual findings with photographs, a thin aluminum sterile foil is pressed into the defect to create a three-dimensional mold, as a complete replica of the defect. Once formed, the foil mold is removed from the defect and placed on the back table of the operating room. Using the measured defect dimensions, the defect surface area was calculated. One package of DeNovo NT graft is used for each 2.5 cm^2 defect. Larger defects require proportionally more packages of DeNovo NT graft.

The DeNovo NT graft, in a specially formulated nutrient preservation medium, is shipped in an aseptic temperature-controlled packaging. The medium is aspirated and the particulated cartilage pieces are transferred to the foil mold and distributed 1–2 mm apart (potentially less separation depending upon the ratio between the implanted tissue volume and the surface area of the defect). Fibrin glued is then added to the cartilage pieces until the foil mold was filled to within 1 mm of its full depth. The glue is allowed to cure (typically 3–10 min) (Fig. 5.11). At that point, the fibrin glue/cartilage tissue construct is gently separated and then lifted from the foil in one piece. Fresh fibrin glue is applied at the base of the patient's cartilage lesion, and the fibrin glue/particulated cartilage construct is pressed into the defect and the glue allowed to cure. It is imperative that the fibrin glue cartilage tissue construct is thinner (average 1 mm) than the surrounding cartilage shoulders (average 2–3 mm), to minimize the potential for shear or direct compressive load.

Results

To date, there are only two clinical studies on the use of DeNovo NT for symptomatic cartilage lesions in the knee that are reported in the literature [27, 42].

The first is a case report on the use of particulated juvenile cartilage tissue for a symptomatic full-thickness patella cartilage defect [43]. At 2-year follow-up, the patient experienced substantial clinical improvement in both pain and function when evaluated with both the IKDC subjective evaluation and the KOOS outcome measures. MRI at final follow-up demonstrates fill of the defect with repair tissue and near-complete resolution of preoperative bony edema.

The second is an early interim report of patients that are a part of an ongoing multicenter, prospective, single arm study of 25 subjects [44]. This study is designed to evaluate clinical outcomes such as IKDC, KOOS, and visual analog scale (VAS) scores, as well as extent and quality of repair with MRI and optional biopsies. To date, 25 patients with one or two chondral lesions on the femoral condyle or trochlea have been enrolled at three study sites. Four patients have completed 24-month follow-up and their outcomes have been recently reported in Cartilage [44]. Detailed results of all 25 patients will be reported once they have all reached the 2-year postoperative follow-up milestone.

Of the four patients with 2-year follow-up, three had nontraumatic cartilage lesions and one had a traumatic cartilage injury. The average age was 43 years and body mass index was 27 lb/in^2. The average lesion size was 2.71 cm^2. Two patients had isolated trochlea lesions, one had an isolated condyle lesion, and one had focal lesions of both the femoral condyle and trochlea. KOOS, IKDC, and VAS scores demonstrate clear improvements in all scores across the 24-month follow-up period. Most of these improvements, especially in KOOS and VAS, were achieved at the 12-month mark and maintained throughout the study period.

Combined Anteromedialization

Overview

Tibial tubercle osteotomy, typically anteromedialization, is often used concurrently with cartilage restoration procedures, particularly ACI, to correct maltracking issues and reduce stress on the regenerating cartilage. Maltracking is primarily assessed with physical exam and calculation of TT–TG values. It is important to confirm that medial cartilage is healthy, as the anteromedialization procedure tends to increase medial stresses and would worsen defects in this area. Also, the chondral disease should be limited in scope as advanced disease may be better served with an arthroplasty procedure as there is a lack of healthy cartilage that can be used to unload the diseased cartilage. The AMZ procedure itself can be customized by changing the slope of the osteotomy to provide more exteriorization in patients with central or proximal lesions or more medialization in patients with lateral lesions [38, 42, 45]. Benefits of AMZ must be weighed against the additional risks of infection, symptomatic hardware, wound complications, nonunion (especially in obese patients, diabetic patients, and smokers), tibial fracture, compartment syndrome, and deep vein thrombosis. Removal of hardware is often necessary [39], and several series have reported tibial fractures with AMZ, which have led to more extensive weight-bearing limitations [46]. Despite these complications, patients who are undergoing patellofemoral cartilage restorative procedures have been shown to benefit from a combined AMZ procedure [34, 36, 39, 40, 47].

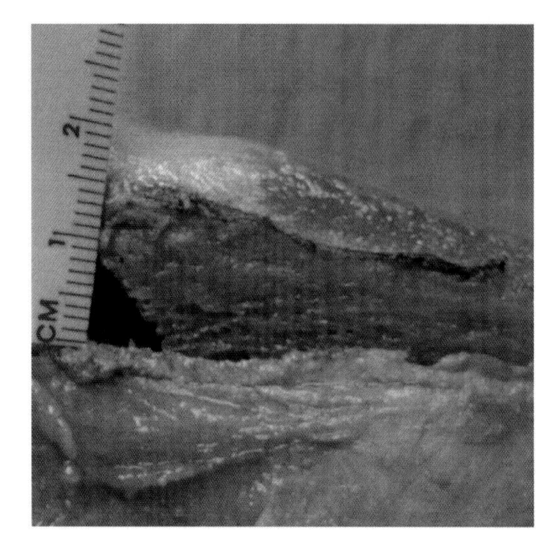

Fig. 5.12 Appropriate amount of anteriorization for the tibial tubercle

Technique

Preoperatively determine the amount of anteriorization and medialization of the tubercle that will be necessary. The goal of the medialization component is to bring the TT–TG distance to within 10–15 mm and to anteriorize around 10–15 mm (Fig. 5.12). By varying the slope and the extent of anteriorization, a variety of medialization distances can be achieved. Position and pad the patient, apply a tourniquet, administer anesthesia, and then perform an exam prior to prepping and draping. The incision should start at the superior aspect of the patella and continue 8–10 cm inferior to the tibial tubercle. Next, identify and release the patellar tendon from the capsule to allow for protection during the case. The incision should extend distally along the lateral margin of the tibial tuberosity and tibial crest to allow for elevation of the anterior compartment musculature and exposure of the tibia. Use a retractor to protect the deep peroneal nerve and anterior tibial artery. Perform the osteotomy with a commercially available system. An initial reference pin is orientated perpendicular to the posterior cortex of the proximal tibia. The reference pin is inserted just distal to the patellar tendon attachment through the tibial tuberosity. Using preoperative calculations for anteriorization and medialization, the desired slope angle guide is assembled with the cutting block and cutting block post. The cutting guide is then placed over the reference pin and the cutting block is positioned immediately medial to the tibial crest beginning directly in line with the medial border of the patella tendon and angled laterally to allow a lateral exit of the osteotomy distally. The desired pedicle length for the osteotomy is approximately 7–10 cm. When correct positioning has been achieved and the entry and exit sites have been confirmed, two breakaway pins secure the cutting block in position. With the retractor still protecting neurovascular structures posteriorly, the cut is made with an oscillating saw that is simultaneously cooled with saline. The cutting block is removed and the oscillating saw is directed towards the distal exit of the osteotomy to finish the distal cut. A small osteotome is used to complete the proximal osteotomy, approaching the tibial tuberosity medially and laterally at the level of the patella tendon insertion. The tuberosity is now free.

A ruler is used to measure the required amount of anteriorization and medialization based on preoperative calculations, and the pedicle position is adjusted along the osteotomy slope. If required, the pedicles can be moved proximally or distally to address patellar height issues. A Kirschner wire is used to temporarily secure the pedicle when correct positioning has been achieved. The tuberosity fragment is then drilled using interfragmentary lag technique and secured using two countersunk 4.5 mm cortical screws. The screws are positioned perpendicular to the osteotomy (angled from the anterolateral aspect of the pedicle to anteromedial tibia) so they are directed away from posterior neurovascular structures (Fig. 5.13). The surgical site is closed in a standard fashion.

Results

Some of the studies already discussed in this chapter have touched upon the beneficial effects of combining an anteromedialization procedure

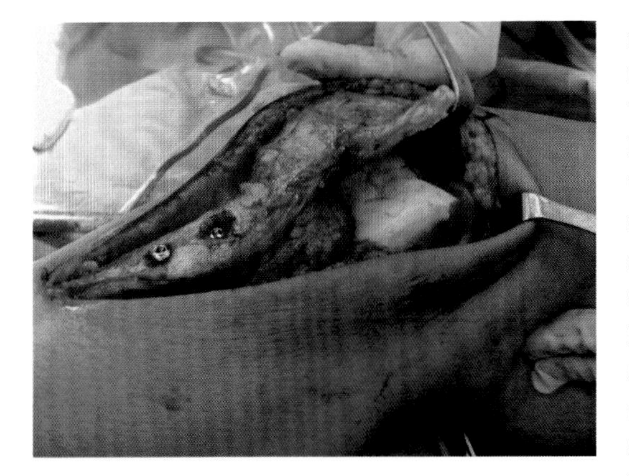

Fig. 5.13 Completed anteromedialization procedure with fixation of the tibial bone cut

with other cartilage restorative procedures. Pascual-Garrido et al. [38] demonstrated that at an average 4-year follow-up, the patients who received anteromedialization with ACI tended to have better results than those with ACI alone. Farr et al. [39] also demonstrated successful results combining biomechanical realignment procedures with ACI. However, it must be noted that 44 % of the reoperations in this series were due to hardware-related pain at the anteromedialization site.

Henderson and Lavigne [47] specifically evaluated the impact of concomitant correction of the extensor mechanism with ACI by comparing 22 patients with realignment and patellar ACI to 22 patients with "normal" patellofemoral tracking and patellar ACI. The group of patients with simultaneous extensor mechanism correction had a greater increase in average modified Cincinnati knee score (4.5 vs. 1.7 points), better function, better SF-36 physical component scores (70.9 vs. 55.4 points), and higher IKDC scores (85.2 vs. 60.6 points) at an average follow-up of 2 years.

Treatment Theory

First, it is critical to correlate a patient's symptoms and presentation with the specific pathology of the knee and not reflexively assume that a cartilage lesion is the source of a patient's pain simply because one is present. The outcomes of cartilage restoration procedures can be unpredictable, and the natural history of these lesions is unknown. Therefore, the simple presence of a cartilage lesion does not necessitate treatment. Understanding and managing patient goals and expectations is also critical to a successful outcome. Patient concerns about progression to arthritis, safety of continuing activity with the lesion, level of improvement to expect, and possible need for subsequent procedures are typical questions. Unfortunately, these are difficult to answer given the lack of data on these subjects. Patient age, body mass index, symptom type (weight-bearing pain, non-weight-bearing pain, swelling, mechanical symptoms, giving way, pain walking on level ground vs. stair climbing), occupation and/or family commitments, risk aversion (desire to avoid current or subsequent surgical procedures), responsiveness and rehabilitation after previous surgical treatments, and the patient's specific concerns related to his or her problem are all important preoperative considerations. Age is a consideration because patients in their 4th of 5th decade often have disease on opposing surfaces, which is a contraindication to cartilage restoration procedures. Further, arthroplasty procedures should be considered in this population given the predictable and successful results. Concomitant pathological conditions in the knee often must be addressed prior to or during the restoration procedure to have a successful outcome. All aspects of the cartilage defect including depth, size, location, number, and geometry must be considered along with the condition of the surrounding cartilage and underlying bone. As noted above, always examine the opposing surface as the presence of disease, which is easily overlooked, may prevent a successful restoration procedure.

Treatment Algorithm

Concomitant conditions such as malalignment, ligament insufficiency, or meniscal deficiency must be treated prior to or during the restoration procedure. Patellofemoral lesions are often treated with simultaneous realignment of the tibial tuberosity. Lateral patellofemoral lesions are treated with anteromedialization while medial lesions are treated with more anteriorization. The treatment algorithm is essentially based on both defect variables (mainly size and location) and patient characteristics (mainly activity level). Primary repair is done for any chondral injury that is amenable to fixation, which includes acute osteochondral fragments or in situ and unstable osteochondritis dissecans lesions. The basic principles for primary repair include elevation of the unstable fragment, debridement of the base, and microfracture, if necessary, to gain access to the subchondral blood supply to promote healing, bone grafting of areas of cystic changes or bone loss, and rigid fixation of the fragment under compression. Headless compression screw fixation may be necessary and these screws can be removed once healing has occurred. Continuous passive motion for 6 h each day is recommended. A second-look arthroscopy may be performed to evaluate the success of the procedure, likely prognosis, and to evaluate for fragment settling, which can expose screws used for fixation.

Lesions not amenable to primary repair may be fixed using cartilage restoration techniques discussed earlier in this chapter. Marrow stimulation techniques are often a first-line treatment in the general population and are used for smaller lesions (<2 cm) or in patients with larger lesions (>3 cm) and decreased activity levels. Small lesions in high-demand patients or those for whom marrow stimulation has failed can be treated with osteochondral autografting. This procedure can be a reasonable option in the athletic population. However, it is challenging at the patellofemoral articulation given the complex geometry in this area. Larger lesions (>2.5 cm) are typically more amenable to osteochondral allografting or autologous chondrocyte implantation. Allografting, however, has the same structural difficulties as autografting does in the patellofemoral joint. Autologous chondrocyte implantation is advised for younger patients with shallow lesions, especially those of the patellofemoral joint. It is often the optimal choice in an athlete with patellofemoral cartilage disease. This method does not violate the subchondral bone and hence minimizes the impact on future treatments. Also, these lesions are typically smaller than those elsewhere in the knee, and for this additional reason, they are better treated with autologous chondrocyte implantation. Deep lesions with associated bone loss, on the other hand, typically require an osteochondral allograft to replace the damaged or missing bone. In general, defects of the femoral condyle are better treated with allografting and those of the patellofemoral joint with autologous chondrocyte implantation.

Return to Sports

Unfortunately, there is limited data on return to sports following knee cartilage restoration, especially in specific regard to the patellofemoral joint. Many individualized factors come into play including desire versus need to play a sport, the lesion size, physiologic and knee-specific comorbidities, age, BMI, expectations, pre-injury level, and level of sport. Return to sport can take a few months for small defects and up to years with an ACI procedure. Many of the recommendations are vague and based on personal experience rather than literature; however, there are some basic concepts. Older patients, in general, require more time as do patients with associated ligamentous repair, meniscal repair, or anteromedialization surgery. Larger patients logically put more stress upon the patellofemoral joint that it typically takes these individuals longer to return as well. If the patient is a lower level athlete, it is often prudent to encourage them to adopt a lower impact sport if possible. Finally, it is important to educate patients and manage expectations as return to high-level athletics for a sustained time, while possible, is often not attainable.

There are, however, some patient- and lesion-specific factors that are prognostic for returning to sport which are supported by literature. Younger age has been associated with more favorable outcomes in several studies [4, 48–51]. Cartilage injuries in adolescent or young adult athletes may occur after an acute traumatic injury or secondary to osteochondritis dissecans (OCD).

These injuries generally result from a shearing force through the zone of provisional calcification in a patient with open physes. However, the fact that these patients have open physes can lead to more healing potential. Mithofer et al. [4] studied 45 soccer players following autologous chondrocyte implantation with average follow-up of 41 months. They noted that that the mean age of patients that returned to sport was 22.3 years versus 27.6 years in patients who did not return to sport. A higher proportion of high-level athletes returned to sport as well as patients with a shorter preoperative duration of symptoms. Patients whose ACI procedure was performed within 1 year of injury had higher likelihood of a return to pre-injury level of competition. Although there are no definitive reasons for lower rate of return with more delayed treatment, chronic cartilage lesions in theory may increase in size, affect the opposite articular surface, and contribute to an unfavorable repair environment. Also, a delay in treatment may decondition the athlete, delay rehabilitation, and thereby negatively affect likelihood of return to competition. An increased number of prior procedures may also negatively affect an athlete's outcome and ability to return to pre-injury athletics [52, 53]. The duration of rehabilitation after ACI varies with regard to specific patient characteristics, lesion location, concomitant procedures, and the type of sport played. The appropriate recommendation for return to play can be difficult to ascertain from the literature because there are multiple factors that may lead an athlete to return to competition. In the previously mentioned Mithofer study, it was reported that while 72 % of subjects reported good to excellent knee function, only 33 % were able to return to soccer; however, 10 of 12 (83 %) high-skill soccer players compared with only 5 of 31 (16 %) recreational soccer players were able to return to the same level of competition. The mean time to return to soccer for high-skill players was 14.2 months. The disproportionate percentage of high-level athletes returning to the same level of competition has also been observed in patients undergoing microfracture surgery, with greater than 76 % returning to play. This figure is obtained from a study by Steadman et al. [54] who evaluated the return to play rates in 25 NFL players following microfracture. While these are promising results, many studies have demonstrated that athletes who underwent ACI as compared to microfracture are able to remain competitively active for a longer period of time [4, 48, 54, 55]. This is not surprising, however, given that the restored cartilage with ACI consists of more durable hyaline cartilage as compared to the fibrocartilage that fills the defect with microfracture. There are several factors likely contributing to an increased percentage of high-level athletes returning to sport, including younger age, shorter duration of symptoms before treatment, improved postoperative rehabilitation, psychological factors, and economic incentives.

Future Directions

The future of patellofemoral cartilage restoration is exciting with much room for development as many of the modern techniques were only recently invented and are constantly evolving. It may become possible to utilize more microbiology and genetics in the diagnosis and treatment of these injuries. On the diagnostic side, creating a genetic profile of a patient's cartilage that could determine the risk of progression or further injury would be instrumental in the operative decision-making process. Genetics may also be used to profile donors of allograft tissue and predict the likelihood of successful implantation based on tissue compatibility. On a histologic level, the ability to grade the quality of donor cartilage would also be helpful for determining prognosis. Prosthetic scaffolds for autologous chondrocyte implantation are already in place; however, the quality of these materials will continue to improve. Biologic growth factor additives may allow for quicker healing, single-stage ACI with an allogeneic source of cells, or microfracture with increased hyaline cartilage as opposed to fibrocartilage content. Saw et al. [56] demonstrated good results in a case series of five patients who were treated with microfracture along with the addition of peripheral blood progenitor cells and hyaluronic acid. This idea was generated based on similar study using a goat model [57] in which the resultant cartilage had a better mix of hyaline cartilage and more histologic features of hyaline cartilage. Overall, cartilage restoration procedures will continue to progress as the current procedures are optimized and new techniques are developed.

References

1. Widuchowski W, et al. Articular cartilage defects: study of 25,124 knee arthroscopies. Knee. 2007;14:3.
2. Curl WW, et al. Cartilage injuries: a review of 31,516 knee arthroscopies. Arthroscopy. 1997;13:4.
3. Walczak BE, et al. Abnormal findings on knee magnetic resonance imaging in asymptomatic NBA players. J Knee Surg. 2008;21:1.
4. Mithofer K, et al. Articular cartilage repair in soccer players with autologous chondrocyte transplantation: functional outcome and return to competition. Am J Sports Med. 2005;33:11.
5. Eckstein F, et al. In vivo cartilage deformation after different types of activity and its dependence on physical training status. Ann Rheum Dis. 2005;64:2.
6. Lane NE. The risk of osteoarthritis with running and aging: a 5-year longitudinal study. J Rheumatol. 1993;20:3.
7. Sohn RS, Micheli LJ. The effect of running on the pathogenesis of osteoarthritis of the hips and knees. Clin Orthop Relat Res. 1985(198):106–9.
8. Marti B. Is excessive running predictive of degenerative hip disease? Controlled study of former elite athletes. BMJ. 1989;299:6691.
9. Flanigan DC, et al. Prevalence of chondral defects in athletes' knees: a systematic review. Med Sci Sports Exerc. 2010;42:10.
10. Shelbourne KD. Outcome of untreated traumatic articular cartilage defects of the knee: a natural history study. J Bone Joint Surg Am. 2003;85-A Suppl 2:8–16.
11. Widuchowski W, et al. Untreated asymptomatic deep cartilage lesions associated with anterior cruciate ligament injury: results at 10- and 15-year follow-up. Am J Sports Med. 2009;37:4.
12. Hunter W. Of the structure and diseases of articulating cartilages. Clin Orthop Relat Res. 1995(317):3–6.
13. Haggart G. Surgical treatment of degenerative arthritis of the knee joint. N Engl J Med. 1947;236:971–3.
14. Bennett GA, Bauer W. Further studies concerning the repair of articular cartilage in dog joints. J Bone Joint Surg. 1935;17:141–50.
15. Pridie K. A method of resurfacing osteoarthritic knee joints. J Bone Joint Surg Br. 1959;41:618–9.
16. Nomura E. Chondral and osteochondral injuries associated with acute patellar dislocation. Arthroscopy. 2003;19:7.
17. Gomoll AH. Treatment of chondral defects in the patellofemoral joint. J Knee Surg. 2006;19:4.
18. Dejour H. Factors of patellar instability: an anatomic radiographic study. Knee Surg Sports Traumatol Arthrosc. 1994;2:1.
19. Schoettle PB. The tibial tuberosity-trochlear groove distance; a comparative study between CT and MRI scanning. Knee. 2006;13:1.
20. Witvrouw E. Open versus closed kinetic chain exercises in patellofemoral pain: a 5-year prospective randomized study. Am J Sports Med. 2004;32:5.
21. Fond J, et al. Arthroscopic debridement for the treatment of osteoarthritis of the knee: 2- and 5-year results. Arthroscopy. 2002;18:8.
22. Shapiro F. Cell origin and differentiation in the repair of full-thickness defects of articular cartilage. J Bone Joint Surg Am. 1993;75:4.
23. Mithoefer K, et al. The microfracture technique for the treatment of articular cartilage lesions in the knee. A prospective cohort study. J Bone Joint Surg Am. 2005;87:9.
24. Kreuz PC, et al. Results after microfracture of full-thickness chondral defects in different compartments in the knee. Osteoarthritis Cartilage. 2006;14:11.
25. Steadman JR, et al. Outcomes of microfracture for traumatic chondral defects of the knee: average 11-year follow-up. Arthroscopy. 2003;19:5.
26. Hangody L, et al. Autologous osteochondral grafting–technique and long-term results. Injury. 2008;39 Suppl 1:S32–9.
27. Bentley G, et al. A prospective, randomised comparison of autologous chondrocyte implantation versus mosaicplasty for osteochondral defects in the knee. J Bone Joint Surg Br. 2003;85:2.
28. Aubin PP. Long-term followup of fresh femoral osteochondral allografts for posttraumatic knee defects. Clin Orthop Relat Res. 2001(391 Suppl): S318–27.
29. Bugbee WD, Convery FR. Osteochondral allograft transplantation. Clin Sports Med. 1999;18:1.
30. Garrett JC. Fresh osteochondral allografts for treatment of articular defects in osteochondritis dissecans of the lateral femoral condyle in adults. Clin Orthop Relat Res. 1994(303):33–7.
31. Torga Spak R, Teitge RA. Fresh osteochondral allografts for patellofemoral arthritis: long-term followup. Clin Orthop Relat Res. 2006;444:193–200.
32. Jamali AA, et al. Fresh osteochondral allografts: results in the patellofemoral joint. Clin Orthop Relat Res. 2005(437):176–85.
33. Krych AJ, et al. Return to athletic activity after osteochondral allograft transplantation in the knee. Am J Sports Med. 2012;40:5.
34. Steinwachs M, Kreuz PC. Autologous chondrocyte implantation in chondral defects of the knee with a type I/III collagen membrane: a prospective study with a 3-year follow-up. Arthroscopy. 2007;23:4.
35. Brittberg M. Treatment of deep cartilage defects in the knee with autologous chondrocyte transplantation. N Engl J Med. 1994;331:14.

36. Minas T, Bryant T. The role of autologous chondrocyte implantation in the patellofemoral joint. Clin Orthop Relat Res. 2005(436):30–9.
37. Yates Jr JW. The effectiveness of autologous chondrocyte implantation for treatment of full-thickness articular cartilage lesions in workers' compensation patients. Orthopedics. 2003;26:3.
38. Pascual-Garrido C, et al. Recommendations and treatment outcomes for patellofemoral articular cartilage defects with autologous chondrocyte implantation: prospective evaluation at average 4-year follow-up. Am J Sports Med. 2009;37 Suppl 1: 33S–41S.
39. Farr J, et al. Autologous chondrocyte implantation improves patellofemoral cartilage treatment outcomes. Clin Orthop Relat Res. 2007;463:187–94.
40. Peterson L, et al. Autologous chondrocyte transplantation. Biomechanics and long-term durability. Am J Sports Med. 2002;30:1.
41. Albrecht F, Roessner A, Zimmermann E. Closure of osteochondral lesions using chondral fragments and fibrin adhesive. Arch Orthop Trauma Surg. 1983; 101(3):213–7.
42. Beck PR. Trochlear contact pressures after anteromedialization of the tibial tubercle. Am J Sports Med. 2005;33:11.
43. Bonner KF, Daner W, Yao JQ. 2-year postoperative evaluation of a patient with a symptomatic full-thickness patellar cartilage defect repaired with particulated juvenile cartilage tissue. J Knee Surg. 2010;23(2):109–14.
44. Farr J, Yao JQ. Chondral defect repair with particulated juvenile cartilage allograft. Cartilage. 2011;2(4): 346–53.
45. Rue JP. Trochlear contact pressures after straight anteriorization of the tibial tuberosity. Am J Sports Med. 2008;36:10.
46. Pidoriano AJ. Correlation of patellar articular lesions with results from anteromedial tibial tubercle transfer. Am J Sports Med. 1997;25:4.
47. Henderson IJ, Lavigne P. Periosteal autologous chondrocyte implantation for patellar chondral defect in patients with normal and abnormal patellar tracking. Knee. 2006;13:4.
48. Blevins FT. Treatment of articular cartilage defects in athletes: an analysis of functional outcome and lesion appearance. Orthopedics. 1998;21:7.
49. Kish G. Osteochondral mosaicplasty for the treatment of focal chondral and osteochondral lesions of the knee and talus in the athlete. Rationale, indications, techniques, and results. Clin Sports Med. 1999;18:1.
50. Kocher MS. Functional and radiographic outcome of juvenile osteochondritis dissecans of the knee treated with transarticular arthroscopic drilling. Am J Sports Med. 2001;29:5.
51. Micheli L. Articular cartilage repair in the adolescent athlete: is autologous chondrocyte implantation the answer? Clin J Sport Med. 2006;16:6.
52. Hefti F. Osteochondritis dissecans: a multicenter study of the European Pediatric Orthopedic Society. J Pediatr Orthop B. 1999;8:4.
53. Peterson L. Treatment of osteochondritis dissecans of the knee with autologous chondrocyte transplantation: results at two to ten years. J Bone Joint Surg Am. 2003;85-A Suppl 2:17–24.
54. Steadman JR, et al. The microfracture technique in the treatment of full-thickness chondral lesions of the knee in National Football League players. J Knee Surg. 2003;16:2.
55. Kon E. Arthroscopic second-generation autologous chondrocyte implantation compared with microfracture for chondral lesions of the knee: prospective nonrandomized study at 5 years. Am J Sports Med. 2009;37:1.
56. Saw KY, et al. Articular cartilage regeneration with autologous peripheral blood progenitor cells and hyaluronic acid after arthroscopic subchondral drilling: a report of 5 cases with histology. Arthroscopy. 2011;27:4.
57. Saw KY. Articular cartilage regeneration with autologous marrow aspirate and hyaluronic acid: an experimental study in a goat model. Arthroscopy. 2009;25:12.

MPFL Repair and Reconstruction

6

Philip B. Schoettle

Introduction

The medial patellofemoral complex, consisting of the medial patellofemoral ligament (MPFL) and the medial patellotibial ligament, is the main passive stabiliser of the patellofemoral joint. Since it has been shown that a rupture of the MPFL occurs after a first-time patellar dislocation [1] and biomechanical studies have demonstrated that the MPFL is the main restraint against lateral patellar displacement, reconstruction (or repair) of the MPFL has become a widespread technique for restoration of patellofemoral stability. MPFL reconstruction (MPFLR) has become increasingly popular since distal realignment procedures have provided inadequate restoration of patellofemoral stability, leading to increased mediolateral instability, increased patellofemoral pressure or arthritic degeneration [2, 3]. Furthermore, it has been shown that lateral release or opening of the lateral retinaculum leads to an increased lateral and medial instability as well as to lateral pain after cicatrisation (AMIS, etc.). Therefore, not the loosening of the lateral but the strengthening of the medial soft tissue complex became the surgical strategy to act against the lateralising force of the quadriceps.

P.B. Schoettle, M.D. (✉)
Isar Medical Center, Sonnenstrasse 24-26, Munich, Bavaria 80331, Germany
e-mail: philip.schoettle@isarkliniken.de

Since medial reefing procedures have shown mixed results, MPFL reconstruction has become the widely accepted surgical technique for the treatment of patellofemoral instability. The reefing technique tightens the vastus medialis, which only stabilises the patellofemoral joint in flexion by increasing the patellofemoral pressure, but not in extension when the lateralising quadriceps vector is the highest. The repair of the MPFL, published mainly as an arthroscopic technique, may be a surgical alternative in patients with a first-time dislocation, enough remaining functional soft tissue and an MR diagnosis, showing the rupture location of the MPFL, so a repair at the femoral or patellar insertion could be performed.

Therefore, numerous techniques for reconstruction of the medial patellofemoral complex have been described with promising clinical results [4]. In this chapter, the anatomy and function of the MPFL as well as the different indications and contraindications for MPFL repair and reconstruction will be explained.

Anatomy and Biomechanics

The MPFL takes an important role in patellofemoral stability as it is the main passive stabiliser, working as a ligamentous restraint against the lateralising force of the quadriceps vector [5]. It is situated in between the second and the third medial patellofemoral layers [6]. The MPFL attaches posterior to the saddle in between the

R.V. West and A.C. Colvin (eds.), *The Patellofemoral Joint in the Athlete*,
DOI 10.1007/978-1-4614-4157-1_6, © Springer Science+Business Media New York 2014

medial epicondyle and the adductor tubercle [7]. At the patella, there is a wider insertion area at the upper and middle third of the patella, covering 40 % of the medial patellar edge [8]. Due to the oblique direction of the MPFL (compare attachment areas, see above), an intact or reconstructed MPFL not only decreases patellar tilt and shift and therefore limits the subjective apprehension, but it also distalises the patella and lowers the risk of a subluxation close to extension. Despite the MPFL being very thin, it had a mean tensile strength of 208 N and has been reported to be the primary passive restraint to patellar lateral displacement [9], occurring most easily at 20° knee flexion. Therefore, the contribution of the MPFL to resisting patellar lateral subluxation is greatest close to extension.

Indication for Surgery: Repair

Indication for an MPFL repair is the acute (traumatic) first-time lateral patellar dislocation. Thereby, MPFL and medial parapatellar retinaculum can be elongated, partially or totally ruptured. A persistent subluxation and a detachment of the VMO as well as a well-defined MPFL rupture localisation after a first-time dislocation are indications for an MPFL repair. A relative indication for a repair may be the first-time dislocation in an athletic individual to return to sports with an improved stability as soon as possible or an early failure after conservative treatment. However, a relative contraindication for a repair may be in patients with underlying risk factors such as a high-grade trochlear dysplasia or a femoral malrotation. These patients may do better with a reconstruction.

For a successful repair, the rupture localisation has to be identified exactly, making an MRI examination mandatory. Overviewing the literature, the rupture localisation of the MPFL after a first-time dislocation shows a big variance, but seems to be mainly at the femoral insertion [10, 11]. However, if a repair is planned, the exact rupture localisation (patellar, femoral or intramural) must be known to address the injury correctly.

Surgical Technique for MPFL Repair

After identifying the rupture localisation, the repair can be done with either sutures (intramural rupture) or suture anchors (femoral or patellar detachment). While intramural sutures can be performed arthroscopically according to a technique described by Yamamoto [12], bony detachments have to be performed in an arthroscopically assisted mini-open technique. In patellar fixation, two little suture anchors can be placed at the proximal and distal MPFL insertion area, and the ruptured MPFL (and VMO retinaculum if indicated) can be re-sutured to the patella. In cases of a femoral detachment, one bigger suture anchor should be inserted into the femoral MPFL insertion area under fluoroscopic control (see later: femoral attachment), and the ruptured fibres can be reattached either by a mini-open or by an arthroscopically assisted technique.

Postoperative treatment should place the knee in a fixed 20° brace to avoid damage to the repair for 2 weeks. The brace is then adjusted to 0°–10°–60° to begin ROM exercises avoiding active quadriceps strengthening in week 3–4 and adjusted to 0°–10°–90° for week 5 and 6. Thereafter, full ROM is allowed. Partial weight bearing is permitted directly after surgery and progressed after 2 weeks as tolerated.

Indication for MPFL Reconstruction

Patients with recurrent PFI tend to have subsequent dislocations with a risk of re-dislocation around 50 % within 2–5 years [13]. In these cases, a surgical intervention is normally recommended, especially if the patient wishes a reduction of the persistent apprehension and to minimise the re-dislocation rate. The concept of stabilising the patellofemoral joint by MPFLR is to reduce the excessive laxity or insufficiency of the medial passive patellar stabiliser.

For a correct indication, patient history and clinical examination as well as additional radiographic diagnostics are required to ensure the lateral instability. In the clinical examination, the lateral apprehension test has to be performed in different degrees of flexion to document if and when the patella gets a good stability and guidance. Furthermore, an MRI helps to define the morphology of the trochlea, tilt and shift of the patella, the height of the patella and, most importantly, the condition of the MPFL. In the history, it is important to know about the age, when the first patella dislocation occurred, if it is bilateral and if other family members are suffering from a similar problem.

The ideal patient does not report additional pain in between the dislocations. If pain is the main problem, even in PFI, the indication for MPFLR has to be taken very carefully. If pain and instability have the same impact on the patient's daily life, the patient has to be counselled beforehand that the stabilisation will not reliably treat pain as well, since MPFLR is increasing patellar constraint and therefore the patellofemoral pressure. Finally, a permanent dislocator or instability up to a flexion of 60° is not due to an isolated lack of the MPFL, but due to a complex entity.

Overall, the ideal patient and indication for an isolated MPFLR is the recurrent dislocator with a positive apprehension up to 30° of knee flexion and a tremendous laxity or insufficiency of the medial retinacular structures and MPFL, being responsible for recurrent lateral dislocations that have not responded to conservative treatment or that have showed an early failure after local repair.

MPFL Reconstruction: Author's Preferred Technique

Since it is known that a nonanatomical reconstruction of the MPFL can lead to non-physiologic patellofemoral loads and kinematics [9], the goal of a surgical intervention must be an anatomical reconstruction. Since the femoral insertion of the MPFL has been evaluated anatomically [9], biomechanically [14] and radiologically [15], the complications of an increased patellofemoral pressure in flexion associated with nonanatomical femoral graft fixation that is too anterior/proximal [9] can be avoided. Upon careful observation of the anatomical shape of the original MPFL, it is apparent that the patellar insertion is much wider than the femoral one. Additionally, Amis et al. have shown that the native MPFL has a double-bundle structure [9]. Respecting this anatomical condition, a double-bundle reconstruction at the patellar side is reasonable to restore native ligamentous morphologic and biomechanical properties; moreover, this method lessens the patellar rotation during flexion–extension movement that may occur during single-bundle reconstruction. Since the MPFL has a tensile strength of 208 N, a gracilis tendon graft has enough strength for MPFLR and, furthermore, has a lower diameter than a semitendinosus graft, making a patellar fixation easier.

When performing an MPFLR, one has to take in consideration that we reconstruct a checkrein which gives a firm stop when the patella is passively lateralised but is not a structure with an active persistent pulling force, since the patella has a physiological gliding towards lateral of 7–9 mm which has to persist even after MPFLR.

Recent studies have described an anatomical double-bundle reconstruction, using an aperture fixation at the femoral insertion [16, 17], while the patellar fixation remains relatively indirect, resulting in the eventual risk of postoperative micromotion and subsequent loosening. Patellar graft fixation has been described with either an anchor system, attaching the graft into a bony rim [18], or by tying the attached graft sutures to each other at the lateral patellar edge [17]; however, this method may potentially result in graft slippage by degloving [19].

On the other hand, other techniques are described with a patellar fixation by looping the graft through a bone tunnel without any additional fixation devices [20]. This technique appears to produce stable fixation at the patella. However, in soft bone, a widening of the tunnel could occur in the long-term results, such as partial patellar bone breakage; moreover, in patients with a short gracilis graft, the tendon length may not be long enough to reach the anatomical femoral insertion.

In the following, the author's preferred technique is described, consisting of a double-bundle technique with an aperture fixation at the patella and the femur, providing a high initial stability on both insertions, resulting in improved bony ingrowth and, consequently, an earlier return to full range of motion and activity.

Set-up

This surgery typically requires between 45 min and 1 h of operation time and can be performed either under general or local anaesthesia. A tourniquet is required, and we use a hydraulic knee support to adjust the knee in the demanded flexion degrees during surgery. Additionally, a fluoroscope is mandatory to identify the correct femoral MPFL insertion. Instruments are very similar to ACL instrumentation and can also be received as a complete package by the industry.

If an additional arthroscopy is performed, the author recommends doing this without water support to avoid soft tissue swelling.

Harvesting and Preparing of the Gracilis Tendon

A 2-cm-long oblique incision is performed at the pes anserinus. After incising the sartorius aponeurosis, the gracilis tendon is harvested after identifying both semi-T and gracilis tendon and when it is free from crural fasciae. The tendonious part of the gracilis should be at least 18 cm long. After determining the doubled tendon diameter, both ends are whipstitched over a short distance, including both very ends of the graft with a #0 absorbable braided suture.

Preparing the Patellar Insertion Side and Tunnels

A 2-cm skin incision is then performed at the medial patellar edge, starting at the superomedial corner of the patella, where the patellar MPFL insertion is located [7, 14] and the bony medial patellar margin is prepared (Fig. 6.1).

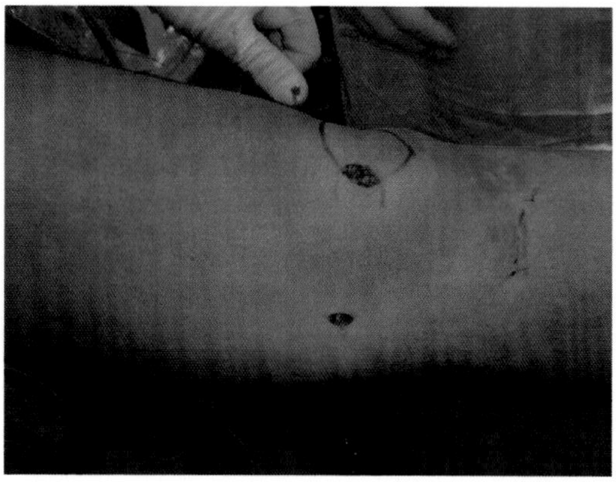

Fig. 6.1 After the anatomical landmarks of the patella are marked, a 2-cm incision from the supermedial corner of the patella to the medial margin is performed

To achieve aperture fixation at the patellar side, the free graft ends have to be fixated directly to the patella. Therefore, two guide wires are into the patella, placing the first at the proximomedial edge with a distolateral drilling direction, and the second one 15 mm distal and parallel to the first one. Then, the guide wires are subsequently overdrilled with a cannulated 4.5-mm drill to a depth of 25 mm. The two free sutured graft ends are fixed into the patellar holes one after each other, using a 4.75×15-mm knotless anchor (SwiveLock, Arthrex), achieving a direct anatomical graft fixation. To accomplish this, the graft sutures are pulled through the PEEK eyelet of the SwiveLock and pushed into the drill holes. Keeping the suture under tension, the graft ends are fixed with the knotless anchors (Fig. 6.2). In this way, a double-bundle aperture fixation at the patellar side is achieved, leaving the graft loop free (Fig. 6.3).

Layer Preparation

As the MPFL is situated central to the vastus medialis obliquus (VMO) in the second layer of the medial patellofemoral complex [7], the central part of the VMO is identified, and a scissor is brought along to the medial femoral epicondyle in between the VMO and the joint capsule, cautiously avoiding any injury to the joint. After the opened

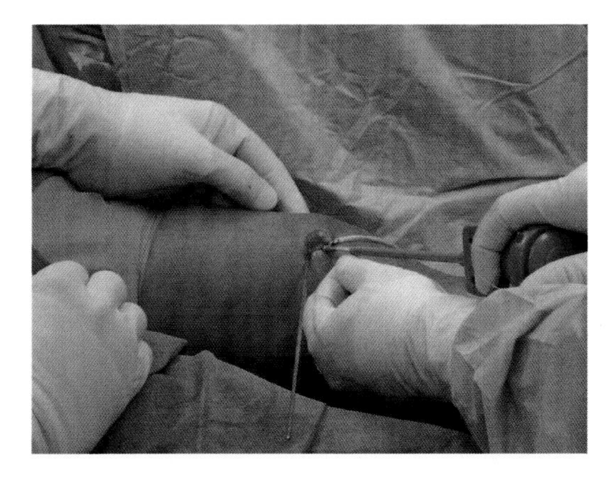

Fig. 6.2 Using two SwiveLock anchors (**a**) the armed graft ends are inserted and fixated into the patella (**b**)

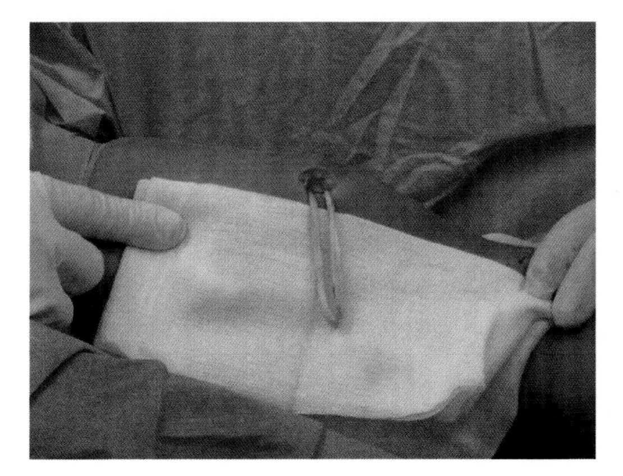

Fig. 6.3 Graft ends are fixed using a 4.75 × 15-mm SwiveLock screw while tensioning the graft

scissors are removed, a right angle clamp is brought into the separated layer, and the tip is directed towards the skin in the area of the adductor tubercle, where the femoral MPFL insertion is located. Then a small longitudinal skin incision is performed over the tip in 30° knee flexion in the femoral MPFL insertion area and a suture loop is inserted in the before-prepared layer.

Preparing the Femoral Insertion Site

To avoid non-physiological patellofemoral forces, the femoral MPFL insertion has to be very accurate. Therefore, a guide wire with an eyelet is placed slightly posterior to the midpoint of the medial epicondyle and the adductor tubercle, and the entering point into the bone is marked by placing a cannulated 6-mm drill over it [7]. Then the probable drill position has to be controlled by a picture intensifier on a straight lateral view to obtain the correct anatomical femoral insertion; if the graft is placed too anterior or proximal, abnormal graft tensioning will lead to increased patellofemoral pressures during flexion [9]. The radiographic landmark of the anatomical MPFL insertion has been shown to be located slightly anterior to an elongation of the posterior femoral cortex in between the proximal origin of the medial condyle and the most posterior point of Blumensaat's line [18] (Fig. 6.4). An anatomical femoral insertion avoids overextension, which occurs if the femoral tunnel is placed too far anterior or proximal. In this case, the insertion point would move towards posterior in flexion, leading to a lengthening of the distance between patellar and femoral insertion, increasing the load onto the graft and, consequently, onto the patellofemoral joint.

If a nonanatomical placement of the drill guide insertion is identified, the guide has to be corrected accordingly. Nowadays, also a special template can be used, where radio-dense lines are adapted according to the findings of an anatomical–radiological study (Fig. 6.5). When the correct insertion is achieved, the guide wire is overdrilled with a 6-mm drill up to the contralateral cortex to achieve enough tunnel length, leaving the drill guide in place.

Graft Fixation

The suture loop is then used to pull the graft from the patellar fixation in between layer 2 and 3 to the femoral insertion. Next, a nitinol wire is inserted into the femoral drill hole along the drill guide, and the suture loop is pulled to the lateral side. Finally, while maintaining equal tension on both bundles, the graft is pulled into the femoral socket. Since biomechanical studies have shown that the MPFL has its maximal length and restraint against patella lateralisation in 30° of flexion (Fig. 6.6) [9].

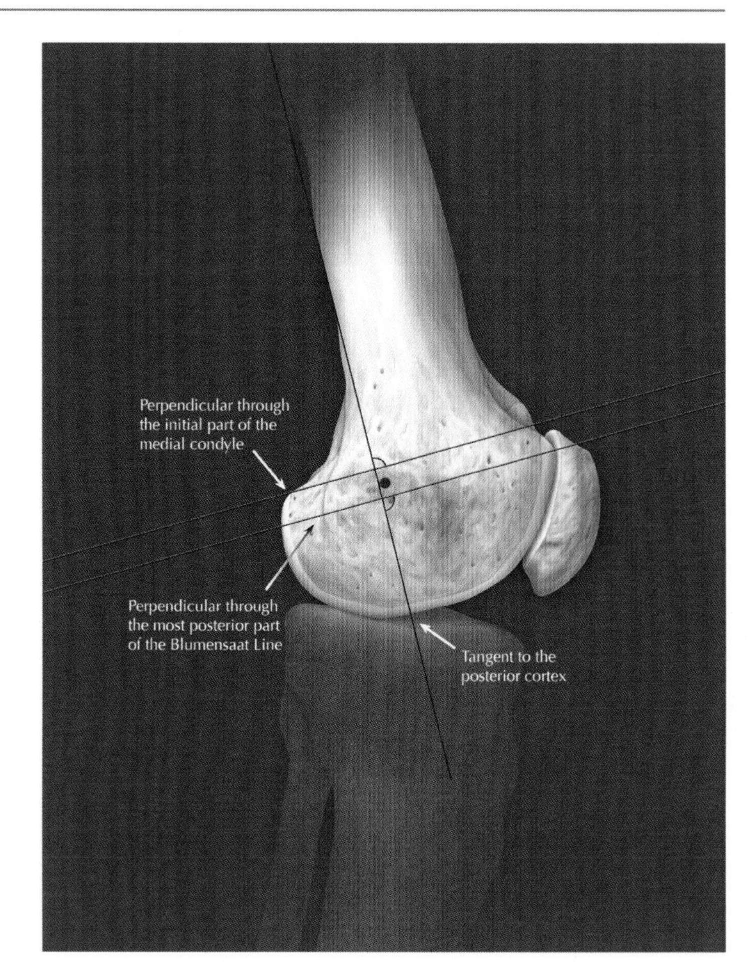

Fig. 6.4 The femoral insertion of the MPFL has been shown to be located slightly anterior to an elongation of the posterior femoral cortex in between the proximal origin of the medial condyle and the most posterior point of Blumensaat's line

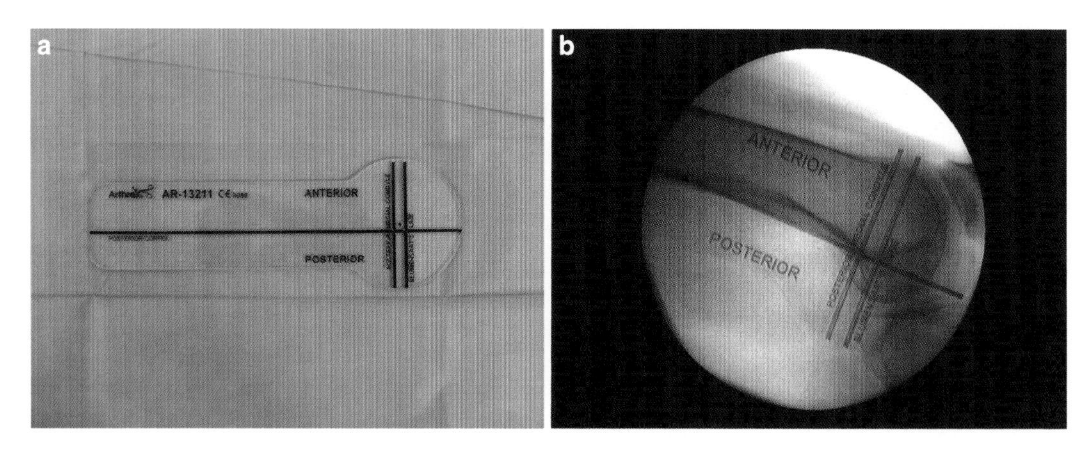

Fig. 6.5 (**a**) Template with radio-dense marking lines to identify the anatomical MPFL insertion. (**b**) The radio-dense lines of the template are placed along the marking points described in Fig. 6.4 under fluoroscopic view, and the guide wire can be drilled through the whole

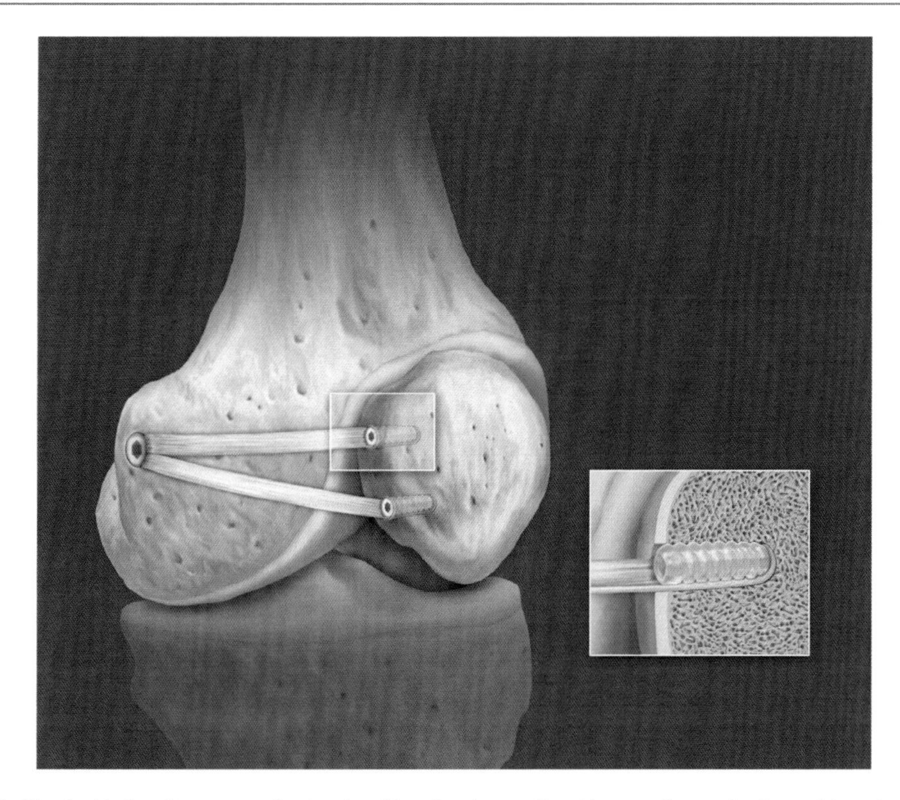

Fig. 6.6 The double-bundle aperture fixation is achieved at the patellar side as well as at the femoral insertion

Femoral fixation is performed in 30° fellows of flexion with the lateral patellar edge positioned in line with the lateral trochlear border using a bioresorbable interference screw with a diameter of 6 mm. If adequate medial restraint has been restored, lateral patellar dislocation should no longer be possible, and routine skin closure is performed after reattaching the aponeurosis of the VMO back to the medial edge of the patella with resorbable sutures.

Postoperative Treatments

This aperture fixation at the patellar and femoral insertion provides an immediate stable tendon to bone fixation with an ultimate load to failure force at the patellar side higher than the 208 N needed to rupture an intact MPFL [9]. Weight bearing is allowed; however, no more than 20 kg until wound healing, while leg raising and quadriceps setting exercises, can be started immediately with a free range of motion as tolerated.

Low-impact activities such as running or cycling are allowed at 6 weeks' post-op; full activity is permitted at 3 months.

Discussion

The benefit of the anatomical graft positioning in ligament reconstruction has been known for a long time and has been clearly demonstrated in ACL reconstruction. Anatomical reconstruction of the MPFL is particularly important as biomechanical studies have demonstrated that the length change pattern of an MPFL reconstruction depends critically on the site of the femoral attachment; moreover, kinematics change significantly when the patellar or the femoral insertion has been off by only 5 mm [14]. Aside from tunnel placement, graft fixation is the another determining factor in ligament reconstruction [19]. Non-aperture fixation at either the femoral or patellar insertion can increase the risk of a delayed or insufficient tendon to bone healing, which may result in early loosening or slackening of the graft. To avoid this, a restricted range of motion is recommended by some surgeons; however, this may lead to arthrofibrosis, potentially necessitating an additional arthroscopic arthrolysis, carrying the additional risk of damage to the graft.

The above described technique gives the possibility of an immediate full range of motion and loading due to an aperture fixation at both insertion sides within an anatomical reconstruction.

In recent studies, a tendon transfer is described either to the patella or to the femur for reconstructing the MPFL [21, 22]. In these techniques, not only is the transferred muscle weakened, but neither the patella nor the femoral insertion can be reconstructed at its anatomical insertion. Also, the graft used is always a single-bundle graft despite the fact that the MPFL consists of a proximal and a distal bundle [9]. This also includes a single-point fixation at the patellar side, increasing the rotational moment of the patella in flexion–extension movement. In terms of the fixation itself, some techniques fix the graft to the surrounding soft tissue [23] and not to the patellar and/or femoral bone even though a ligament is a structure in between bones, and recent studies have proven the high resistance to failure of tendon–bone interfaces.

Since tendon to bone healing showed excellent results in ACL reconstruction with hamstring tendon grafts, the same fixation is used at both the femoral and the patellar sides in our preferred technique [24].

Another technique, looping the graft through the patella, provides a very high initial fixation strength, and preliminary results are promising [20]. However, if micromotion in the patellar tunnels develops, it may lead to a slackening of the graft at later follow-up. However, if the graft is very short, the femoral insertion cannot be reached and a too anterior nonanatomical femoral fixation has to be accepted, leading eventually to an increased patellofemoral pressure, loss of flexion or graft rupture.

The use of a three-point fixation allows us to place the graft at the anatomical insertion with a sufficient length and to recreate the double-bundle structure of the MPFL as it was described in an anatomical study by Amis [9]. According to these findings, this simulates the anatomical situation as close as possible, since the proximal bundle stabilises in extension, while the distal bundle stabilises in flexion. Furthermore, the double-bundle reconstruction decreases patellar rotation in contrast to techniques where only a single-point fixation is performed or the middle part of the quadriceps tendon is flipped medially [14]. Reproducing the anatomy of the native MPFL enables the reconstructed ligament to have an isometric function and therefore avoids increased patellofemoral pressure in higher degrees of knee flexion [18]. We also estimate that in long-term follow-up, slackening of the graft will not occur due to an improved tendon to bone healing by using direct fixation at the femoral as well as at the patellar insertion.

References

1. Desio SM, Burks RT, Bachus KN. Soft tissue restraints to lateral patellar translation in the human knee. Am J Sports Med. 1998;26:59–65. Christoforakis, 2006 http://www.ncbi.nlm.nih.gov/entrez/query.fcgi?cmd=Retrieve&db=PubMed&dopt=Citation&list_uids=16311766; Merican, 2009, http://www.ncbi.nlm.nih.gov/entrez/query.fcgi?cmd=Retrieve&db=PubMed&dopt=Citation&list_uids=18925647.
2. Elias JJ, Cech JA, Weinstein DM, Cosgrea AJ. Reducing the lateral force acting on the patella does not consistently decrease patellofemoral pressures. Am J Sports Med. 2004;32:1202–8.
3. Elias JJ, Wilson DR, Adamson R, Cosgarea AJ. Evaluation of a computational model used to predict the patellofemoral contact pressure distribution. J Biomech. 2004;37:295–302.
4. Nomura E, Inoue M. Surgical technique and rationale for medial patellofemoral ligament reconstruction for recurrent patellar dislocation. Arthroscopy. 2003; 19:E47.
5. Hautamaa PV, Fithian DC, Kaufman KR, Daniel DM, Pohlmeyer AM. Medial soft tissue restraints in lateral patellar instability and repair. Clin Orthop. 1998; 174–182.
6. Warren LA, Marshall JL, Girgis F. The prime static stabilizer of the medical side of the knee. J Bone Joint Surg Am. 1974;56:665–74.
7. Nomura E, Inoue M, Osada N. Anatomical analysis of the medial patellofemoral ligament of the knee, espe-

cially the femoral attachment. Knee Surg Sports Traumatol Arthrosc. 2005;13:510–5.
8. LaPrade RF, Engebretsen AH, Ly TV, Johansen S, Wentorf FA, Engebretsen L. The anatomy of the medial part of the knee. J Bone Joint Surg Am. 2007; 89:2000–10.
9. Amis AA, Firer P, Mountney J, Senavongse W, Thomas NP. Anatomy and biomechanics of the medial patellofemoral ligament. Knee. 2003;10:215–20.
10. Sillanpaa PJ, Peltola E, Mattila VM, Kiuru M, Visuri T, Pihlajamaki H. Femoral avulsion of the medial patellofemoral ligament after primary traumatic patellar dislocation predicts subsequent instability in men: a mean 7-year nonoperative follow-up study. Am J Sports Med. 2009;37:1513–21.
11. Weber-Spickschen TS, Spang J, Kohn L, Imhoff AB, Schottle PB. The relationship between trochlear dysplasia and medial patellofemoral ligament rupture location after patellar dislocation: an MRI evaluation. Knee. 2011;18:185–8.
12. Yamamoto RK. Arthroscopic repair of the medial retinaculum and capsule in acute patellar dislocations. Arthroscopy. 1986;2:125–31.
13. Fithian DC, Paxton EW, Stone ML, Silva P, Davis DK, Elias DA, White LM. Epidemiology and natural history of acute patellar dislocation. Am J Sports Med. 2004;32:1114–21.
14. Steensen RN, Dopirak RM, McDonald 3rd WG. The anatomy and isometry of the medial patellofemoral ligament: implications for reconstruction. Am J Sports Med. 2004;32:1509–13.
15. Schottle PB, Schmeling A, Rosenstiel N, Weiler A. Radiographic landmarks for femoral tunnel placement in medial patellofemoral ligament reconstruction. Am J Sports Med. 2007;35:801–4.
16. Schottle PB, Weiler A. Technique for anatomical reconstruction of the medial patellofemoral ligament. Tuttlingen: EndoWorld; 2007. p. 1–13.
17. Thaunat M, Erasmus PJ. The favourable anisometry: an original concept for medial patellofemoral ligament reconstruction. Knee. 2007;14:424–8.
18. Schottle PB, Romero J, Schmeling A, Weiler A. Technical note: anatomical reconstruction of the medial patellofemoral ligament using a free gracilis autograft. Arch Orthop Trauma Surg. 2008;128:479–84.
19. Brand Jr J, Weiler A, Caborn DN, Brown Jr CH, Johnson DL. Graft fixation in cruciate ligament reconstruction. Am J Sports Med. 2000;28:761–74.
20. Christiansen SE, Jacobsen BW, Lund B, Lind M. Reconstruction of the medial patellofemoral ligament with gracilis tendon autograft in transverse patellar drill holes. Arthroscopy. 2008;24:82–7.
21. Ostermeier S, Stukenborg-Colsman C, Wirth CJ, Bohnsack M. Reconstruction of the medial patellofemoral ligament by tunnel transfer of the semitendinosus tendon. Oper Orthop Traumatol. 2007;19:489–501.
22. Steensen RN, Dopirak RM, Maurus PB. A simple technique for reconstruction of the medial patellofemoral ligament using a quadriceps tendon graft. Arthroscopy. 2005;21:365–70.
23. Ellera Gomes JL, Stigler Marczyk LR, Cesar de Cesar P, Jungblut CF. Medial patellofemoral ligament reconstruction with semitendinosus autograft for chronic patellar instability: a follow-up study. Arthroscopy. 2004;20:147–51.
24. Weiler A, Hoffmann RF, Bail HJ, Rehm O, Sudkamp NP. Tendon healing in a bone tunnel. Part II: histologic analysis after biodegradable interference fit fixation in a model of anterior cruciate ligament reconstruction in sheep. Arthroscopy. 2002;18:124–35.

Tibial Tubercle Osteotomies

7

Cory Edgar, Matthew Bollier, and John P. Fulkerson

Introduction

Anterior knee pain is a common complaint among athletes. Although the etiology of the knee pain is not always clearly delineated, it is often associated with patellofemoral anatomic abnormalities. Common examples are abnormal lateral patella tracking leading to increased joint reactive forces resulting in pain, with or without chondral wear. Traumatic patella dislocations can lead to painful and debilitating lateral laxity resulting in recurrent subluxations with a patella "jump" when entering the trochlea or even chronic instability. Chronic patella instability is not common with a single traumatic patella dislocation, but with certain risk factors, recurrent instability can occur: patella alta, trochlea dysplasia, rotational malalignment, and extensor mechanism valgus (as represented by increased *Q* angle or elevated TT–TG distance). In patients with "anterior knee pain," it is very important to systematically delineate activity-related pain from patella instability as the primary complaint in order to appropriately treat the pathology. Unfortunately, it is not uncommon for the two to be found concurrently.

The tibia tubercle osteotomy has the ability to change the orientation of the extensor mechanism by which it can be a powerful tool to treat multiple complaints within the patellofemoral compartment. The power of this osteotomy is related to the ease of surgical exposure and the multiplanar corrections possible. Osteotomy cuts can be made to accommodate alignment changes within the coronal, axial, and sagittal planes. Consequently, osteotomy has a variety of functions; it can alter the area and amount of joint contact pressures, decrease the patella height to allow for earlier patella capture, and decrease the lateral displacement force vector. Understanding the effects each plan has on the function and forces within the patellofemoral joint during activity allows the surgeon to treat both pain and instability in this population. There are subtle complexities with this type of surgery that requires an understanding of the pathophysiology of the condition and knowledge of the effects of a given surgical treatment on the mechanics and biology of patellofemoral function for optimal outcomes.

Fortunately, nonoperative treatments are very effective and should be exhausted prior to surgical intervention. The described measures include quadriceps and hip flexor/external rotator strengthening, extensor mechanism stretching,

C. Edgar, M.D., Ph.D. (✉)
Assistant Professor and Team Physician
Department of Orthopedic Surgery,
University of Connecticut, Farmington, CT, USA
e-mail: cm.edgar71@gmail.com

M. Bollier, M.D.
Department of Orthopaedic Surgery, University of Iowa Hospitals and Clinics, Iowa City, IA, USA

J.P. Fulkerson, M.D.
Department of Orthopedic Surgery, Orthopedic Associates of Hartford, P.C., Hartford, CT, USA

University of Connecticut Medical School, Farmington, CT, USA

R.V. West and A.C. Colvin (eds.), *The Patellofemoral Joint in the Athlete*,
DOI 10.1007/978-1-4614-4157-1_7, © Springer Science+Business Media New York 2014

core stability training, McConnell taping, and patella bracing.

The purpose of this chapter is to define the situations in which tibial tubercle transfer is indicated for anterior knee pain and/or patellar instability. In this chapter, we will attempt to present a brief overview of the anatomic and biomechanical factors important to decision-making and then present techniques for the treatment of these issues with osteotomies about the tibia tubercle.

Patient Selection and Osteotomy Selection

Patients presenting with patellofemoral pain may or may not have instability. Anterior knee pain can be generated by a variety of factors that may not be addressed by adjusting the position of the tibia tubercle. Patient selection and workup are critical to successful treatment. Quadriceps weakness is one of the most common causes of anterior knee pain as joint forces are increased in the setting of weak and/or stiff extensor mechanism that has a clear function in absorbing energy during gait [1]. In the athletic population, flexibility imbalance, iliotibial band friction syndrome, vastus lateralis tendinitis, lateral retinacular strain or contracture, patellar or quadriceps insertional tendinitis, and plica or fat pad syndrome have all been described and would need to be treated conservatively [2, 3]. The workup of patients with activity-related anterior knee pain and chronic injury to the posterior cruciate ligament must also be ruled out. Posterior tibia laxity can lead to retropatellar pain as the extensor mechanism holds the tibia from posterior subluxation and leads to increased patellofemoral contact pressures resulting in pain [4, 5]. It is important to take a rational approach to patellofemoral disorders that require an understanding that various problems may be related to combinations of articular pain, soft tissue pain, and pain resulting from lateral instability of the joint. Therefore, a careful examination is indispensable for an accurate diagnosis of patellofemoral disorders. We feel it is imperative that a diagnosis of patellofemoral pain is dependent on the physician's ability to reproduce the patient's complaints by physical examination. The examination can suggest or determine an underlying malalignment pattern, abnormally tight soft tissue structures, generalized ligamentous laxity, or patterns of tenderness, which are all critical to understanding the pathophysiology of each individual and thus the correct application of an osteotomy to correct a malalignment or alter the patellofemoral joint contact pressures.

Understanding the *Q* Angle or Lateral Force Vector

The quadriceps angle (*Q* angle) is a clinical assessment of the angle made by the attachment vector of the extensor mechanism and the relationship of the quadriceps tendon to the tibia tubercle (Fig. 7.1). The angle is classically measured in extension from the anterior superior iliac spine to the midpoint of the patella that forms the angle between patella tendons force vector to the tibial tuberosity (Fig. 7.1). An increased angle leads to an increase in the lateral vector of quadriceps force, which may increase tension in the medial soft tissue restraints and may lead to an increased tendency toward lateral patellar translation or subluxation, especially in the patient with a concomitant dysplasia of the trochlea [6]. Measurements of the *Q* angle have been made while the patient is supine and standing. We favor the standing measurement because it includes physiologic loading. Unfortunately, the *Q* angle also has not been proved to correlate with the incidence of pain or the results of treatment [7]. Although the importance of understanding the lateral extensor moment and its potential effects on patellar alignment is undeniable, the role of *Q* angle measurement is less clear. It should be noted that there is significant variability within populations and differences between males and females. Ranges have been reported to be 14–23° within a normal, asymptomatic population [3, 7–9]. There is a dynamic component, and thus, examine the patient while standing and ambulating for evidence of an increased *Q* angle, torsional deformities of the femur or tibia, knee

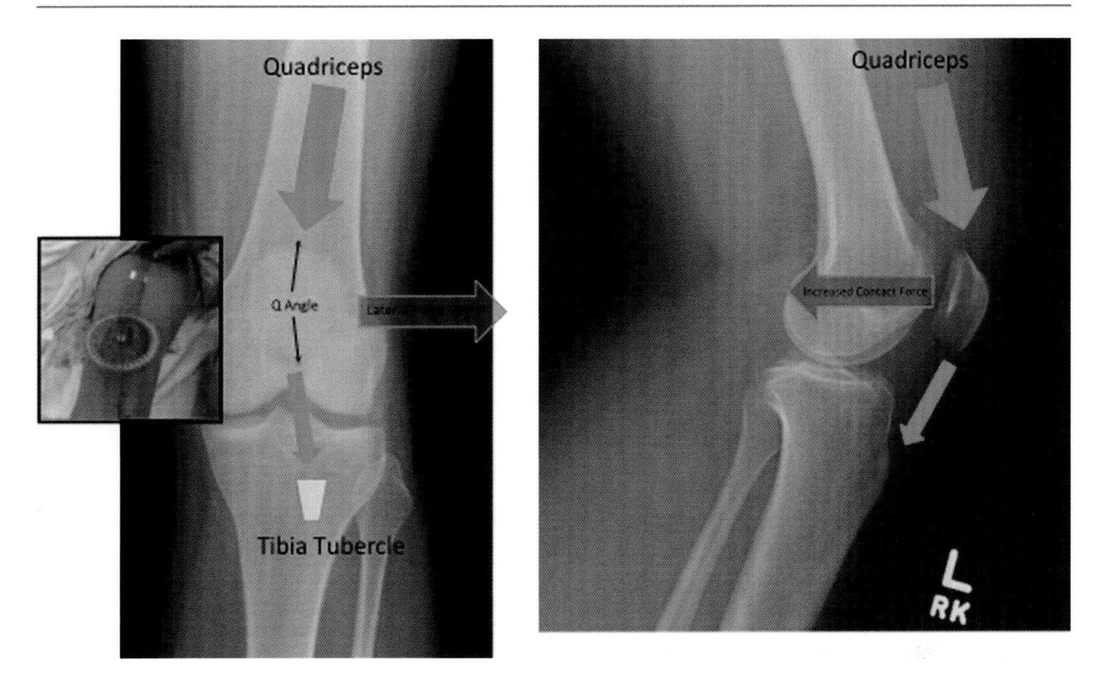

Fig. 7.1 Graphical representation of the measurement of the quadriceps angle or *Q* angle in the supine position. Important force vectors are drawn on radiographic images to delineate the effects of malalignment of patellofemoral joint during quadriceps activation and flexion

varus/valgus, pronation of the hindfoot, leg length discrepancy, ankle deformity, scars, and other factors that may affect patellar alignment. One clinical test to examine function changes in *Q* angle related to poor proximal muscular control and hip external rotator weakness is to have the patient perform a single-leg knee bend while you watch from the front. A positive test results in the knee rolling inward, increasing valgus and suggesting weakness of external rotation at the hip, a known and important variable leading to torsional changes and anterior knee pain [10, 11].

A better estimation of the functional malalignment is measuring the distance between the tibia tubercle and the trochlea groove (TT–TG distance) on CT scan or MRI as it directly estimates the correctable static distance between the points of articulation and attachment of the extensor mechanism [12]. Dejour and associates first described this measurement and found, upon comparing normal patients with those with patellar instability, that the threshold for normal was 20 mm [13]. This measurement is done by measuring the lateral distance of the tibial tuberosity from the most posterior point in the femoral sulcus, along a line parallel to the axis of the posterior femoral condyles (Fig. 7.2). Certainly there is a spectrum of anatomic malalignment in the form of increased TT–TG distances. These increased distances have been associated and found in patients with recurrent patella instability [3, 13, 14]. A recent report looking at patients with instability or anterior knee pain associated with "pathologic" TT–TG malalignment determined to be 15 mm or greater. The authors concluded that both stability and pain were corrected with isolated anteromedialization osteotomy procedures [15]. Based on expert opinion from the Patellofemoral Society Members [16], a TT-TG distance of 20 mm or greater is considered "severely abnormal" and blue bone needs to be addressed surgically a re-adjustment osteotomy to correct the increased lateral vector. The amount of medialization needed can also be estimated from this measurement, and the most often targeted goal for postoperative TT–TG distance is less than approximately 10 mm. Measurement of the TT–TG is helpful in confirming that tuberosity

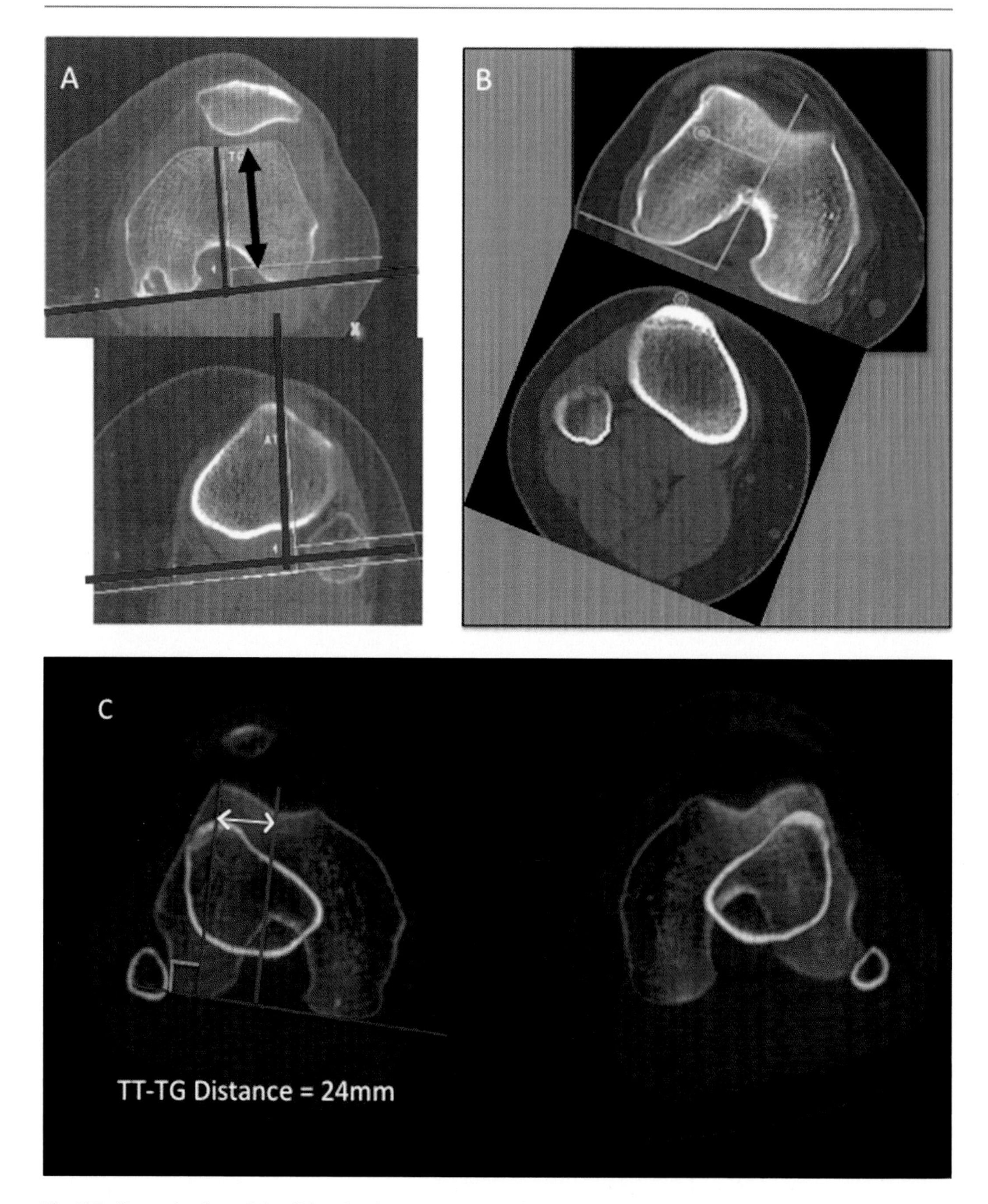

Fig. 7.2 Determination of the tibia tubercle to trochlea groove (TT–TG) distance on a CT scan axial in which cuts at the deepest section of the trochlea groove are measured to the highest point on the tibia tubercle. Representation of three techniques to determine distance; (**a**) posterior condyle axis is used as reference to ensure no rotational effect and perpendicular line is drawn in center of groove and tubercle. (**b**) On a free software package OsiriX© a reference point can be placed and "fixed" as the axial cuts are scrolled to the groove and distance measured. (**c**) During CT reformatting, the axial cuts can be superimposed to allow for a direct measurement. *Note*: The TT–TG distance should represent a true lateral distance and not have a rotational or radius component

medialization is appropriate in a clinical situation that otherwise warrants medial or anteromedial transfer.

Standing anteroposterior films are important to search for confounding sources of pain such as arthrosis or mechanical axis abnormalities, which need to be confirmed by measurements from a standing hip to ankle X-ray. The true lateral knee image provides the most information as it can delineate patella alta and estimate trochlea dysplasia; both are important variables in determining the need and type of tubercle osteotomy to perform. A normal ratio of patellar tendon length to patellar length of less than 1.2 has been described by Insall and Salvati [17]. However, we prefer the Blackburne and Peel [18] method as it accounts for changes in patella osteology and imperfect lateral X-rays better. The measurement represents the ratio of the articular length of the patella to the height of the lower pole of the patellar articular cartilage above the tibial articular surface (normal, <1.0). If patella alta is present, a distalization osteotomy may be considered to allow for "earlier" capture of the patella during flexion that can lead to increased stability if significant dysplasia is not present.

Axial tangential views of the patellofemoral joint, such the one described by Merchant et al. [19], may be used as screening tests for malalignment but can be difficult to interpret because of image overlap (unless the image is precisely tangential to the joint). Other radiographic variables that may affect the decision to perform a distal osteotomy include the congruence angle of Merchant and Mercer and the lateral patellofemoral angle of Laurin and Dussault (both are estimations of lateral subluxation and tilt, respectively). The symmetry of subchondral sclerosis of the patellar facets should also be evaluated for signs of localized sclerosis (indicating unbalanced stress) [6]. Kujala and Kormano [20] emphasized imaging of the patellofemoral joint in early flexion. They found greater magnetic resonance imaging (MRI) differences in tilt and lateral subluxation on views with less than 30° of flexion in a group of patients with recurrent patellar dislocations than in a normal control group. Computed tomography (CT) provides a fast, low-cost way of determining amount of dysplasia, flexion angle at which the patella is captured, and helps to define malalignment in the form of increased distance from the tibia tubercle to the center of the trochlea groove (TT–TG distance) which serves as a anatomic *Q* angle. The use of CT scans was first suggested by Delgado-Martins [21] in 1979 as he described its use in a series of 24 patients looking at patella–trochlea contact with increasing knee flexion angles. These studies are not used for diagnosis but in patients being considered for surgical correction to understand the anatomy needed to be corrected to provide stability. We are currently utilizing a CT tracking study protocol in which the patients have four sections taken at 5 mm through the patellofemoral articulation at 0, 10, 20, 30, 40, and 50° of knee flexion followed by a full scan at 1.25 mm in extension (Fig. 7.3). This provides information regarding the articulation of the patella during knee flexion and identifies the flexion angle at which the patella is fully captured and allows us to quantify the amount of trochlea dysplasia present.

Anterior Knee Pain and Chondral Pressures

Vague anterior knee pain is common in the athlete and can be associated with overuse that leads to soft tissue inflammation and pain within the peripatellar tissue or fat pad. These typically respond to activity modification in addition to stretching and strengthening of the fatigued and tight muscle groups, quadriceps. However, pain can also develop from an imbalance created from malalignment within the quadriceps–patella–tibia tubercle relationship which affects lateral facet contact pressures. This lateral malalignment, or elevated *Q* angle, can produce increased contact pressures within the lateral facet of the patella and degradation of the overloaded cartilage [22–26]. Through a concept of "edge" loading and repeated motion, cartilage lesions can lead to increase the pressure applied to the surrounding cartilage, which can overload the subchondral bone and activate the nociceptive fibers in the bone, causing pain [27]. By moving the

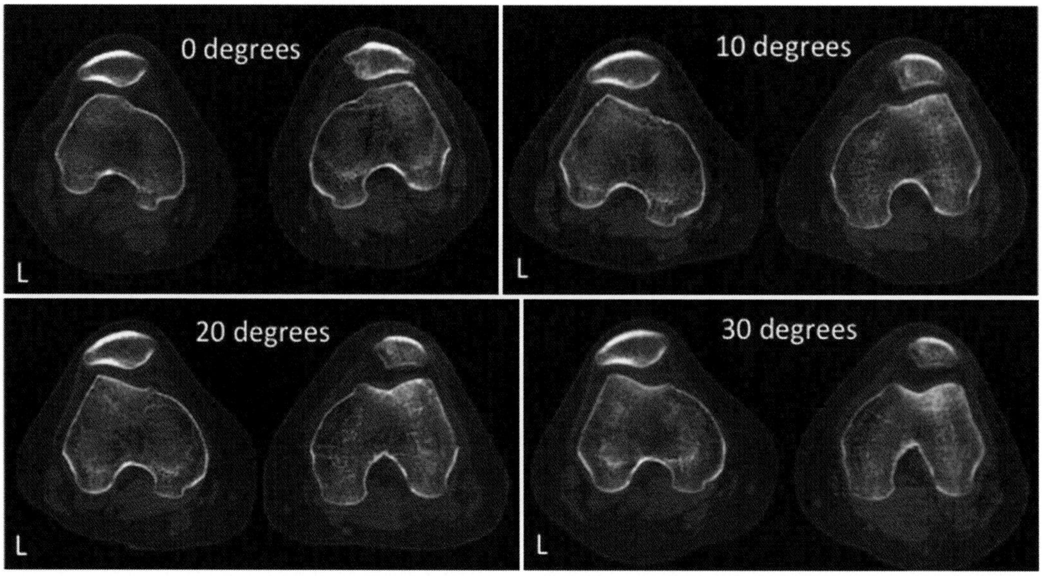

Fig. 7.3 An example of CT tracking images, bilateral axial cuts at 0, 10, 20, and 30° of knee flexion, in a patient with right recurrent patella instability and demonstrates Dejour C dysplasia (based on lateral X-ray, not included). Images show lateral patella tracking with incomplete patella capture even at 30° of knee flexion

tibia tubercle 10 mm medial, a reduction of 15 % of the contact pressures can be observed at knee flexion angles of 60 and 80° [24].

Approach to Distal Realignment Procedures (Fig. 7.4)

Medialization of the Tibia Tubercle

Roux in 1888 was the first to report tibia tubercle realignment osteotomy coupled with lateral release and medial plication in the treatment of recurrent patellar dislocation [3]. Later this technique to treat patella instability was adapted and described by Hauser in 1938. Medial transfer of the tubercle has the effect of decreasing the lateral extensor vector [28]. This procedure moved the tubercle distal and medial with an effective posterior displacement of the tubercle that leads to an increased incidence (~70 %) of patellofemoral arthrosis at 7.3, 16, and 18 years after the procedure [29–31]. The Roux–Elmslie–Trillat procedure is a pure distal realignment technique because it provides isolated medialization without transferring the tibial tubercle anteriorly [3]. The Roux–Elmslie–Trillat procedure involves a lateral retinacular release of the knee, medial capsular reefing, and medial displacement of the infrapatellar tendon hinged on a distal periosteal attachment. This procedure has been shown to demonstrate maintained correction of the extensor angle and has been reported with good results to control patella stability [32] especially if combined with a proximal procedure [33]. This procedure has limited use as it can only produce pure medial realignment, and there does exist the risk of painful hardware and osteotomy nonunion as the osteotomy surface area is limited.

Recommendations: Pure medialization procedure is reserved for patients with mild elevation in quadriceps angle as minimal correction can be obtained. Bone contact is minimal with more medialization as the medial cortex curves posterior.

Distalization of the Tibia Tubercle

The role for distalizing the tibia tubercle in isolation is very limited. It can be used to correct anterior knee pain associated with patella alta [34]. In patients without instability and mild grade 2

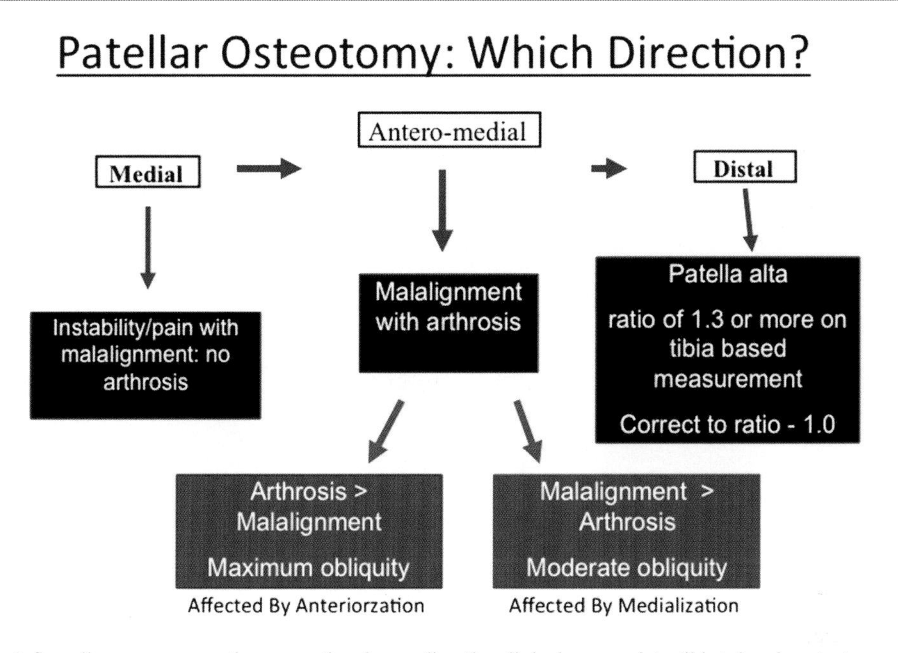

Fig. 7.4 A flow diagram representing one rational regarding the clinical approach to tibia tubercle osteotomy, compliments of Tony Schepsis, MD

chondromalacia at greater than 2 years, there were improved Kujala scores compared to baseline or preoperative values [34]. However, in patients with higher grades of patella chondromalacia, their scores did not demonstrate significant improvement.

Patella alta is rarely an isolated finding and it is most often a symptom of a regional patellofemoral dysplasia with four major instability factors, i.e., trochlear dysplasia, patella alta, excessive TT–TG, and patellar tilt all contributing to the pain and instability. In patients with abnormal patella height leading to late trochlear capture, stability and pain are improved with a combined osteotomy to distalize and medialize the tubercle. Caton and Dejour describe having a 75 % success rate with a combined procedure to produce a stable patellofemoral articulation in a series of 50 patients with chronic instability with young age [35].

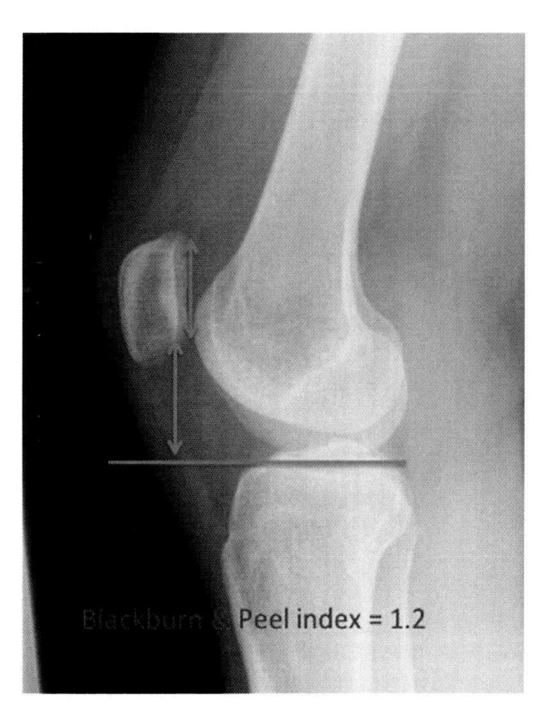

Fig. 7.5 Measurement of patella height: example of Blackburne and Peel index. Measurement and the upper limit of normal: 1.2

Recommendations: A pure distalization osteotomy procedure is rarely indicated. In the clinical setting of a patient with chronic patella instability and elevated Blackburne–Peel (Fig. 7.5) or Caton–Deschamps index, then a distalizing tubercle osteotomy in addition to medialization or anteromedialization should be strongly considered.

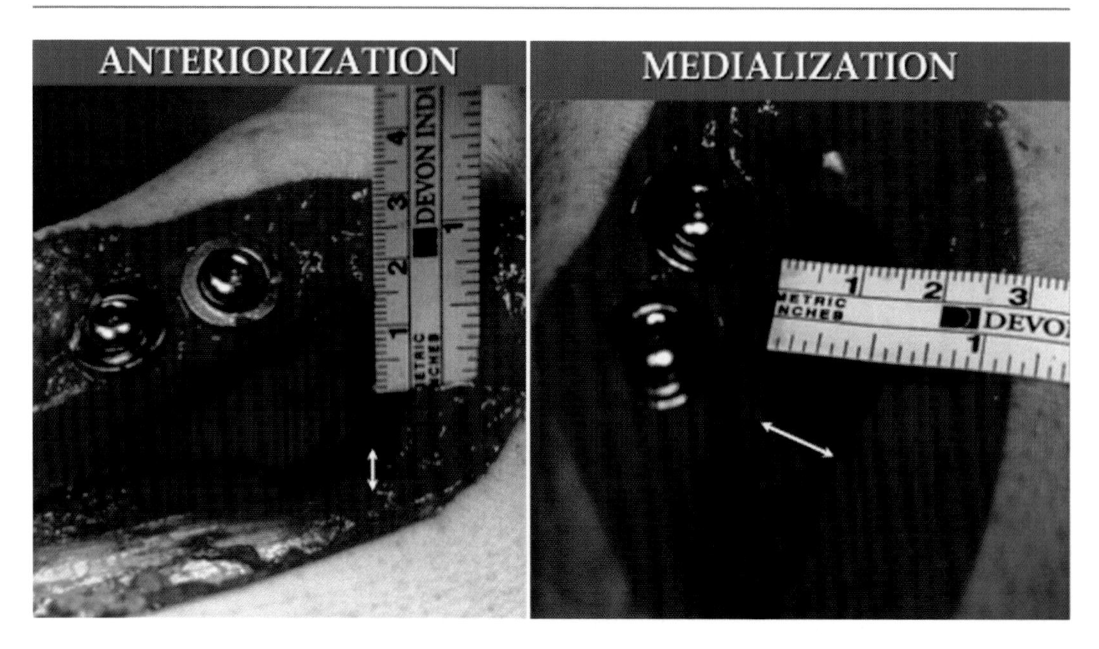

Fig. 7.6 An intraoperative picture as an example of the final osteotomy position and effect of the cut produced by an oblique proximal tibia osteotomy. Note the direction of tubercle position change is anterior and medial, case example of Fulkerson AMZ osteotomy

Anteriorization of the Tibia Tubercle

In 1990, Fulkerson et al. (Fulkerson JP) reported a tubercle osteotomy known as anteromedialization to achieve dual plan realignment and address some of the complications associated with the Maquet procedure [36]. Specifically this osteotomy (AMZ) technique is designed to address patellofemoral pain found in conjunction with patellar maltracking. The osteotomy is made in an oblique fashion that allows for simultaneous anteriorization and medialization of the tibial tubercle (Fig. 7.6). Additionally, it produces a large surface area for healing of the osteotomy and to accommodate multiple bi-cortical screws to be placed in compression to optimize healing of the osteotomy. One advantage of this osteotomy is the variability that can be produced by varying the angle of the osteotomy. Therefore, the tubercle can be biased to a more anterior or more medial position and be "dialed" to the patients needs. Over the last 15 years, the indications for this procedure have evolved significantly. It is now commonly used in conjunction with patellofemoral cartilage resurfacing procedures as well as improved objective measures of patellar alignment, contact area, and forces. Results combining AMZ with PF cartilage restorative procedures such as autologous chondrocyte implantation and osteoarticular grafting procedures within the PF compartment have demonstrated superior results to either procedure performed independently [37–40].

Indications for Anteromedialization of the Tibial Tubercle

Osteotomies to the tibia tubercle can be performed in isolation or in combination with a proximal procedure when patella instability or lateral patella instability is the primary patient complaint. It can produce excellent clinical results in patients with lateral tracking and arthritis wear secondary to increased contact pressures in deeper knee flexion.

For the treatment of anterior knee pain associated with lateral facet chondral wear, an anteromedialization (AMZ) of the tibial tubercle is a powerful surgical technique. It will reduce loading of the lateral and distal PF joint by transferring load medially and proximally on the patella [3, 24, 25]. Therefore, the procedure is most appropriate and beneficial for those patients with symptomatic lateral tracking of the patella, usually because the patella alignment vector is abnormally lateral; this leads to excessive loading of the distal patella cartilage. In patients with malalignment, the lateral facet strikes the lateral trochlea as the patella engages the trochlea and receives accentuated contact pressures until it becomes fully centered within the trochlea deeper knee flexion. These patients may or may not have instability, but pain is the primary complaint.

In some patients, this abnormal tracking pattern may be difficult to identify without computerized tomography with mid patella transverse images at 0, 15, 30, and 45° knee flexion to prove that the patella is entering the central trochlea late in knee flexion, thereby resulting in prolonged and excessive lateral and distal articular loading of the patella. An osteotomy that can anteriorize the tubercle reduces load on the distal and lateral facet joint that has become painful as a result of the chronic, abnormal overload [3, 24, 25].

Because of the reduced contact pressures produced with this technique, AMZ has proven useful in conjunction with articular cartilage resurfacing procedures [37–41]. The obliquity of the AMZ osteotomy should be designed to optimally unload the resurfaced area. A short, steep AMZ can provide substantial and even complete relief of pain in the patient with distal patella articular softening related to late entry of the patella into the trochlea.

Another advantage of the AMZ osteotomy is correction of extensor malalignment and secondary rotational abnormalities that can lead to increased lateral force during active knee flexion. In the patient with attenuated medial restraints and with a shorted, dysplastic trochlea, it can help to obtain stability and protect the proximal reconstruction. Typically it is indicated in the treatment of patella instability in patients in whom the TT–TG relationship is grossly abnormal (>20 mm), the *Q* angle is abnormally high (>20), and the distal/lateral patella will benefit from reduced load. In patients with patella alta, the patella may be moved distally by removing a predetermined amount of bone distally from the osteotomy fragment.

In patients with patella baja and infrapatellar contracture, a steep AMZ may be used to distract the released contracture and also slide the extensor mechanism proximally as needed before screw fixation of the transferred tubercle.

Case Examples

Case 1: Isolated Lateral Patellofemoral Arthrosis

This is a case very common of a 38-year-old woman who has mild malalignment and history of obesity, now 1 year out from a gastric bypass procedure with 145 lb weight loss and progressive anterior knee pain. She has attempted physical therapy for extensor mechanism stretching and strengthening with some success. She wishes to be more active but retropatellar knee pain with stairs and prolonged sitting is becoming very limiting to her. Her current weight is 190 lb. Radiographs demonstrate lateral tracking and arthrosis with large osteophyte (Fig. 7.7a, b) and MRI demonstrates bone edema from increased pressure and bone–bone articulation (Fig. 7.7c). Arthroscopy confirms the lateral compartment bone loss (Fig. 7.7d) and minimal cartilage loss in medial trochlea wall and in the medial/lateral knee compartments. Patient was treated with open osteophyte removal, lateral release and AMZ (native TT–TG was 10), and subchondral drilling of patella and lateral trochlea. Postoperative radiographs demonstrate AMZ (Fig. 7.8). Patient is allowed to immediately start motion postoperative and electrical stimulation is done for quadriceps activation. At 3 months she is almost pain free but with much improved function. This is an example of an intermediate procedure for arthrosis in a younger patient or in a patient with higher activity demands for which arthroplasty is not an option, either isolated patellofemoral or total knee arthroplasty.

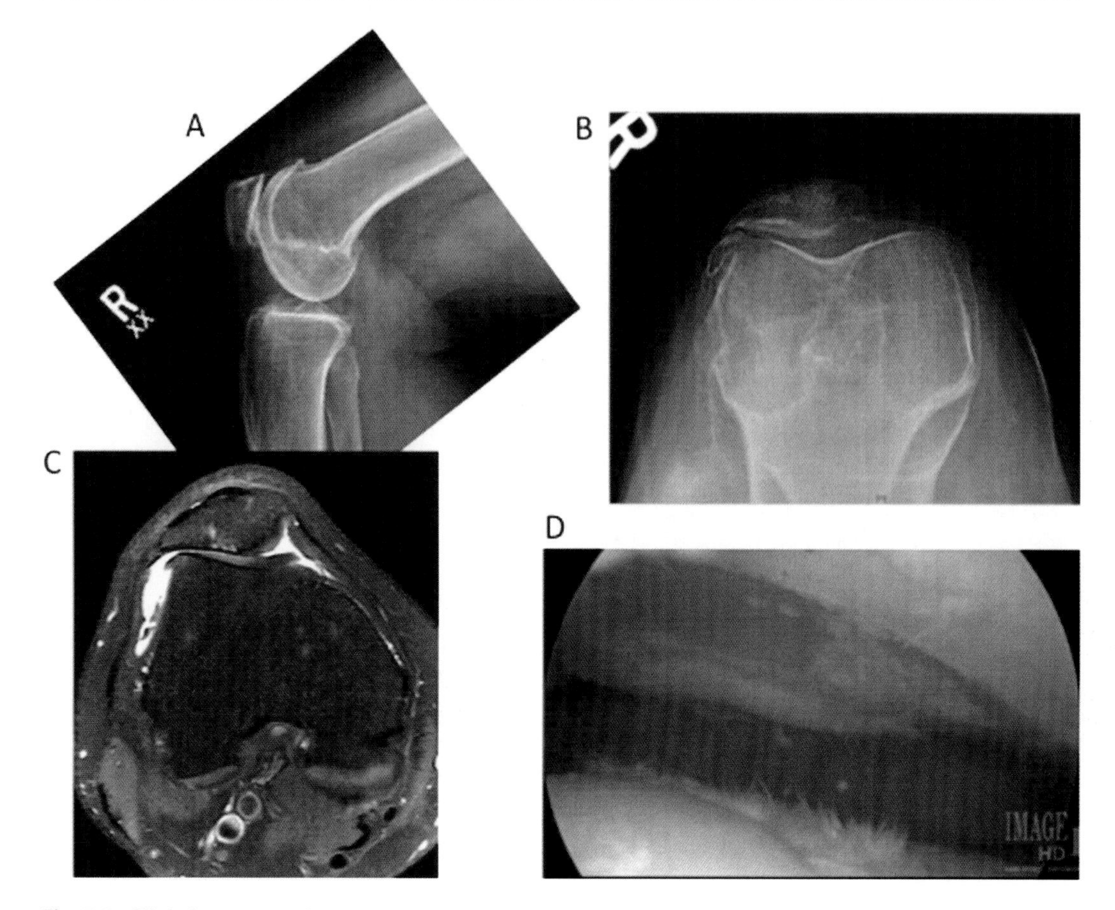

Fig. 7.7 Clinical case example 1: (**a**) lateral radiograph demonstrating isolated patellofemoral arthritis. (**b**) Merchant view demonstrating a lateral tracking patella with osteophyte and subchondral sclerosis but normal patella tilt angle of Laurin or congruence angle of Merchant. (**c**) MRI of the same patient noting the lateral facet bone edema with cystic changes present secondary to increased contact pressures and arthritis. (**d**) Intraoperative arthroscopic image of isolated lateral patellofemoral compartment grade IV cartilage loss and arthritis

Case 2: Recurrent Patella Instability

This is a case example of a 22-year-old college senior with multiple patella dislocations after her first dislocation at age 14. Her first dislocation occurred while running and turning while playing soccer. She currently significantly limits her activities secondary to patella instability and intermittent pain with effusions following subluxation events which occur one to two times per week. She does have decreased symptoms with lateral stabilization brace and mild obesity and has attempted physical therapy on several occasions with a focus on hip external rotators and gait training. Her exam demonstrates clear apprehension with lateral directed patella force in extension, 3+ quadrant glide before she removes your hand, J tracking, pain with patella load, and measured *Q* angle of 19–20 with 20° of flexion. Knee series and CT tracking studies demonstrate patella alta (ratio 1.8) and type C trochlea dysplasia (Fig. 7.9), and her TT–TG distance is measured to be 24 (Fig. 7.10). This case demonstrates the situation where a proximal MPFL procedure was done in addition to combining a distalization of 8 mm to the AMZ tibia tubercle osteotomy secondary to her dysplasia and alta (Fig. 7.11). Postoperative course was excellent with no reported instability at 6 M; repeat radiographs demonstrate correction of patella alta with distalization/AMZ osteotomy (Fig. 7.12).

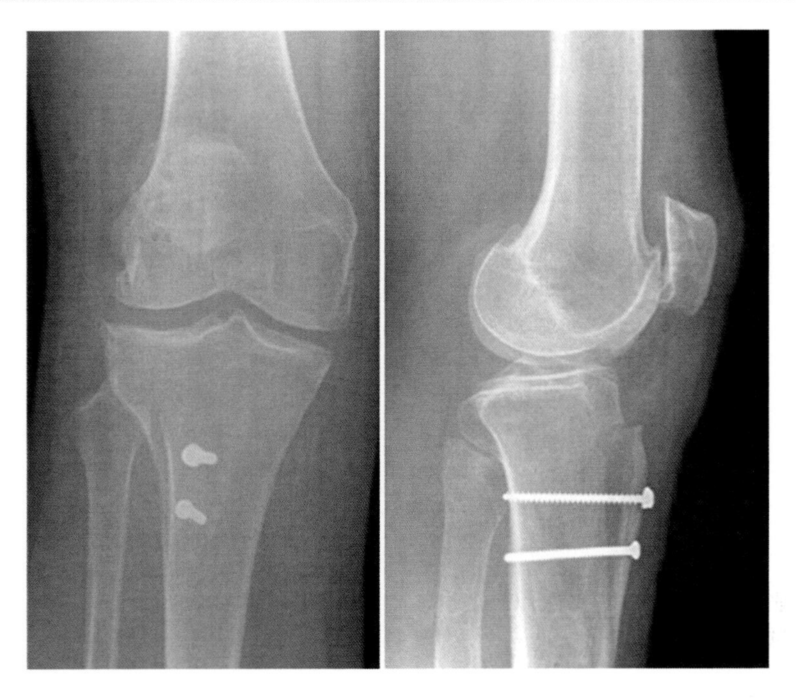

Fig. 7.8 Clinical case example 1: postoperative AP and lateral radiograph of knee following AMZ (Fulkerson) osteotomy for isolated lateral patellofemoral compartment arthritis

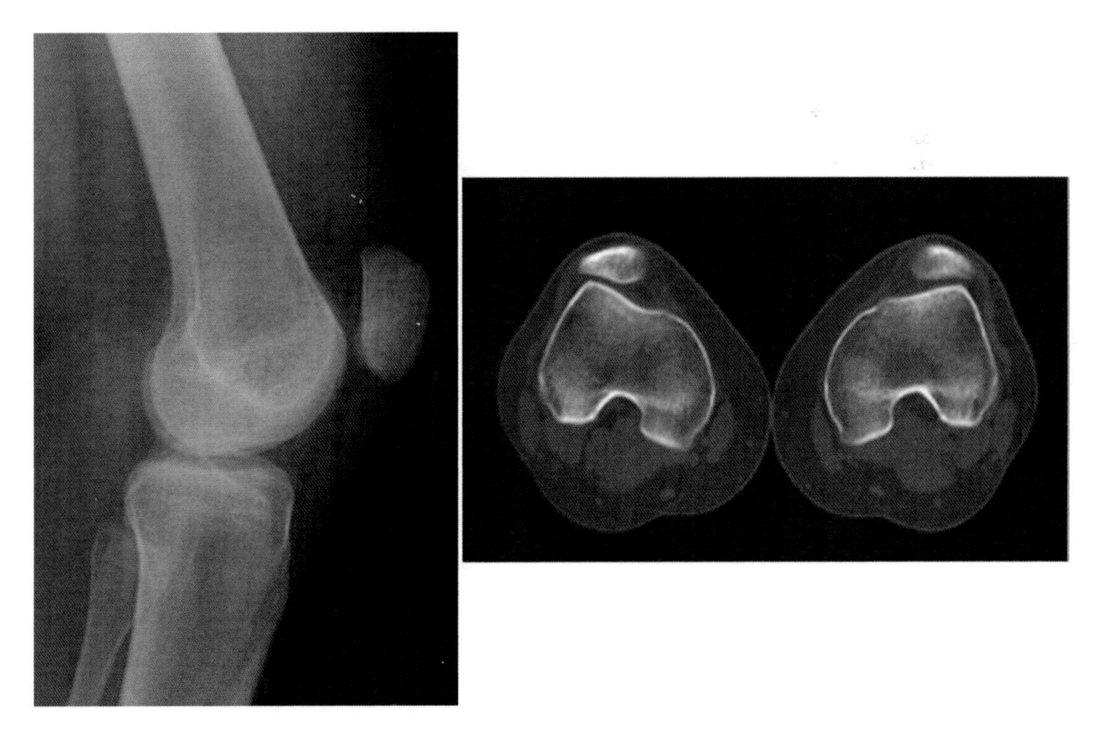

Fig. 7.9 Clinical case example 2: lateral radiograph demonstrating mild type C trochlea dysplasia with patella alta and axia bilateral CT cuts in full extension demonstrating lateral patella tracking. Dysplasia is moderate and present on both lateral X-ray and CT axial cuts

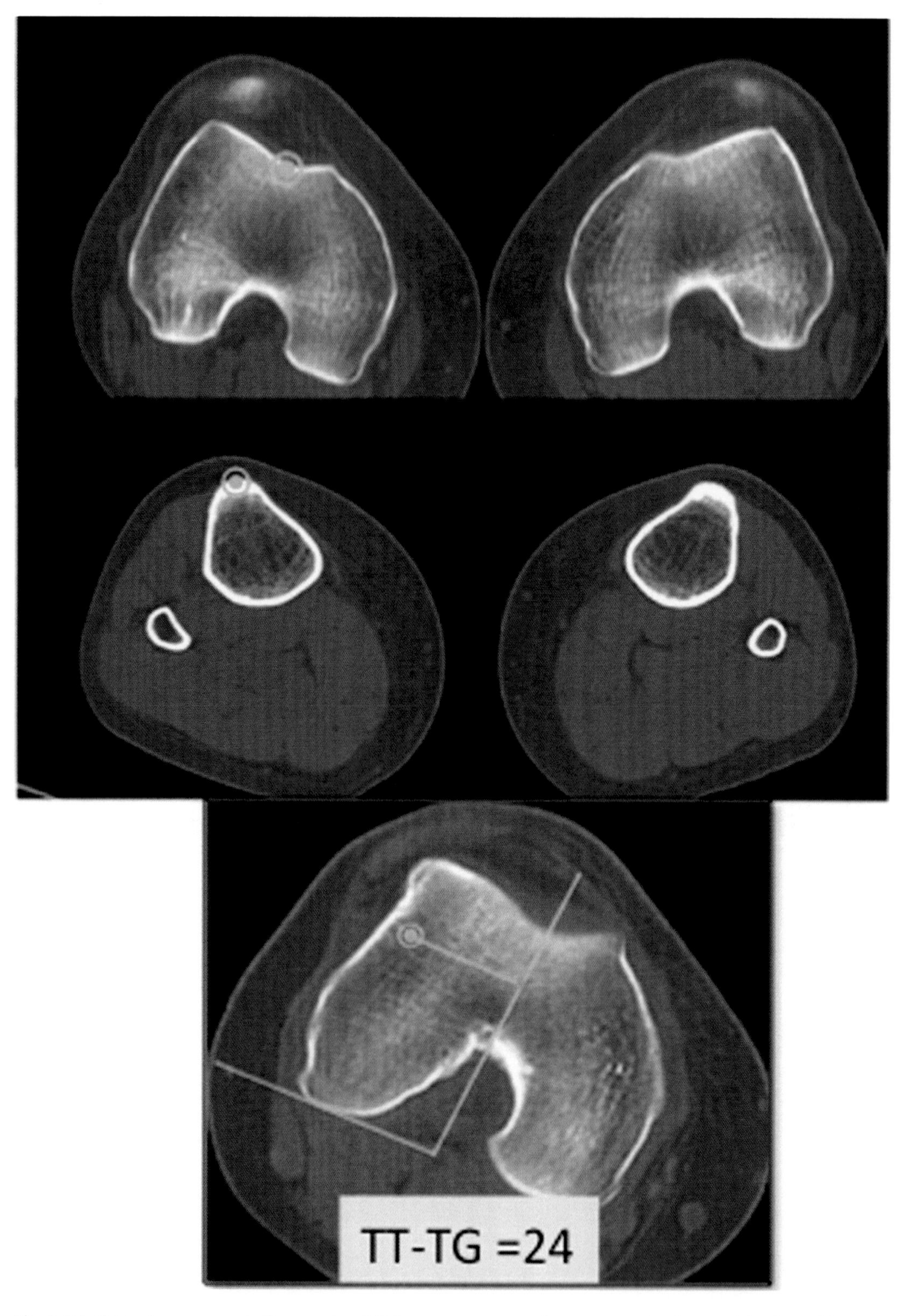

Fig. 7.10 Clinical case example 2: example of CT scan axial cut overlays measurements of TT–TG distance with OsiriX program, measuring 24 mm on this patient and corresponding to a grossly abnormal level requiring correction with tubercle medialization osteotomy

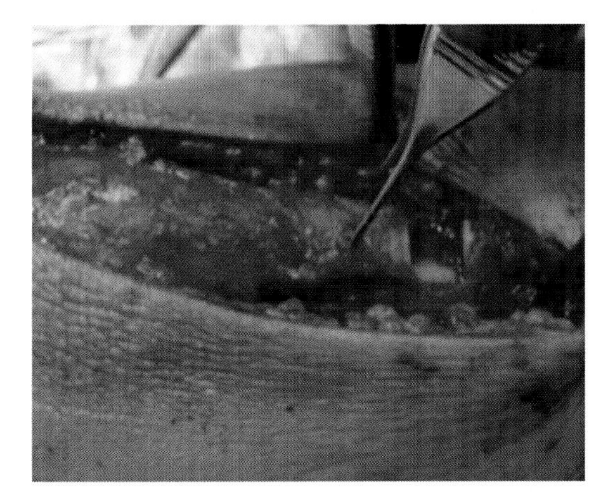

Fig. 7.11 Clinical case example 2: secondary to the patella alta in this patient with increased TT–TG distance and exposure and moderate trochlea dysplasia, the tubercle osteotomy incorporated a 10 mm resection of cortical bone and flat cut distalization osteotomy as seen here in this intraoperative picture

Author's Preferred Techniques

Technique of AMZ

Preoperative planning provides the critical information needed to design an AMZ osteotomy. Since the operation involves moving the tibial tubercle medially as well as anteriorly, the preoperative indication is lateral patella tracking with excessive pressure on the lateral patella and trochlea facets. Distal patella articular damage will also benefit from unloading following and anteriorization osteotomy. Suffice it to say that the AMZ procedure should provide improved tracking of the patella (putting it into a balanced, centered, mechanically desirable relationship with the trochlea throughout flexion and extension of

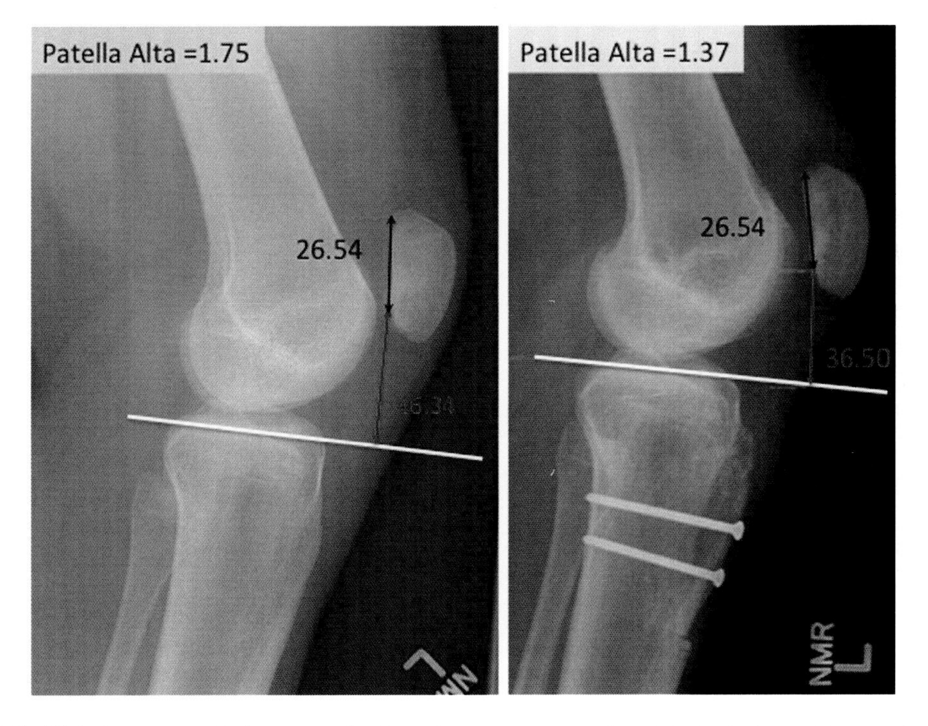

Fig. 7.12 Clinical case example 2: preoperative to postoperative comparison lateral radiograph demonstrating the patella alta correction and new measurement by Blackburne–Peel index. *Note*: The goal is not a complete or over correction, but simply to provide enough correction to affect "earlier" entrance of the patella into the trochlea

the knee) while optimizing articular contact in the patellofemoral joint by shifting the patella off of damaged and/or painful articular surfaces and onto better cartilage more medially and proximally on the patella.

Anteromedial tibial tubercle transfer starts with an arthroscopy using low anteromedial and lateral portals to fully examine the knee. Patellofemoral tracking and alignment, with and without fluid in the knee, dysplasia, displaceability of the patella, and documentation of location and extent of articular damage should be assessed. The surgeon may then determine how much anteriorization and medialization are appropriate when designing the osteotomy. A more oblique osteotomy will achieve anteriorization, thereby unloading or reduce the contact pressures within the distal articular cartilage; a more flat osteotomy will produce a more medial translation of the patella tendon resulting in a medial shift within the patella–trochlea articular contact. During the history, chief complaint, clinical examination, and lastly with imaging, the balance of medial and anterior transfer is considered and decided preoperatively, which is implemented by designing the osteotomy obliqueness according to each patient's need. Of note, the concomitant problem of excessive patella alta can be addressed by planning some amount osteotomy bone removal that produced a distal displacement of the tubercle to allow for patella alta normalization.

Limited lateral release at the time of arthroscopy is helpful in many cases, particularly releasing any infrapatellar scar or abnormal tether that will restrict the desired patella displacement. Because the osteotomy will create some anteriorization, the release is distracted and therefore scarring down is very uncommon.

The skin incision placement is important and is positioned just lateral to the tubercle, so when the osteotomy is medialized, it is away from the incision site (Fig. 7.13). It extends usually for a length of 5–6 cm depending on how long the surgeon wises to make the osteotomy and should be made judiciously during the first 10–20 procedures, and a shorted skin incision places the patient at risk for damage to the skin during osteotomy creation that can impact healing or cosmetics of the wound (Fig. 7.13).

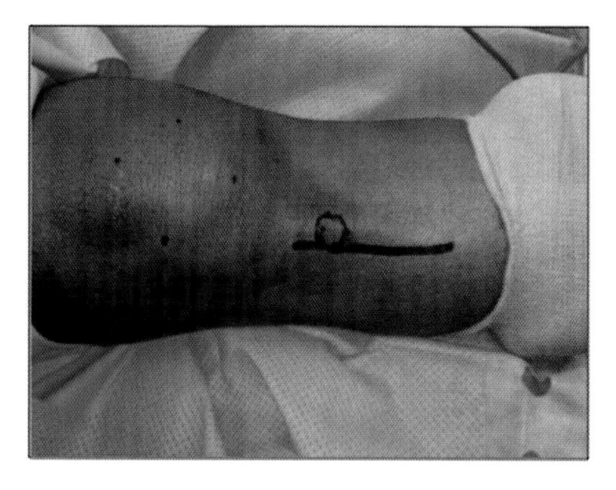

Fig. 7.13 Clinical example of the placement of the skin incision for Fulkerson osteotomy

The distal patella tendon is exposed such that a hemostat may be placed behind the tendon (Fig. 7.14). The anterior compartment is then incised along its anterior edge and reflected off of the lateral tibia with a large periosteal elevator. This careful elevation should expose the junction of the lateral and posterior tibia, and then a large retractor exposes the entire lateral tibia over the extent of the planned osteotomy before starting the osteotomy itself. Thereby, the surgeon will have a complete exposure of the saw blade as it comes through the lateral tibia and avoid any possibility of neurovascular injury (the anterior tibial artery and the deep peroneal nerve run just behind the posterolateral tibia at the osteotomy level).

The obliquity of the osteotomy may be determined in several ways and guides are available for this purpose. My preferred technique however requires a free hand cut after studying the proximal tibia geometry using an oscillating saw. First the line along the anteromedial tibia where the osteotomy will be medial is defined and marked with the electrocautery. Important: the osteotomy line must be drawn such that the osteotomy is tapered to the anterior tibial cortex at the osteotomy's distal extent (Fig. 7.15). For osteotomies intended to provide mainly medial translation with a flat cut, less obliquity, the osteotomy starts more posteriorly, often a centimeter medial to the medial patella tendon insertion. For a steeper

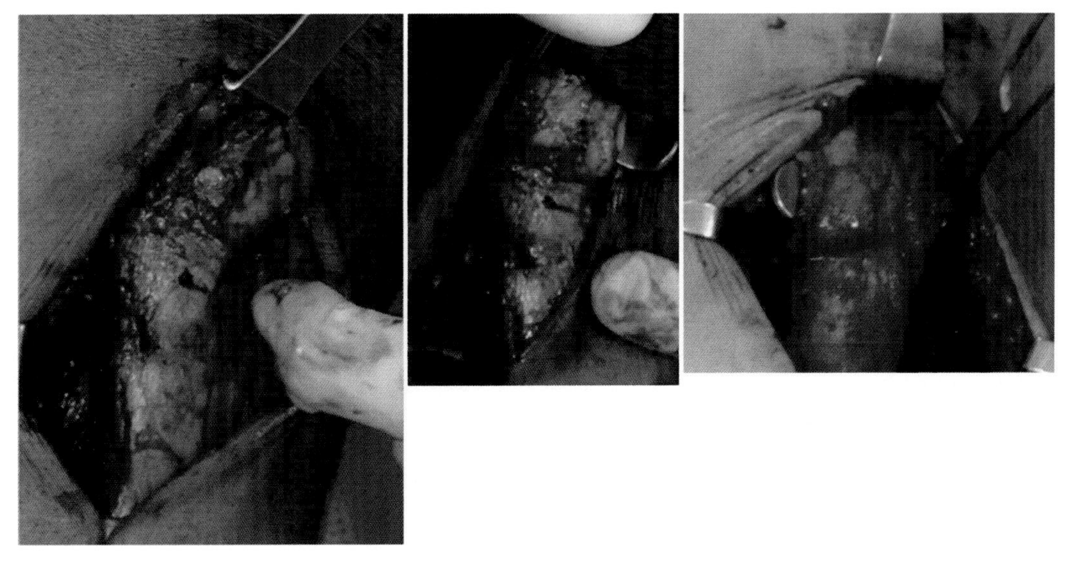

Fig. 7.14 Intraoperative pictures of the isolation of the patella tendon insertion and protection with retractor behind tendon. Also note the length of skin incision and exposure medial and lateral

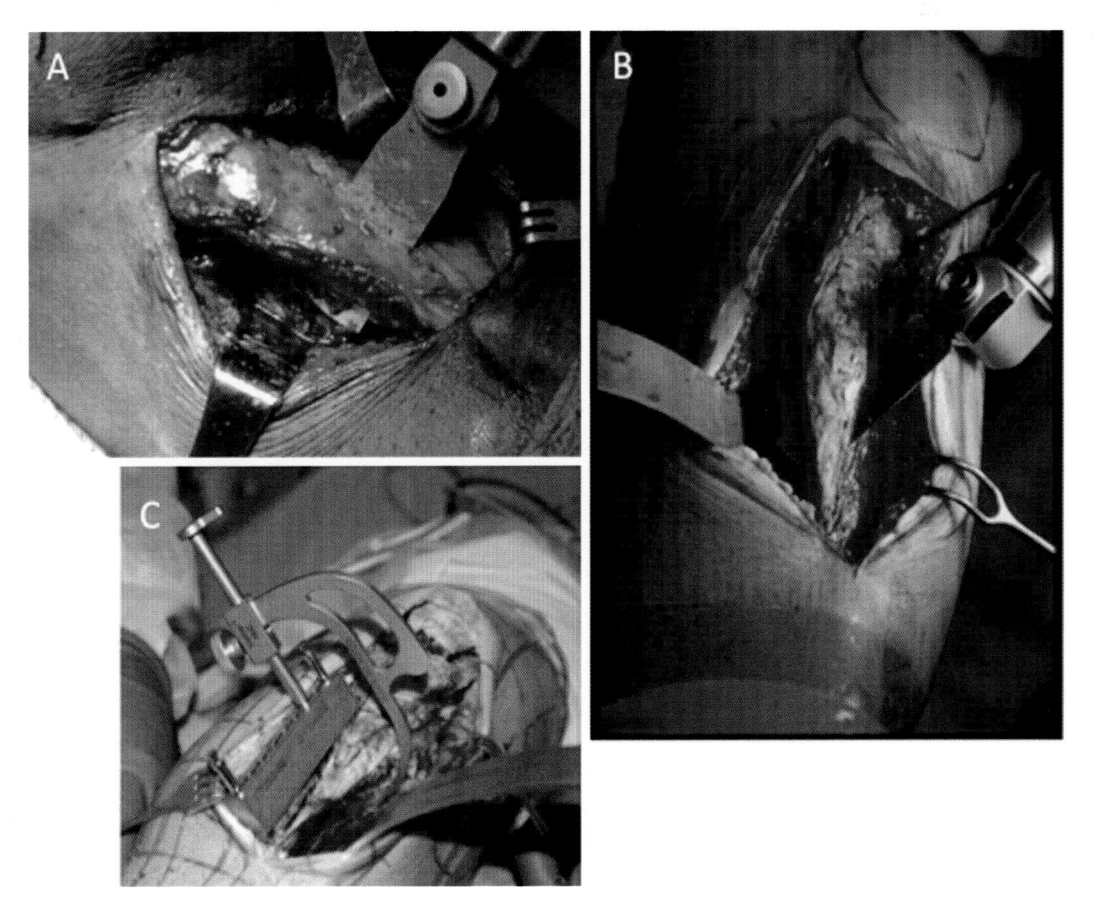

Fig. 7.15 Intraoperative pictures of freehand creation of the osteotomy (**a**, **b**) with the saw blade cutting from medial to lateral in a sloped position. The more shallow the slope (**a**) and the more medial and less anterior the osteotomy created, the steeper the cut an increase in anterior tubercle placement is made (**c**). A few systems designed to help "guide" the cut angle with more precise measurement are available; the system demonstrated is the AMZ Tracker System©

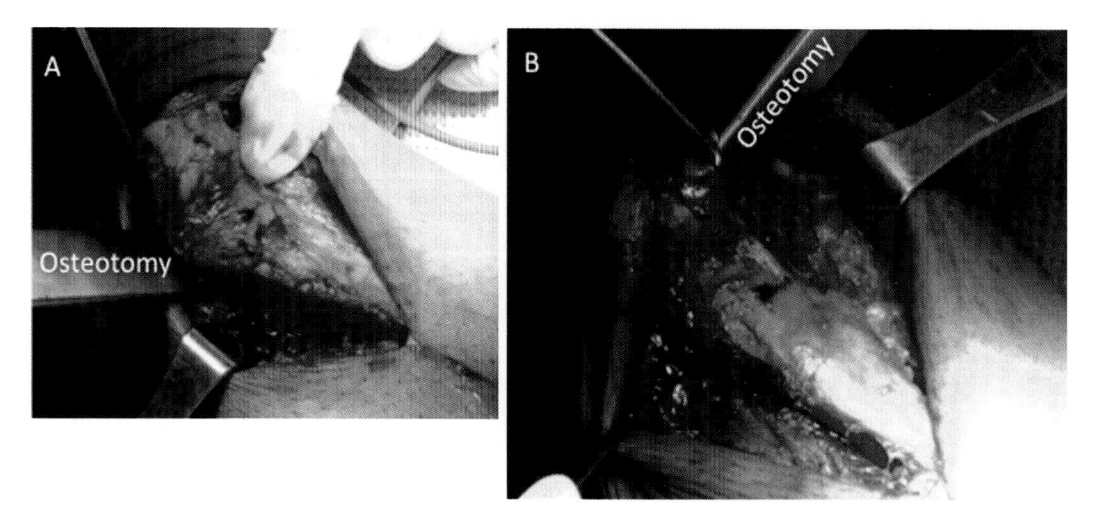

Fig. 7.16 Intraoperative image of the use of the osteotome to complete the osteotomy connecting the plateau cut to the cortex cut on either side of the patella tendon. Use of osteotomy to complete lateral (**a**) and medial (**b**) cuts at the saw is under to create major osteotomy cut is anterior tibial

osteotomy, the bone cut will start very close to the medial patella tendon insertion (Fig. 7.15b).

The osteotomy cut is created slowly such that the surgeon visualizes the desired obliquity, watching the saw blade from above and below and assuring that the saw will exit the lateral tibia at the desired level of the lateral tibial cortex (Fig. 7.15a, b). The saw should always exit the lateral tibia first at the most distal aspect of the osteotomy which is the most anterior and therefore safest part of the bone cut. The remainder of the cut then is watched by direct vision as the saw cuts more proximally and therefore exits the lateral tibia more posteriorly at its most proximal extent. The saw blade exit must be watched at all times.

At this point, I prefer to use a large Lambotte osteotome to connect the lateral, proximal extent of the osteotomy, at its posterior extent, to a point just proximal to the lateral patella tendon insertion (Fig. 7.16).

The final cut is made with a ½ in. osteotome by retracting the patella tendon anteriorly and then cutting straight across to meet the medial proximal extent of the osteotomy.

Once these cuts have been completed, it is typically easy to complete the osteotomy by placing a large osteotome into the osteotomy. The osteotomy fragment is elevated anteriorly, thereby creating a small greenstick fracture at its distal extent so that the released osteotomy fragment may be rotated anteromedially using the distal end as the pivot point (Fig. 7.17). At this point, it is imperative to assess the patella by fixing the osteotomy transiently with a drill bit or two K-wires and taking the knee through a flexion arc. I like to use the arthroscope for this purpose to visualize under direct the improvement and more medial tracking that should be noticed in flexion ranges from 20 to 60°. The patella should never be placed into a medial tracking configuration by which the lateral trochlea wall is not contacted. The potential for over correction medial is real, especially if a medial chondral lesion is present and the procedure is being done for instability.

The osteotomy is then secured in the desired position with two fully threaded cortical screws, using lag technique (Fig. 7.18). Typically use 4.5 mm self-tapping screws, overdrilled to provide compression (lag mode) within the near cortex or entry hole to 4.5, and then drill the posterior cortex to 3.2 mm. To prevent fracture, the screws should be placed a minimum of one distal to the patella tendon insertion and a minimum of 2 cm apart from each other. If the size of the osteotomy will not accommodate this spacing, a larger screw can be used, but we would favor using smaller

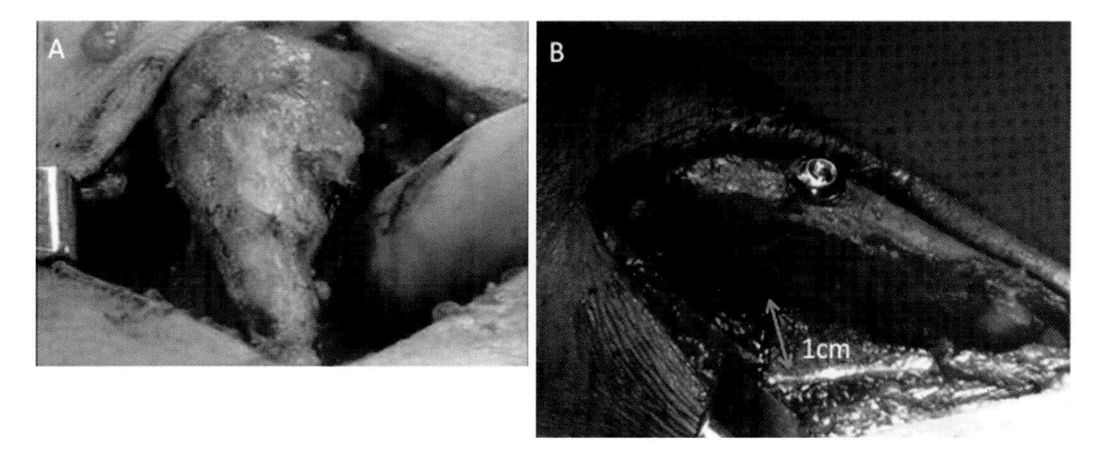

Fig. 7.17 (**a, b**) Intraoperative image of a completed osteotomy and the amount typically translated in the medial direction (1 cm) (**b**) and showing the plane of osteotomy (**a**) cut on the lateral cortex

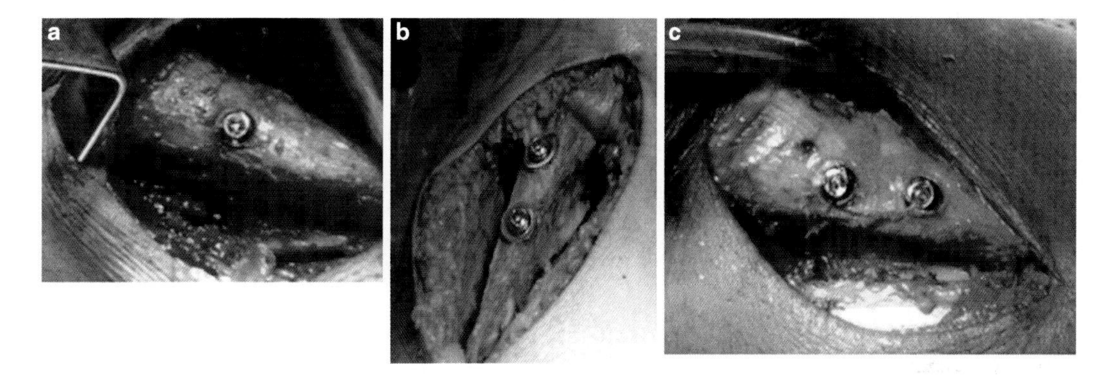

Fig. 7.18 Intraoperative image of various fixations for osteotomy after translation. (**a**) Smaller osteotomy with single bi-cortical 4.5 cortical screw in lag mode with countersink. (**b**) Two 3.5 bi-cortical screws with washer—typically used for an older patient with concerns of softer bone and need for increased surface area contact on the near cortex. (**c**) Typical fixation of two 3.5 bi-cortical placed with overdrilling of the near cortex to get compression of osteotomy and countersink of the near cortex to decrease the screwhead prominence

screw and two points of fixation to prevent rotation around a central fixation point. Assuming the fragment has been moved accurately along the osteotomy plane, the fixation of this displaced fragment is very secure. Nonunion is very rare when this is done properly.

After release of the tourniquet, one should control any soft tissue bleeding and do a final evaluation of the patella tracking arthroscopically. This is a critical step as it is extremely important to avoid any medial tracking as this will lead to problems.

Following AMZ, the retinacular tissues both medially and laterally must be evaluated, and reconstruction, restoration, or release is performed as needed. In patients with trochlea dysplasia increases, the need for balanced retinacular restoration is important as the risk of recurrent instability is greater. In all cases, it is imperative to avoid excessive lateral release and to restore lateral as well as medial retinacular restraints to prevent medial as well as lateral instability. Examination on the OR table after AMZ is the ideal time to determine if the patella may be excessively displaceable as a result of deficient retinacular restraints. In some cases, all that is needed are a few imbrications sutures to restore normal balance.

Postoperative Management

Postoperatively, all patients should start a single arc of knee flexion daily within a few days of surgery. Most patients can achieve a 90 bend within 2–3 weeks. They should use a knee immobilizer for 5 weeks and crutches for 6–8 weeks in most case. Physical therapy for further motion, strength, and progressive weight bearing starts at 5–6 weeks postoperative. Many patients are off crutches by the eighth postoperative week.

References

1. Winter DA. Energy generation and absorption at the ankle and knee during fast, natural, and slow cadences. Clin Orthop Relat Res. 1983;175:147–54.
2. Fulkerson JP. Evaluation of the peripatellar soft tissues and retinaculum in patients with patellofemoral pain. Clin Sports Med. 1989;8:197–202.
3. Post WR, Fulkerson JP. Distal realignment of the patellofemoral joint: indications, effects, results, and recommendations, Chapter 61. In: Insall JN, Scott WN, editors. Surgery of the knee. 5th ed. Amsterdam: Elsevier; 2012.
4. Keller PM, Shelbourne KD, McCarroll JR, Rettig AC. Nonoperatively treated isolated posterior cruciate ligament injuries. Am J Sports Med. 1993;21:132–6.
5. Gill TJ, DeFrate LE, Wang C, Carey CT, Zayontz S, Zarins B, Li G. The effect of posterior cruciate ligament reconstruction on patellofemoral contact pressures in the knee joint under simulated muscle loads. Am J Sports Med. 2004;32(1):109–15.
6. Bicos J, Carofino B, Andersen M, Schepsis AA, Fulkerson JP, Mazzocca A. Patellofemoral forces after medial patellofemoral ligament reconstruction: a biomechanical analysis. J Knee Surg. 2006;19(4):317–26.
7. Post W. History and physical examination of patients with patellofemoral disorders. In: Fulkerson J, editor. Disorders of the patellofemoral joint. Baltimore, MD: Williams & Wilkins; 1997.
8. Insall J, Falvo KA, Wise DW. Chondromalacia patellae: a prospective study. J Bone Joint Surg Am. 1976;58:1.
9. Fairbank JCT, Pynsent PB, van Poortvliet JA, et al. Mechanical factors in the incidence of knee pain in adolescents and young adults. J Bone Joint Surg Am. 1984;66:685.
10. Piva SR, Goodnite EA, Childs JD. Strength around the hip and flexibility of soft tissues in individuals with and without patellofemoral pain syndrome. J Orthop Sports Phys Ther. 2005;35(12):793–801.
11. Willson JD, Binder-Macleod S, Davis IS. Lower extremity jumping mechanics of female athletes with and without patellofemoral pain before and after exertion. Am J Sports Med. 2008;36(8):1587–96.
12. Schoettle PB, Zanetti M, Seifert B, Pfirrmann CW, Fucentese SF, Romero J. The tibial tuberosity-trochlear groove distance; a comparative study between CT and MRI scanning. Knee. 2006;13(1):26–31.
13. Dejour H, Walch G, Nove-Josserand L, Guier C. Factors of patellar instability: an anatomic radiographic study. Knee Surg Sports Traumatol Arthrosc. 1994;2:19–26.
14. Balcarek P, Jung K, Frosch KH, Stürmer KM. Value of the tibial tuberosity-trochlear groove distance in patellar instability in the young athlete. Am J Sports Med. 2011;39(8):1756–61.
15. Koëter S, Diks MJ, Anderson PG, Wymenga AB. A modified tibial tubercle osteotomy for patellar maltracking: results at two years. J Bone Joint Surg Br. 2007;89(2):180–5.
16. Farr J, Cole B, Kercher J, Lachlan B, Sarvottam B. Anterior tibial tubercle osteotomy (Fulkerson osteotomy), Chapter 40. In: Vicente Sanchis-Alfonso, editor. Anterior knee pain and patellar instability. 2nd ed. Berlin: Springer; 2011.
17. Insall J, Salvati E. Patella position in the normal knee joint. Radiology. 1971;101:101–4.
18. Blackburne JS, Peel TE. A new method of measuring patellar height. J Bone Joint Surg Br. 1977;59:241–2.
19. Merchant AC, Mercer RL, Jacobsen RH, Cool CR. Roentgenographic analysis of patellofemoral congruence. J Bone Joint Surg Am. 1974;56:1391–6.
20. Kujala UM, Kormano OK. Patellofemoral relationships in recurrent patellar dislocation. J Bone Joint Surg Br. 1979;71:788–92.
21. Delgado-Martins H. A study of the position of the patella using computerized tomography. J Bone Joint Surg Br. 1979;61:443–4.
22. Elias JJ, Kilambi S, Goerke DR, Cosgarea AJ. Improving vastus medialis obliquus function reduces pressure applied to lateral patellofemoral cartilage. J Orthop Res. 2009;27:578–83.
23. Ramappa AJ, Apreleva M, Harrold FR, Fitzgibbons PG, Wilson DR, Gill TJ. The effects of medialization and anteromedialization of the tibial tubercle on patellofemoral mechanics and kinematics. Am J Sports Med. 2006;34:749–56.
24. Saranathan A, Kirkpatrick MS, Mani S, Smith LG, Cosgarea AJ, Tan JS, Elias JJ. The effect of tibial tuberosity realignment procedures on the patellofemoral pressure distribution. Knee Surg Sports Traumatol Arthrosc. 2012;20(10):2054–61.
25. Fulkerson JP, Shea KP. Disorders of patellofemoral alignment. J Bone Joint Surg Am. 1990;72:1424–9.
26. Saleh KJ, Arendt EA, Eldridge J, Fulkerson JP, Minas T, Mulhall KJ. Operative treatment of patellofemoral arthritis. J Bone Joint Surg Am. 2005;87:659–71.

27. Fulkerson JP. Diagnosis and treatment of patients with patellofemoral pain. Am J Sports Med. 2002;30: 447–56.
28. Hauser EW. Total tendon transplant for slipping patella. Surg Gynecol Obstet. 1938;66:199–214.
29. DeCesare WF. Late results of Hauser procedure for recurrent dislocation of the patella. Clin Orthop Relat Res. 1979;140:137–44.
30. Hampson WGJ, Hill P. Late results of transfer of the tibial tubercle for recurrent dislocation of the patella. J Bone Joint Surg Am. 1975;57:209–13.
31. Juliusson R, Markhede G. A modified Hauser procedure for recurrent dislocation of the patella: a long-term follow-up study with special reference to osteoarthritis. Arch Orthop Trauma Surg. 1984;103:42–6.
32. Carney JR, Mologne TS, Muldoon M, Cox JS. Long-term evaluation of the Roux-Elmslie-Trillat procedure for patellar instability: a 26-year follow-up. Am J Sports Med. 2005;33(8):1220–3.
33. Barber FA, McGarry JE. Elmslie-Trillat procedure for the treatment of recurrent patellar instability. Arthroscopy. 2008;24(1):77–81.
34. Al-Sayyad MJ, Cameron JC. Functional outcome after tibial tubercle transfer for the painful patella alta. Clin Orthop Relat Res. 2002;396:152–62.
35. Caton JH, Dejour D. Tibial tubercle osteotomy in patello-femoral instability and in patellar height abnormality. Int Orthop. 2010;34(2):305–9.
36. Fulkerson JP, Becker GJ, Meaney JA, et al. Anteromedial tibial tubercle transfer without bone graft. Am J Sports Med. 1990;18:490–6.
37. Farr J. Autologous chondrocyte implantation improves patellofemoral cartilage treatment outcomes. Clin Orthop Relat Res. 2007;463:187–94.
38. Minas T, Bryant T. The role of autologous chondrocyte implantation in the patellofemoral joint. Clin Orthop Relat Res. 2005;436:30–9.
39. Peterson L, Brittberg M, Kiviranta I, et al. Autologous chondrocyte transplantation. Biomechanics and long-term durability. Am J Sports Med. 2002;30:2–12.
40. Pascual-Garrido C, Slabaugh MA, L'Heureux DR, Friel NA, Cole BJ. Recommendations and treatment outcomes for patellofemoral articular cartilage defects with autologous chondrocyte implantation: prospective evaluation at average 4-year follow-up. Am J Sports Med. 2009;37 Suppl 1:33S–41.
41. Gomoll AH, Farr J, Gillogly SD, Kercher JS, Minas T. Surgical management of articular cartilage defects of the knee. Instr Course Lect. 2011;60:461–83.

Patellofemoral Resurfacing Arthroplasty in the Active Patient

8

Jack Farr II, Ronald P. Grelsamer, Andreas B. Imhoff, Willem M. van der Merwe, Matthias Cotic, Elizabeth A. Arendt, and Diane L. Dahm

Introduction

Isolated PF arthritis is more common than often assumed. Several authors have evaluated patients presenting for arthroplasty and have found that up to 20 % had isolated PF arthritis [1]. Obviously, nonoperative treatment is the first approach, but over time this will fail. For the younger patients, cartilage restoration is a viable option. In certain situations, however, the extent of the chondrosis or arthrosis may exceed the capabilities of cell therapy, marrow stimulation, and autograft osteochondral plugs. Treatment options for these patients are patellectomy, tuberosity osteotomy, bipolar osteochondral allograft transplantation, TKA, and PFA.

Patellectomy was once a popular option not only for PF arthritis but persistent PF pain as well. It is now recognized that the loss of the mechanical advantage that the patella affords the knee results in permanent weakness often at a clinically significant level. For the active patient, this is problematic. In addition, the increased muscle forces required for any activity involving the knee often result in medial compartment wear. As these patients often have both patella *and* trochlear wear, the pain from the trochlea is obviously not addressed. As a result, patellectomy is now relegated to the treatment of highly comminuted patellar fractures and not pain, chondrosis, or arthrosis.

Tibial tuberosity osteotomy for the treatment of knee pain and arthrosis was first popularized by Maquet [2]. With his procedure of straight anteriorization, the patella is rotated proximally in the sagittal plan: distal lesions are unloaded and the contact areas during range of motion are altered. In addition, the PF resultant forces are decreased by changing the force vectors. The decrease in forces, as noted by modern means (Tekscan® Boston, MA) direct force/pressure transducers and Fujifilm Prescale® (Tokyo, Japan) pressure-sensitive paper directly or finite element analysis (FEA) mathematically, is closer to a 20–25 % reduction as opposed to the 50 % reduction suggested by Maquet using two-dimensional vector analysis [3–5]. Fulkerson modified the

J. Farr II, M.D. (✉)
Orthopaedic Surgery, Cartilage Restoration Center of Indiana, 1260 Innovation Pkwy Ste 100, Greenwood, IN 46143, USA
e-mail: indyknee@hotmail.com

R.P. Grelsamer, M.D.
Patellofemoral Reconstruction, Mount Sinai Medical Center, New York, NY, USA

A.B. Imhoff, M.D. • M. Cotic, M.Sc.
Department of Orthopedic Sports Medicine, Technical University Munich, Munich, Germany

W.M. van der Merwe, M.D.
Orthopaedics Division, Sport Science Institute, University of Cape Town, Cape Town, South Africa

E.A. Arendt, M.D.
Department of Orthopaedic Surgery, University of Minnesota, 2450 Riverside Avenue, Suite R200, Minneapolis, MN 55454, USA
e-mail: arend001@uwn.edu

D.L. Dahm, M.D.
Orthopaedic Surgery, Sports Medicine, Mayo Clinic, Rochester, MN, USA

R.V. West and A.C. Colvin (eds.), *The Patellofemoral Joint in the Athlete*,
DOI 10.1007/978-1-4614-4157-1_8, © Springer Science+Business Media New York 2014

straight anteriorization to add a component of medialization (thus anteromedialization or AMZ) [6]. This has been shown to be effective for distal lateral patellar chondrosis/arthrosis, yet it is much less effective for other areas of the patella especially if the trochlea is involved [7].

For extensive bipolar PF arthrosis, there is one biological option: bipolar osteochondral allograft. Procurement of pristine bipolar donor grafts is extremely difficult because of very limited availability. While transplantation is rather straightforward and initial transplant to host bone healing occurs, the current "stored fresh" grafts have only 50 % survival at 5 years per Bugbee and coworkers [8] compared to the 11 of 13 survivorship up to 10 years reported by Teitge using truly fresh grafts (no longer available) [9]. As a result, this technique is typically reserved for young patients in an attempt to avoid joint replacement surgery and the inherent eventual revisions.

Total knee arthroplasty remains a treatment option for isolated patellofemoral degenerative joint disease. This has been vigorously argued in the literature between total knee proponent Dr. Michael Mont and patellofemoral arthroplasty proponent Dr. Alan Merchant [10, 11]. The basis for the total knee arthroplasty argument was superior long-term results and reliability of total knee arthroplasty versus the historical results after patellofemoral arthroplasty. However, the large majority of patellofemoral arthroplasty series since 1995 have demonstrated that a properly implanted modern generation patellofemoral arthroplasty can be reliable and durable [12]. Even the older generation implants typically did not loosen, but had problems with stability or pain. With these issues largely resolved, the major factor in reliability is surgical technique which depends upon a thorough understanding of patellofemoral biomechanics.

Patellofemoral Biomechanics

Current patellofemoral arthroplasties are resurfacing arthroplasties and thus have the potential to maintain normal kinematics. With normal kinematics reestablished, the knee can "feel" natural to the patient, which is very important for a return to athletics. To achieve this outcome, the forces acting on the patella need to be normalized at the time of implant placement. For the trochlea, it is necessary to appreciate that the trochlear implant is not one-third of a total knee arthroplasty, but rather shaped in a somewhat "normal"-appearing trochlear groove appearance. As the normal trochlear groove has higher lateral facets than medial facets, placing the trochlea implant anatomically yields the appearance (to a total knee arthroplasty surgeon) that the implant is in internal rotation relative to the posterior condylar axis or trans-epicondylar axis. Once again, the goal is to establish a trochlear implant similar in position to a normal trochlea, not to reference to the tibiofemoral compartment. (For a TKA the reason for cutting the trochlea in mild external rotation is to balance the flexion-extension gaps noting the inherent coronal plane joint tibiofemoral alignment, which dictates this external rotation cut.)

With normal lateral to central tracking of the patella during flexion, the soft tissues must duplicate this after PFA. It is very common for the isolated patellofemoral arthritis patient to have excessive contracture in the lateral tissues, loss of lateral bone (when resized to "normal thickness," these lateral tissues will be tensioned), and/or lateral subluxation. To balance these lateral tissues during PFA, there will be a much higher incidence of lateral release or lateral lengthening associated with patellofemoral arthroplasties than total knee arthroplasty. This balancing of the lateral soft tissue is the most common surgery performed concomitant with patellofemoral arthroplasty. If these lateral soft tissues are neglected, the postoperative result may be lateral soft tissue pain or a markedly tilted patella that could lead to uneven stress in the implant.

A subset of patients (especially the dysplastic subset) will have a remote history of recurrent dislocations. They may no longer have dislocations because of the high friction associated with degenerative change. However, when the compartment is resurfaced with low-friction materials, the inadequacy of the medial patellofemoral ligament (MPFL) may be quite evident postoperatively. Therefore, it is important to obtain a thorough history regarding recurrent dislocations in the past and then intraoperatively testing the adequacy of the remaining MPFL tissues. At times it may be possible to shorten the MPFL during the medial arthrotomy repair, but in patients where the tear never fully healed (especially near the femoral attachment), shortening the MPFL will not reestablish the checkrein restraint. In these cases, formal MPFL reconstruction will be necessary. Obviously, in most cases there will be a polyethylene button and thus thinner patellar bone stock. As a result, soft tissue or anchoring in trough techniques would be preferable to bone tunnel techniques [13]. The same principles of MPFL reconstruction for non-arthroplasty patients must be followed. That is, the femoral attachment site is critical for an anatomometric graft. With proper placement the distance between the attachment sites is longest at 20–30° of flexion and becomes closer with flexion. This allows a checkrein at lower flexion angles (such as with sporting activities), and the MPFL becomes lax in flexion as stability is maintained by the intercondylar notch.

The position of the tibial tuberosity affects the quadriceps vector and the timing of entrance into the trochlear groove (e.g., patellar alta delays entrance during early flexion). If it is too lateral (20 mm or greater), there will be a high probability of lateral patella tracking, which may result in either a subluxed appearance or in some cases abnormal tracking with abrupt patellar movement changes [14]. Both of these occurrences may contribute to patient dissatisfaction as well as to polyethylene wear. In these cases straight medialization of the tuberosity would be performed after the implants were in position with a goal of normalizing the tuberosity distance in the range of 10–13 mm [14, 15]. Distal osteoclasis and fixation with inter-fragmentary screws will allow range of motion, weight bearing, and exercise to be unaltered from a standard PFA postoperative protocol. With newer implants having proximal extension of the trochlear component (relative to the native trochlea), even with mild patellar alta, the patella will be engaged in the trochlea at full extension of the knee. In cases of extreme alta, if the patella does not engage at full extension, then a tibial tuberosity distalization will be necessary.

The PFA patella is typically resurfaced in a similar manner to total knee arthroplasty and most implants are either full resurfacing (dome or oval dome) or an inset (dome). These implants allow maintenance of a high level of the contact area even with subtle malpositioning of the patella compared to the trochlea. As PFA is being used not infrequently in the younger patient (40s), it is important to consider that at some point revision may be necessary. With properly positioned patellar buttons, the patellar component may be maintained, if there is no wear or evidence of loosening. In the cases where the button will need to be revised, it is important to have adequate remaining bone stock. Therefore, thicker patellar bone preservation is preferred (compared to TKA). Scott demonstrated that the concept of "overstuffing" the patellofemoral compartment does not occur with maintenance of moderately more patellar bone [16].

Authors' Experiences with Specific Implants

As PFA reports are typically level of evidence 4, we will present the outcomes at five centers that perform a relatively high volume of PFAs. There are many different implants available to surgeons. To give an overview of the broad categories, the following implants will be highlighted:

1. Focal "inlay" patellofemoral resurfacing
2. Regional "inlay" patellofemoral resurfacing
3. Custom patient-specific patellofemoral resurfacing
4. Second-generation symmetrical "onlay" patellofemoral resurfacing
5. Third-generation asymmetrical "onlay or inlay" patellofemoral resurfacing

Focal "Inlay" Patellofemoral Resurfacing (PF HemiCAP)

Personal Experience of Willem van der Merwe, M.D.

PF HemiCAP (Arthrosurface, Franklin, MA) is indicated in patients with localized patellofemoral osteochondral damage that have failed bone marrow stimulation techniques, mosaicplasty, or other focal cartilage restoration/repair. The advantage of the procedure is that the recovery time is short and the joint can be loaded from day 1. The disadvantage is obviously that the knee now has metal (and, at times, plastic) with the associated problems of wear potential and revision surgery.

The procedure really restores the contour of the joint. The rationale for the implant is that by creating a smooth and congruent surface, there will be minimal friction and improved contact area and thus a reduction in pain. The surgery is performed open to get adequate access to allow bone and cartilage preparation with precise instruments, which were designed to afford flush and congruent fit.

The keys for success of the procedure are following the correct indications and meticulous attention to following the precise surgical implantation. The positive aspects of the implant I have observed are the predictable results, a rapid postoperative rehabilitation, and there is no limit to the activity level that these patients can resume. This is not typically a first-line surgery, but in certain cases I will consider it in patients that are unable to adhere to the long rehabilitation with the bone marrow stimulation techniques.

Technique

Figures 8.1, 8.2, 8.3, 8.4, and 8.5 illustrate the HemiCAP implant.

Activity Levels

Provided that the indications were correct, I place no restriction on the activity level of patients receiving only the metal trochlear implant. Seventeen patients have been implanted: 11 with trochlea on and 6 with trochlear and focal polyethylene patellar implant. The only problem that

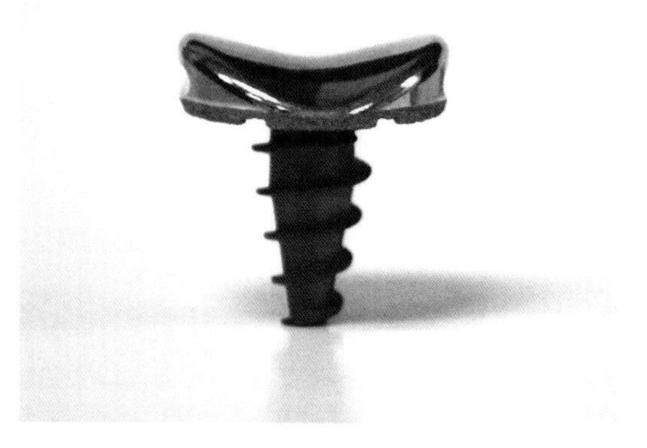

Fig. 8.1 Trochlear implant

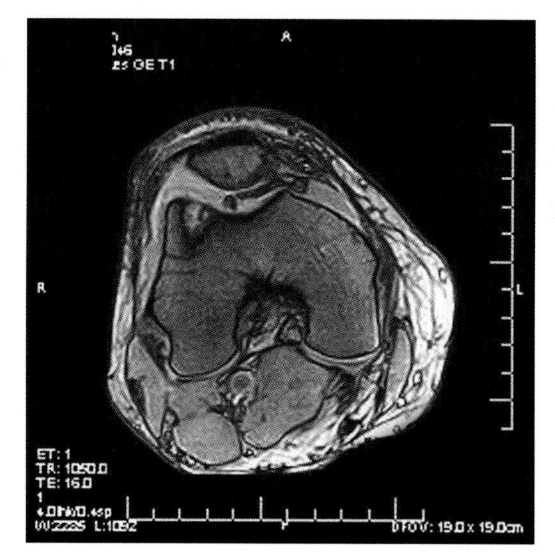

Fig. 8.2 Focal trochlear osteochondral lesion

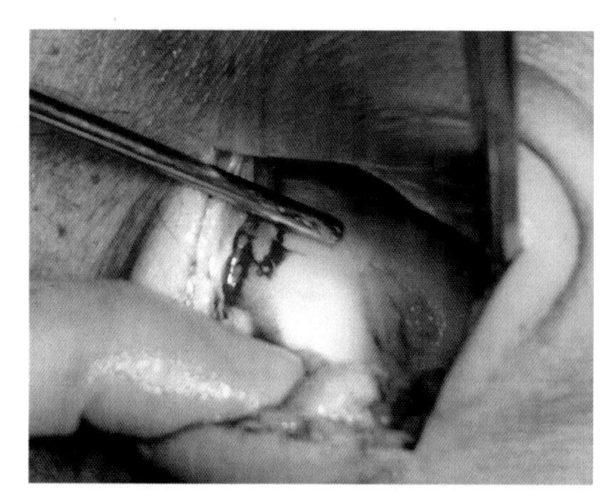

Fig. 8.3 Open appearance of osteochondral lesion

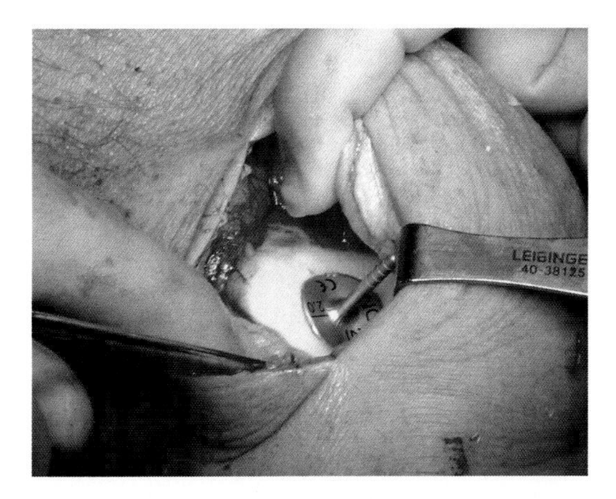

Fig. 8.4 Trail demonstrates flush fit

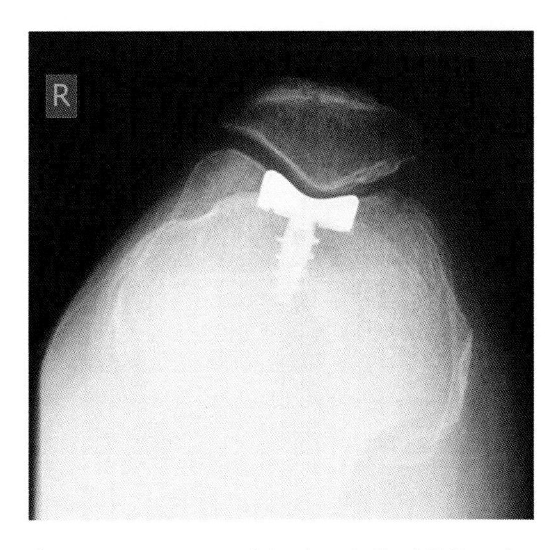

Fig. 8.5 Radiograph of implanted HemiCAP noting metal is flush with the trochlear cartilage, not bone, and thus the "proud" appearance

I found was when we did focal patella resurfacing with polyethylene. Some of those patients had effusions and discomfort. Thus, my use has been primarily to treat focal trochlear lesions with the metal HemiCAP. Trochlea-only patients have gone back to marathon running, cutting, and rotational sports with no deterioration of the knee or function in 5 years.

We have had two failures:

1. Patient had ongoing effusion and pain was diagnosed with RA and had to be converted to TKR.
2. Patient developed medial compartment OA not appreciated during initial evaluation and had to be converted to TKR.

Regional Inlay Patellofemoral Resurfacing (The Wave)

Personal Experiences of Matthias Cotic, M.Sc., and Andreas Imhoff, M.D.

Indication

The HemiCAP Wave (Arthrosurface, Franklin, MA) prosthesis is indicated in patients with symptomatic high-grade OA of the patellofemoral compartment (PFA grades III and IV according to the Kellgren classification), osteochondral lesions (ICRS grades III and IV) and failed conservative treatment (anti-inflammatory drugs/injections, stretching of the quadriceps muscle, and functional training of leg axis), or other failed focal cartilage restoration/repair. Compared to other implants, the advantage of this implant is its inlay design which fits optimally into the trochlea groove of the femur. By leaving the congruent surface of the trochlea, there will be less overstuffing compared to onlay implants, and thus there will be an anatomical surface with minimal friction in the patellofemoral joint involving reduced subchondral pressure. The disadvantage is that this prosthesis does not fit optimally in every kind of trochlea. For example, for patients having a convex or even "bumped" trochlea (type D), we do not recommend to implant the HemiCAP Wave isolated and would implant another implant with an onlay design, which creates a deepened trochlea groove. The key for success of the procedure is to accurately differentiate between the indications for a combined or isolated procedure. Indications for an isolated procedure are severe PFA due to trauma or ongoing hyperpressure due to overload. The decision for a combined procedure is based on our clinical algorithm for treatment of secondary overload and degeneration due to symptomatic patellofemoral instability (PFI).

If the patient's history and clinical examination (positive apprehension sign in 0–30° of flexion) are consistent with instability in early degrees of flexion, PFI is addressed with a concomitant double-bundle MPFL reconstruction. If radiographic (X-ray, CT scan) imaging shows valgus malalignment and/or increased femoral internal torsion, we perform supracondylarosteotomy to either straighten the leg axis or perform a detorsion of the femur. In cases of valgus malalignment, we perform high tibial osteotomy with the aim to set the mechanical axis through 50 % of the proximal tibia plateau width. In patients with a TT-TG>20 mm, we do tibial tubercle osteotomy and a medialization, whereas in patients with a TT-TG<8 mm and medial pain, we do tibial tubercle osteotomy and a lateralization with the aim to reach a normal TT-TG between 10 and 12 mm (range 8–20 mm). Due to the specific inlay design of the implant, we can address mild to moderate trochlea dysplasia. In cases of a type A or B trochlea, we perform an isolated procedure, whereas in patients with a type C trochlea, we do an additional MPFL reconstruction. We do not recommend implantation of the HemiCAP Wave as described above to patients having a type D trochlea.

Technique

In the symptomatic (high-grade OA) patellofemoral compartment of a 36-year-old female patient (Fig. 8.6), the Wave was implanted via an open procedure. The superoinferior curvature and the depth of the preexisting trochlear groove were determined via template (Fig. 8.7).

Then the manufacturer's guiding instruments (Fig. 8.8) were used to develop a working axis normal to the central trochlear articular surface and to cut the cartilage out of the defect of the trochlea (Fig. 8.9).

After satisfying patellar alignment without femoral overstuffing, which was tested with the trial implant (Fig. 8.10), the final implant was inserted and fixed via pilot drill/central screw (Fig. 8.11). Figure 8.12 shows a patient's implant after 2 years.

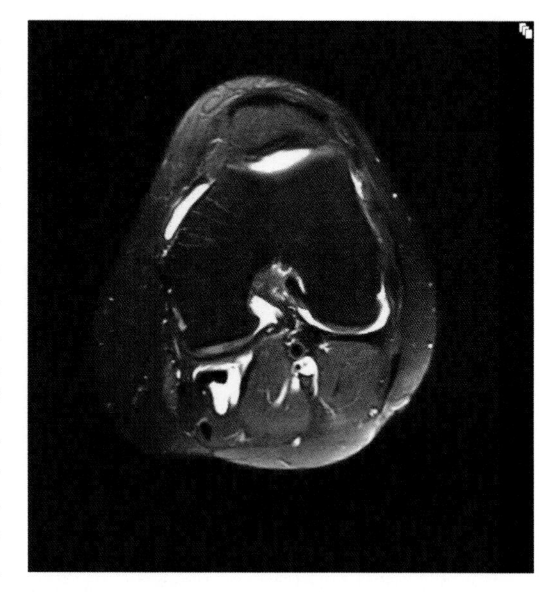

Fig. 8.6 Preop MRI demonstrating OA in the patellofemoral compartment

Demographics of Operated Patients

From October 2009 to July 2010, we implanted 28 HemiCAP Wave prosthesis (Arthrosurface, Franklin, MA) in 27 patients, 18 knees with an isolated and 10 knees with a combined procedure. It was about 14 women and 13 men with a mean age of 41.0 ± 12.4 years at surgery. Seventeen patients with the isolated procedure had a history of previous patellofemoral surgeries (6× retropatellar debridement/shaving, 1× microfracture, 1× OATS), and previous patellar fractures were found in one patient. In four of these isolated cases, patellar resurfacing was performed concomitantly.

Of those undergoing the combined procedures, four had reconstructions of the MPFL, one MPFL in combination with a tibial tubercle osteotomy, two high tibial osteotomies (HTO), one distal femoral osteotomy (DFO), one tibial tubercle osteotomy, and one MPFL in combination with a DFO and a tibial tubercle osteotomy. Previous patellofemoral surgeries in these patients included 4× retropatellar debridement/shaving, 1× microfracture, and one patient had a history of previous patellar fracture. In none of these combined cases was patellar resurfacing performed.

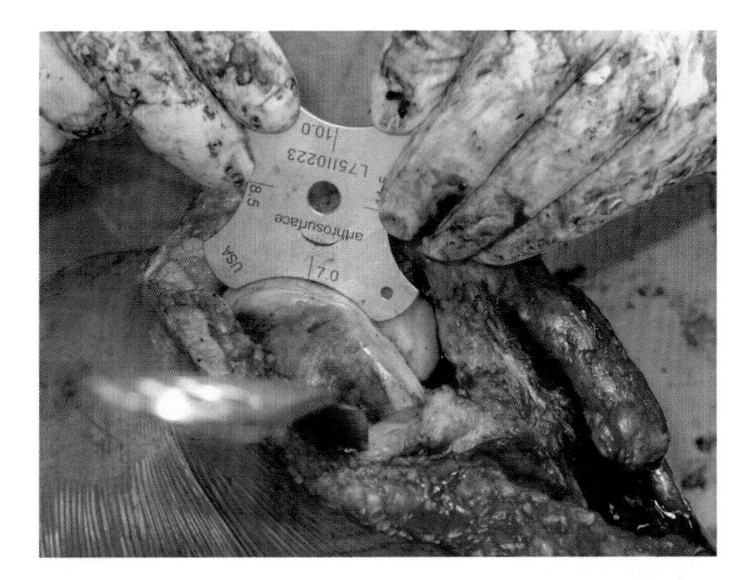

Fig. 8.7 A template is used to measure the depth and curvature of the trochlear groove

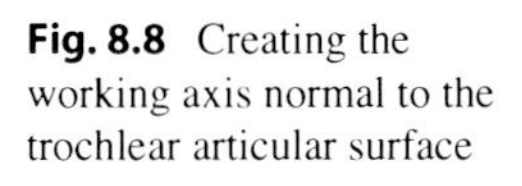

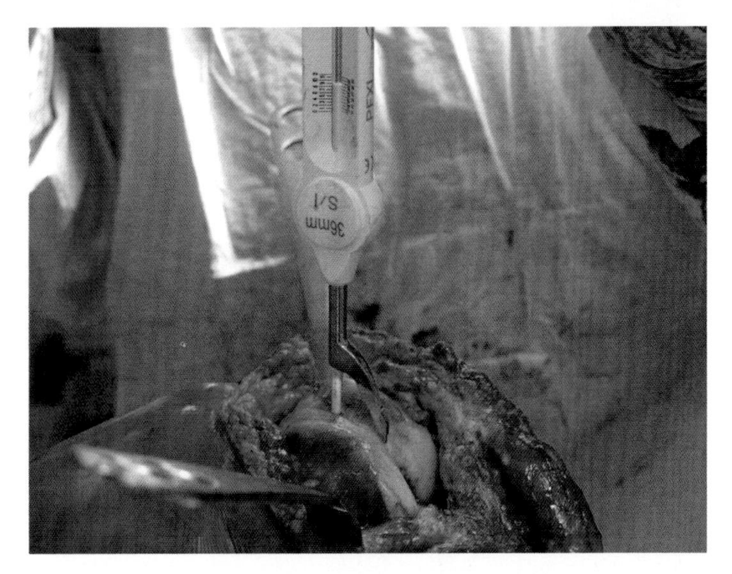

Fig. 8.8 Creating the working axis normal to the trochlear articular surface

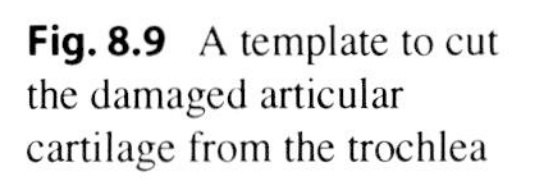

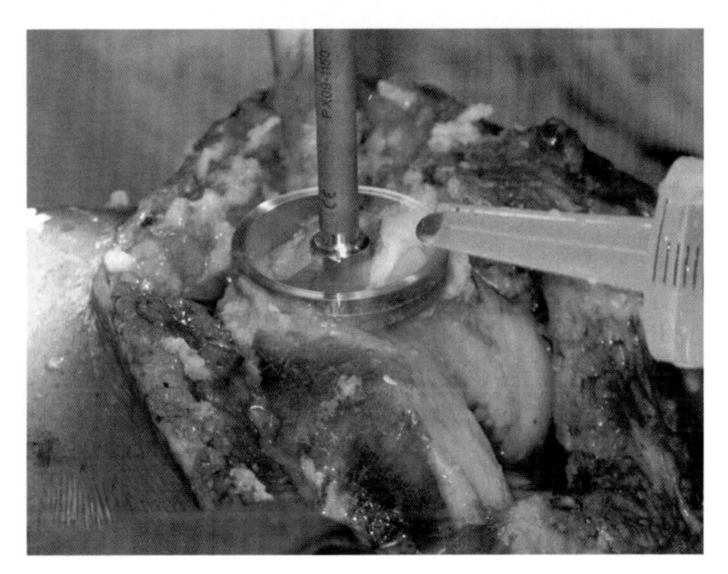

Fig. 8.9 A template to cut the damaged articular cartilage from the trochlea

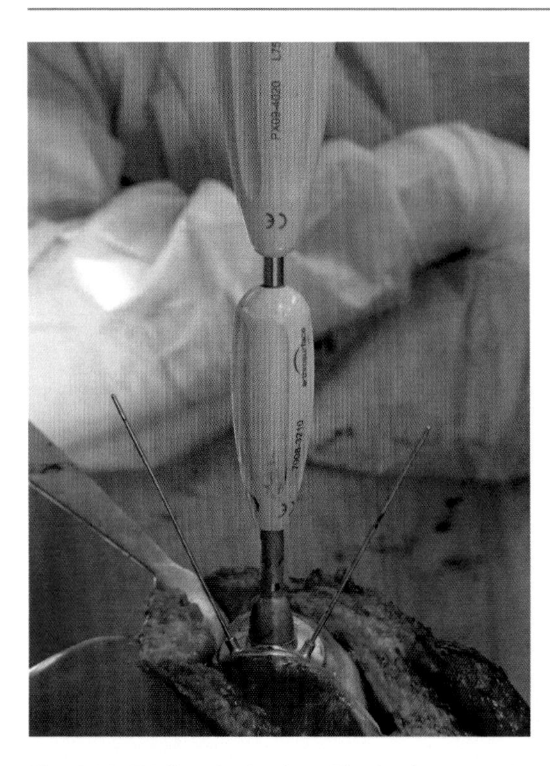

Fig. 8.10 Trialing the implant. The implant must be tested for overstuffing of the patellofemoral compartment

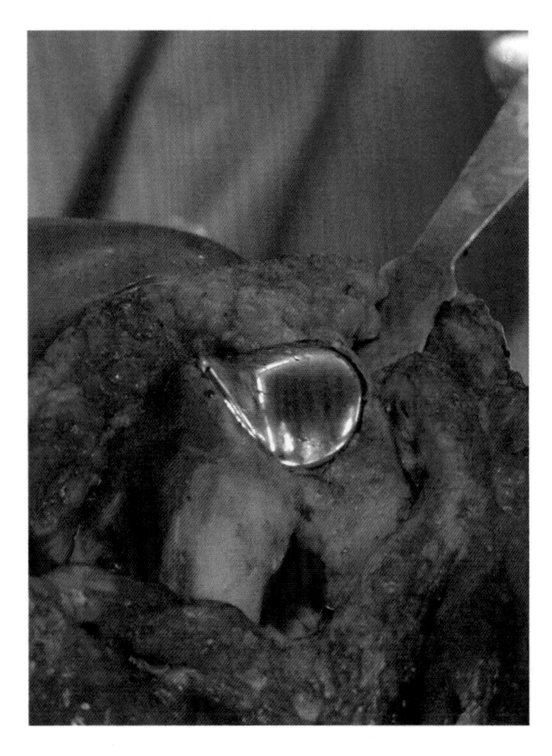

Fig. 8.11 The implant secured in the trochlear groove

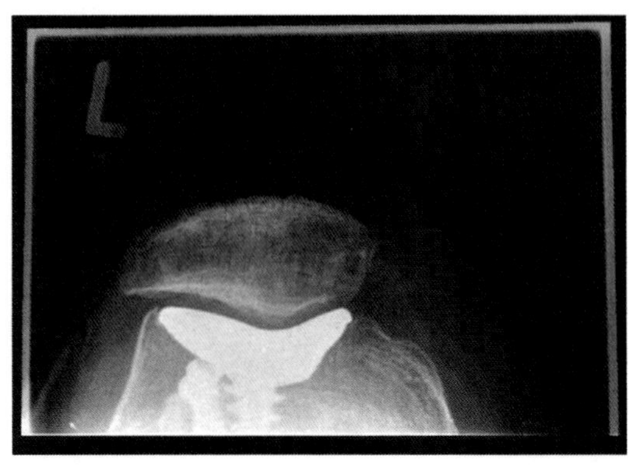

Fig. 8.12 Radiographic axial control 2 years after HemiCAP Wave implantation combined with a MPFL and a tibial tubercle osteotomy

Pain, Functional, Osteoarthritic, and Activity Levels

For the clinical program Visual Analog Scale for knee pain (0 = no pain, 10 = extreme amount of pain), Lysholm, Tegner, and WOMAC scores were recorded preoperatively and at 24 months postoperatively (Table 8.1, Figs. 8.13, 8.14, 8.15, and 8.16) [17–19]. Two patients did not complete the questionnaire and one patient was converted to TKA 1 year after surgery (see revision surgeries below). Therefore, 24 patients (25 knees) were included for statistical analysis. The Wilcoxon signed-rank test for two related samples revealed that all patients showed significant improvement (*, $p < 0.05$) 2 years after surgery based on the following medians:

Sport Participation

To avoid deteriorations of the knee or function, we generally recommend our patients after HemiCAP Wave implantation to do low- to moderate-impact sport activities. Mean time of sport participation per week was 2.1 h (SD ± 1.9) before surgery and 2.9 h (SD ± 2.7) 24 months postoperatively. The number of sport participations increased from 20 (preoperative) to 33 (postoperative status) (Fig. 8.17).

Whether patients received patellar resurfacing or not, we did not place any different limitations on their activity levels. However, we observed in the isolated cases that patients who received patellar resurfacing do have a tendency of higher activity

Table 8.1 Pre- and postoperative scores of patients implanted with the HemiCAP Wave prosthesis

	VAS_pre	VAS_24mo	Lysholm_pre	Lysholm_24mo	WOMAC_pre	WOMAC_24m	Tegner_pre	Tegner_24m
N Valid	25	25	25	25	25	25	25	25
N Missing	3	3	3	3	3	3	3	3
Median	6	3	34	75	40	10	2	3
Standard deviation	2.02731	2.41523	12.56317	19.31735	17.37604	16.12586	1.15470	2.24944
Minimum	3	0	15	20	5	2	0	0
Maximum	10	10	70	95	70	80	5	8

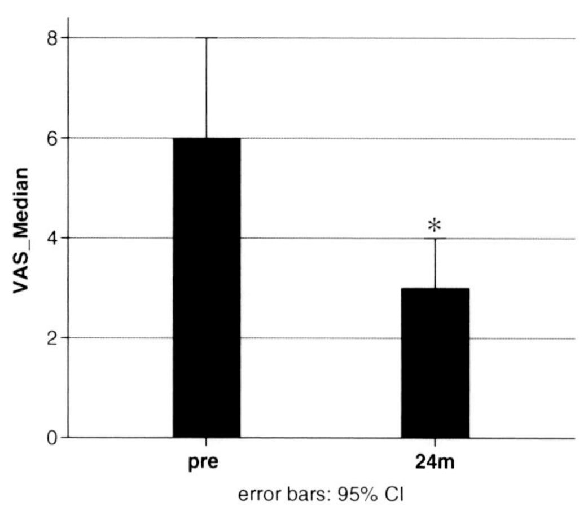

Fig. 8.13 Median VAS (Visual Analog Scale) scores show an improvement at 24 months

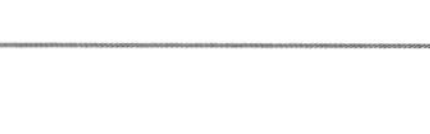
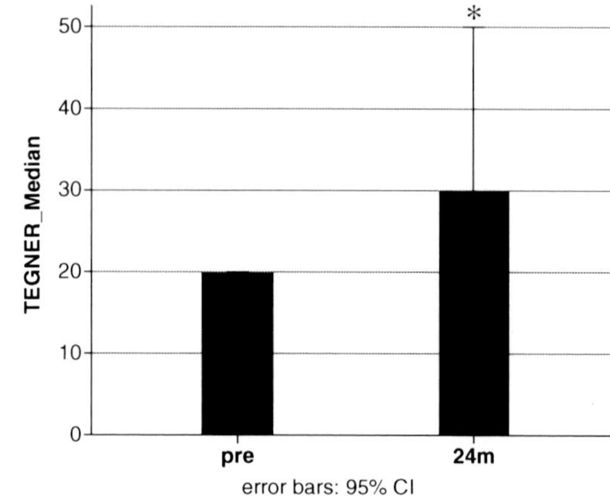

Fig. 8.16 Tegner scores show improvement over a 24-month period

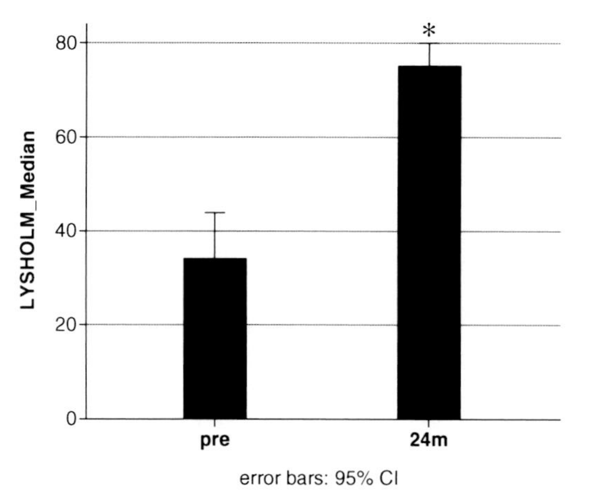

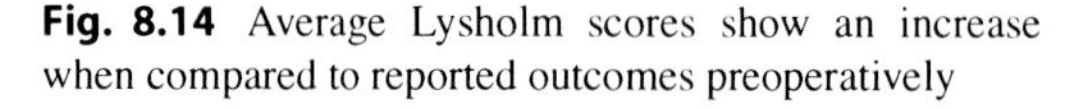

Fig. 8.14 Average Lysholm scores show an increase when compared to reported outcomes preoperatively

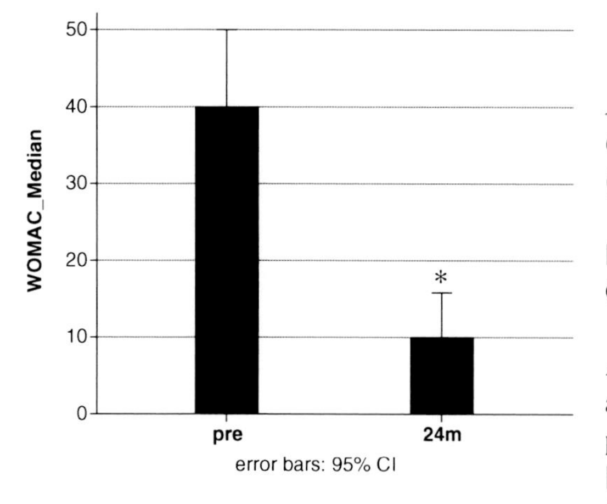

Fig. 8.15 Median WOMAC scores improved from pre- to post-op

status (mean Tegner score: 4.5, SD ± 2.5) than patients without patellar resurfacing (mean Tegner score: 2.5, SD ± 1.8) 24 months after surgery.

We have had three revision surgeries:

- After 1 year, one patient with ongoing effusion and pain was allergic to chrome and nickel and had to be converted to oxinium-coated TKA.
- In one patient we diagnosed a loosening of the central screw 5 days postoperative which had to be repositioned in the revision surgery.
- Two months postoperative, one patient with a combined MPFL reconstruction showed ongoing effusion and pain after spontaneous hyperflexion. We diagnosed a graft slippage at the femur insertion of the MPFL through a screw loosening and refixed the graft with a new screw.

Custom Patellofemoral Resurfacing (Kinamed® Camarillo, CA)

Personal Experience of Ronald Grelsamer, M.D.

A custom PFA is an attractive option for the active patient. Compared to other forms of patellofemoral arthroplasty, a custom PFA offers [20, 21]:

1. Greatly diminished operative time
2. An intact femur upon revision

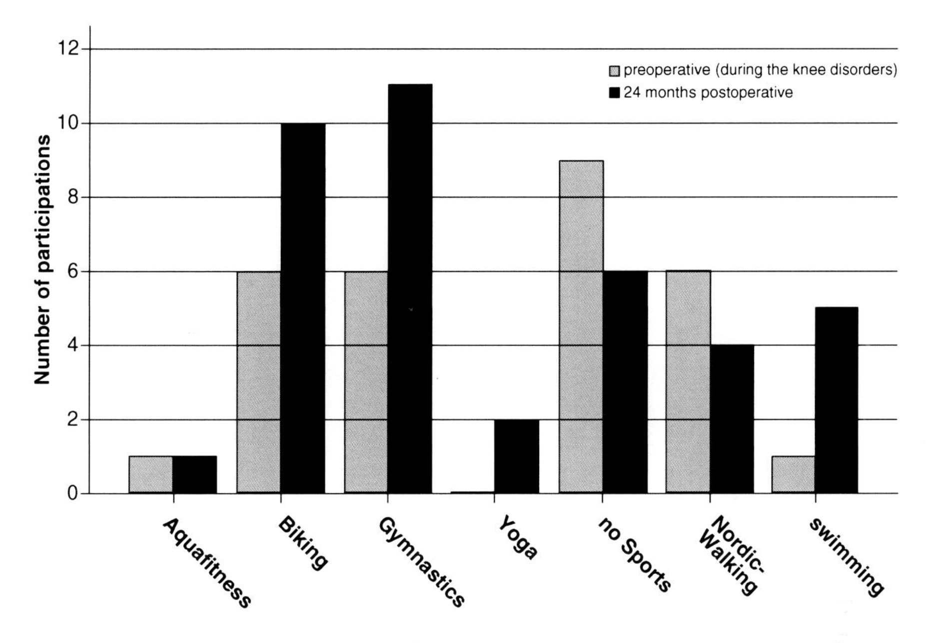

Fig. 8.17 Sport participation before and after HemiCAP Wave implantation

The diminished operative time is the result of the preoperative work performed by the surgeon and the manufacturer. The intact femur upon revision is the result of the onlay aspect of the (trochlear) implant (no bone is removed from the trochlea). There are two components to a custom PFR: the patellar button which is round (and no different from that of a TKR or other PFA) and the metallic trochlear component—the custom piece.

Design Rationale

Despite all attempts to screen out patients at risk for developing tibiofemoral arthritis, a patient receiving a PFA stands a chance of requiring a TKA at some point in the future. When an anterior cut has to be made, the subsequent surgeon will have to address this anterior cut; the inclination of that cut relative to the desired rotation of the new femoral component will determine the ease or difficulty of this step. On the other hand, with the exception of the anchoring drill holes, the femur upon removal of the custom trochlear component will be intact.

Trochleas present a remarkable variety of shapes and sizes. Some appear wide while others are narrow. Off-the-shelf implants can address sizing issues but not morphologies. The quality of the off-the-shelf fit will therefore vary from patient to patient; the long-term effects of this have yet to be determined. A custom trochlea, by definition, will fit every patient. Contrary to first incarnation of custom trochleas (Techmedica®), this custom implant features two differing surfaces: the surface facing the trochlea, which is a *negative* of the trochlea, and the surface facing the patella which *always* matches the patellar button; this concavity provides a measure of stability even in the setting of dysplasia.

Implant Creation and Implantation

A thin-slice CT scan of the distal femur is obtained. From the CT scan pictures, a plaster model is made on which the manufacturer (Kinamed) will outline the contours of the anticipated implant. The surgeon can accept or modify the contour. When all parties agree, the manufacturer creates both a custom drill guide and a custom trochlea (Fig. 8.18). At the time of surgery, the surgeon applies the custom drill guide to the trochlea and outlines it with methylene blue. (At this point, the fit is imperfect due

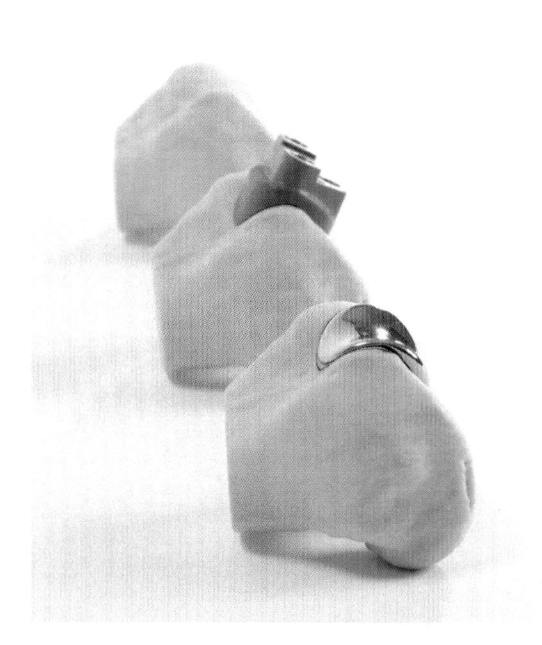

Fig. 8.18 After the contours of a patient's trochlea are outlined, a custom guide and trochlear implant from Kinamed are created. From Sisto DJ, Grelsamer RP, Sarin VK (2012) Patient-Specific Patellofemoral Arthroplasty. In: *Recent Advances in Hip and Knee Arthroplasty*, Edited by S.K. Fokter. InTech Publishing. Rijeka, Croatia. Open Access: http://www.kinamed.com/pdf/Sisto-Grelsamer-Sarin%20-%20Patient%20Specific%20PFR%20-%20Recent%20Adv%20in%20Hip%20and%20Knee%20Arth%20-%20InTech%20%202011.pdf

to the remaining cartilage.) The surgeon removes this cartilage within the outline. The drill guide is reapplied and three holes are created.

The real trochlear implant is applied to the trochlea; the patella is resurfaced. Care is now taken to insure proper tracking of the patella. If the patella is malaligned, the realignment options are the same as for any unstable patella (lateral release, medial imbrication, MPFL reconstruction, tibial tuberosity transfer, etc.).

The following issues have been raised in relation to this implant:

(a) In the setting of dysplastic trochleas, is there overstuffing of the patellofemoral compartment?
   - The recent literature has tended to refute the concept of overstuffing as a cause of limited flexion [16].
   - Trochlear dysplasia is most pronounced proximally; yet it is the *distal* portion of the trochlea that is in contact with the patella during flexion. The patellofemoral compartment is not overstuffed during flexion regardless of any proximal dysplasia.

   A surgeon nevertheless concerned with overstuffing can fashion the plaster model *any way* he/she wishes. The dysplasia can be removed from the plaster model, and an implant will be created to fit this "new" trochlea.

(b) The implant does not extend far enough proximally.
   - The surgeon can ask for the implant to be extended proximally beyond the native trochlea.

(c) The implant is expensive.
   - The cost of the implant is in line with other PFAs, and the implant may be considered less expensive when operating time is factored in.

Athletics

The custom PFA has not been formally investigated in the setting of sports. A distinction has to be made between a patient's ability to perform a given sport and the wisdom of performing such a sport. I define the "Bo Jackson" syndrome as a person's ability to perform a sport—only to see the implant worn or loosened as a result of that activity (Bo Jackson returned to baseball with a hip replacement—and promptly needed a revision).

A number of my patients have resumed athletic activities; I discourage activities involving repeated knee bends and, in patients with poor VMOs, uncontrolled twisting. Barring these restrictions, I allow patients a return to sports, with the understanding that we (the patients and I) are in unchartered waters.

Second-Generation Onlay Patellofemoral Arthroplasty

Two Surgeons' Experience with the Avon™ (Kalamazoo, MI) PFA

Elizabeth A. Arendt, M.D., and Diane L. Dahm, M.D.

Partial knee replacements by design are indicated for patients who have preservation of two joints with isolated arthritis in the third compartment. An ideal patellofemoral arthroplasty (PFA) patient is somebody with a functioning aligned patellofemoral (PF) joint or one that can be realigned surgically. The disease is isolated to the PF joint with minimal to no coexisting arthritis in the tibiofemoral joint. Although some patients may have a mild valgus alignment of the limb, it is important that there is no narrowing of the lateral joint space, suggesting early lateral compartment wear. Mild valgus limb alignment due to varying degrees of hypoplasia of the lateral femoral condyle is common with PF arthrosis; often the joint line remaining parallel to the floor and the tibiofemoral compartment is not compromised. Trochlear dysplasia is often present as a morphologic feature [22]. Ideally there should be no systemic arthropathies.

Design Features

The prosthesis of choice for the authors has been the Avon™ prosthesis, which is a second-generation implant developed in 1996. Early (5 years) results have been published and are encouraging for improvement in function with essentially no incidence of loosening [23].

The characteristics of the design of the trochlea come from the Kinemax total knee. There are four sizing options on the femur, no left or right differences. There are two options for the patella: a domed polyethylene symmetric button and an asymmetric button. Both are compatible with revision knee systems. The design of the trochlea is an onlay-style prosthesis that is implanted flush with the anterior cortex. It offers a broad trochlea upon which to capture the patella, making it one of the least constraining trochleas on the market.

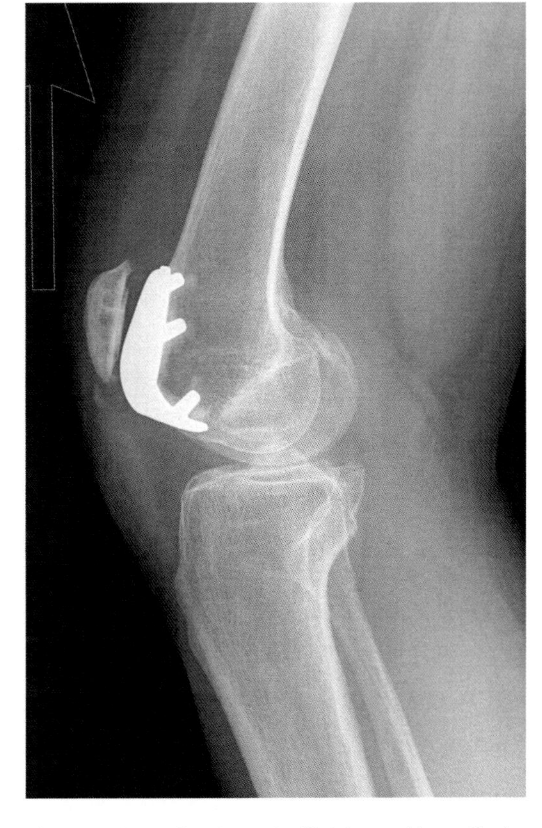

Fig. 8.19 Lateral radiograph of left knee with patella alta (Insall/Salvati ratio >1.6), S/P Avon PFA. The kneecap remains contained in the flange of the femoral prosthesis

The length of the anterior flange is designed to have the patella component articulate with the trochlear component in extension, eliminating the potential to have the patella component catch on the superior extent of the trochlea component in early flexion. This longer trochlear design is useful, as patella alta is often associated with isolated patellofemoral arthritis (Fig. 8.19) [22]. Another advantage of this design is the initial femoral cut, which is an anterior cut, similar to that of a total knee. This anterior cut essentially removes the condylar deformity that is associated with trochlear dysplasia. The surgeon can then place the "normalized" trochlear component in the appropriate anatomic position.

In our hands it is rare that formal patella realignment is necessary. This is due in part to the trochlear design being very forgiving. In addition, the lateral patella tilt which is often present

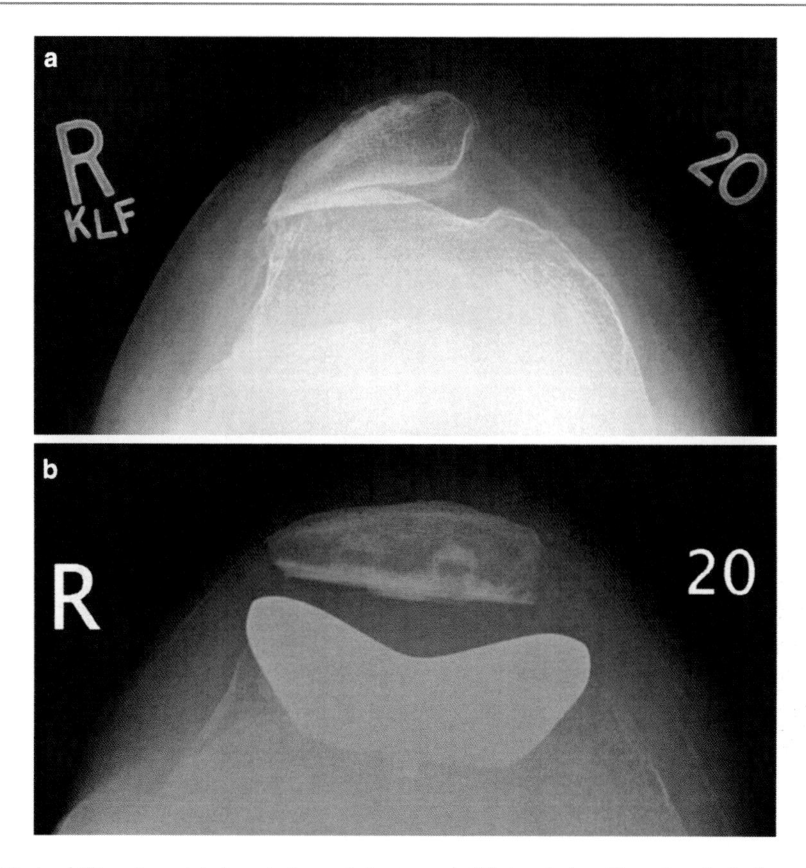

Fig. 8.20 (**a**) Lateral tilt on the axial views is (in part) due to grade IV chondral and bone loss in the lateral PF compartment. (**b**) Prosthetic restoration of the trochlear and lateral facet surface volume recreates more normal tracking

in patients with PF arthritis is in part due to wear of the lateral patella compartment (loss of bone and cartilage) (Fig. 8.20). This volume loss is "restored" with the arthroplasty resurfacing. Lateral soft tissue tightness can be managed with a peri-retinacular release (Ackroyd, CE, personal communication) [24]. At times, a formal lateral retinacular release or lengthening is performed. There may be medial retinacular tissue redundancy that can be imbricated.

This brief review outlines the collective experience of two surgeons with separate but similar practices. They have collectively performed over 220 (113; DD plus 111; EAA) patellofemoral arthroplasties from 2003 to June 2012.

To date there has been no concomitant medial tibial tubercle osteotomy associated with this procedure in our patient cohort, though some have had this procedure previously to treat PF instability. There have been two cases (EAA) that have had excessive patella alta, with the patella not being contained within the anterior flange of the trochlear design. A patella tendon imbrication was performed in both cases. Alternatively a distal tibial tubercle osteotomy can be performed provided adequate proximal tibial bone is present.

Activity Levels

The incidence of isolated patellofemoral joint arthritis is more common in females, with trochlear dysplasia commonly seen in this population [22]. The PF complaints are frequently bilateral and coupled with a long-standing history of patellofemoral pathology. As such, many patients have reduced their activity levels over time; even as teenagers they typically did not get involved in traditional jumping and pivoting sports. Therefore, many patients that are appropriate for a PFA are not involved in sporting or athletic activities that involve running, jumping, and/or pivoting.

At times, a patient may present with PF symptoms due to PF arthritis that occur only with high-level sporting activities (e.g., running), and their day-to-day activities are not compromised. Since we have little information on activity levels after a patellofemoral arthroplasty, we cannot encourage the use of a PFA for this surgical indication. The authors believe that to advise a patellofemoral resurfacing for the *sole indication* of returning a person to a high-level impact activities is not recommended.

We place no absolute restrictions on the patient's postoperative activity but discourage dedicated running defined as one's primary exercise with daily or near daily frequency. To date there is little information about the effect of running on prosthetic wear and loosening over the long term.

In one patient cohort (DD), Knee Society Score (KSS) was used as the outcome tool. In a follow-up of 61 patients operated on between 2003 and 2009, 59 have complete follow-up (minimum 2 years, mean 3.5 years). The Tegner [19] and UCLA activity scores [25] were used to gauge activities. The UCLA scale is a simple scale ranging from 1 to 10. The patient indicates her or his most appropriate activity level, with 1 defined as "no physical activity, dependent on others" and 10 defined as "regular participation in impact sports." The Tegner score is similar to the UCLA scale, a simple scale ranging from 0 to 10, and the patient has to indicate the most appropriate activity level, with 0 defined as "no physical activity, disabled," and 10 defined as "participation in competitive soccer—national and international elite."

Pre- and postoperative means are presented below (Table 8.2). There is improvement in their scores, with mean values in both activity scores representing a moderately active population.

In a previous review comparing total knee arthroplasty patients to PFA patients in 50 matched pairs, specific sporting activity was requested [26]. This is reported in Table 8.3.

In a second patient cohort (EAA), Knee injury and Osteoarthritis Outcome Score (KOOS) was used. Of the 55 knees, 50 knees (91 %) have >2-year follow-up. KOOS subset data included averages of presurgery and 2+ years postoperatively, respectively: pain 50.0 and 74.8, symptoms 39.9 and 54.7, ADL 53.2 and 79.5, sports 26.3 and 53.7, and QOL 18.2 and 53.2. Though sporting activity has significantly improved postoperatively, it remains low compared to a young and active population.

Marx activity scale is designed for knee-injured athletic patients [27, 28]. This scale consists of four questions asking the frequency the patient performs activities such as "running, cutting, decelerating, and pivoting." Each question can be scored from 0 (less than one time per month) to 4 (four times per week or more often) and ranges from 0 to 16 points. Impact activities that are done less than once a month or not at all receive a score of zero. Review of Marx activity scales in a similar cohort of Avon PFA patients reveals a mean preoperative score of 1.94 (range 0–12) and a postoperative mean 2.17 (range 0–12). This indicates that our PFA population on

Table 8.2 Pre- and postoperative means of a cohort of Avon™ patients

	Preoperative mean (SD)	Postoperative mean (SD)
ROM arc	122.7 (9.8)	124.2 (6.6)
KSS Pain	51.4 (7.4)	89.9 (13.6)
KSS function	56.0 (10.9)	77.6 (20.6)
KSS stairs	26.9 (6.7)	38.8 (10.2)
Tegner	2.3 (0.9)	3.8 (1.2)
UCLA	3.4 (0.6)	5.8 (1.8)

Table 8.3 Sporting activities after PFA/TKA

Sporting activity	PFA group	TKA group
Walking	20 (87 %)	18 (81 %)
Swimming/water aerobics	7 (30 %)	1 (5 %)
Running	3 (13 %)	0
Bicycling	7 (30 %)	1 (5 %)
Hiking	3 (13 %)	0
Square dancing	1 (4 %)	0
Camping/fishing	1 (4 %)	0
Racquetball	0	1 (5 %)
No sports	2 (9 %)	2 (9 %)

PFA patellofemoral arthroplasty, *TKA* total knee arthroplasty average does not partake in high-impact and pivoting activity. Four patients specifically mentioned running as a desired postoperative goal and were able to go back to running activity at some level postoperatively.

In review of our collective experience to date, the authors are encouraged that PFA is a good option for the patient with isolated grade 4 arthritis. It is our impression that the typical PFA patient returns to moderate activity levels, primarily partaking in low-impact aerobic activities. They typically return to these activities postoperatively with less pain and greater frequency than their preoperative situation.

Third-Generation Asymmetrical Onlay PFA Sigma High-Performance Partial Knee Replacement® (DePuy Synthes, Warsaw, IN)

Personal Experience of Jack Farr, M.D.

Several manufacturers now have a third-generation option. The means to optimizing a PFA are detailed in another article [29]. In this third generation, the patella remains an oval or oval dome as with second-generation implants. The trochleas are commonly asymmetrical to allow a narrower component for a specific size of femur in an attempt to decrease soft tissue impingement. With this narrower size, it is therefore possible to insert these implants in an "inlay" technique for those patients with near normal trochleas and use the same implant as on "onlay" for those with more advanced dysplasia. The trochlear aspect is lengthened proximally past the native trochlea, to allow for PF contact in full extension even with mild amounts of patellar alta. As a design surgeon (Farr is a DePuy Synthes consultant, design surgeon for the Sigma HP PKR PFA, and receives royalties), it would be somewhat disingenuous to present results in this article format as lead author. Therefore, the techniques of other authors are outlined, followed by their patients' sports activity levels. The technique for the Sigma HP PFA is demonstrated in

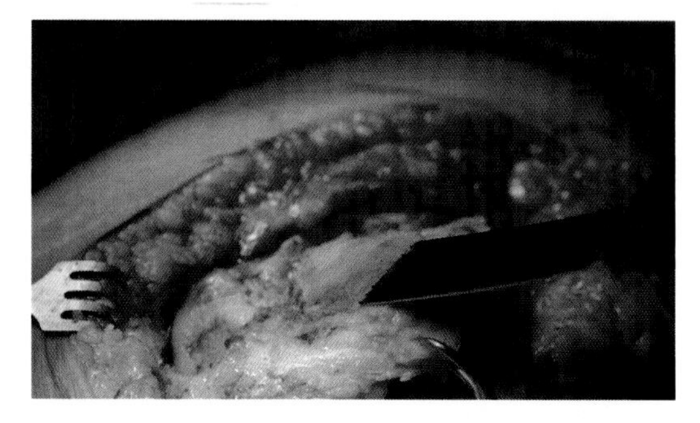

Fig. 8.21 Standard flat cut patella maintaining approximately 15 mm thickness

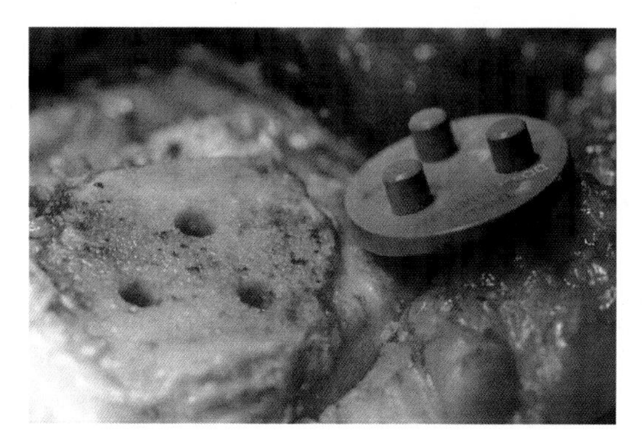

Fig. 8.22 A size 3 peg oval dome trial as would be used for TKA

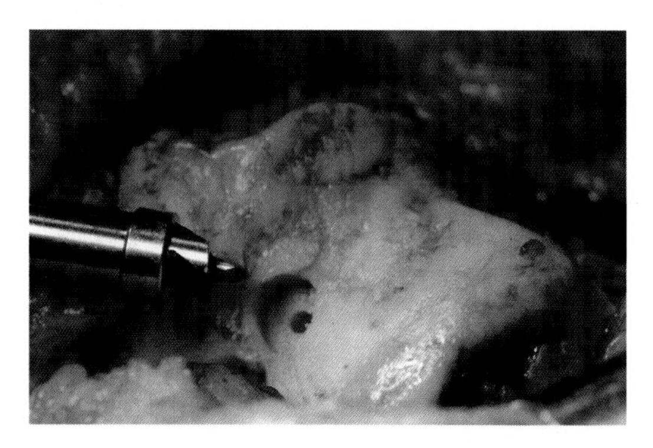

Fig. 8.23 Collared drill bit creates socket with radius same as implant tip and depth to reference all further cuts

Figs. 8.21, 8.22, 8.23, 8.24, 8.25, 8.26, 8.27, and 8.28. Figures 8.29 and 8.30 show a patient's radiographs implanted with a Sigma HP PFA.

Sports After Sigma HP PFA

Of the 213 patients undergoing this PFA from 2008 to 2012, 78 % of patients were either unable

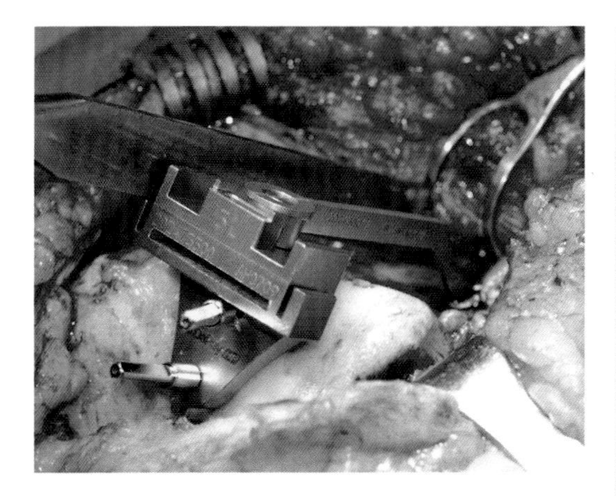

Fig. 8.24 Anterior cutting guide reference distal socket and anterior femoral cortex. Rotation matches anatomy of "normal" trochlea with higher lateral trochlea than medial. Vertical slots may be used when an inset trochlea is desired; otherwise, the horizontal slot captures the saw blade which removes all anterior bone

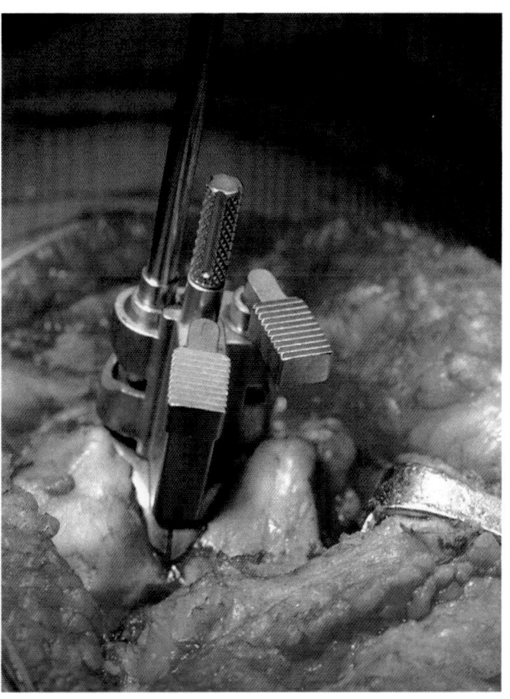

Fig. 8.26 With trial trochlear implant seated flush to adjacent cartilage of distal trochlea, a drilling guide is used to create three holes for trochlear component lugs

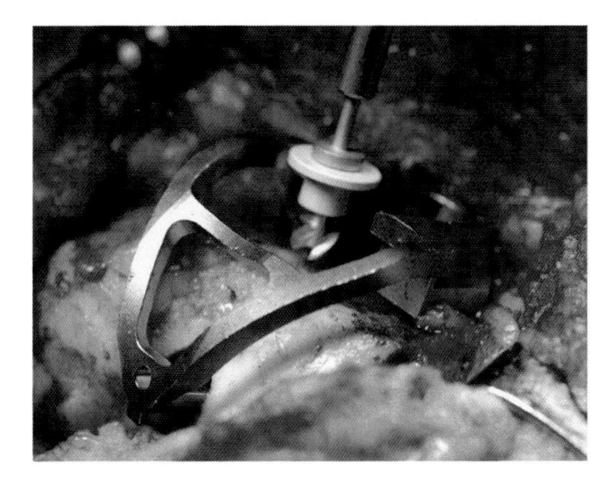

Fig. 8.25 End-cutting mill tracks on guide set in distal reference socket and anterior cut, which creates a depth equal to final trochlear component

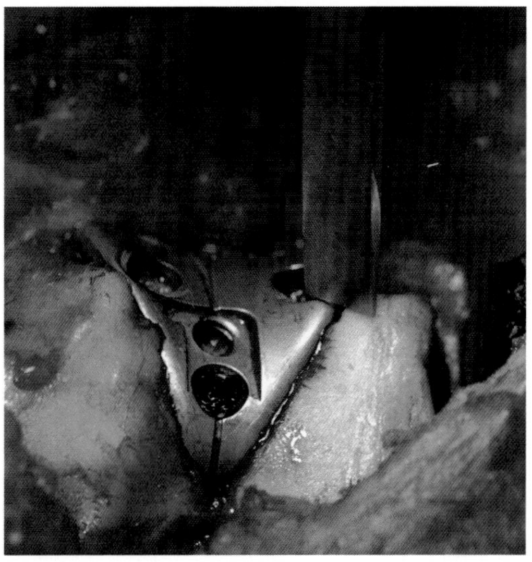

Fig. 8.27 Checking to assure the trochlear trial is flush with adjacent cartilage

or not interested in participating in sports. This group of tertiary referral patient had predominantly patients with long-standing PF degenerative arthritis in conjunction with dysplasia and thus had moderated their activity over many years. All patients who desired to return to "sport" were able to, but in this patient population, there were no high-level athletes who participated in high-demand activities except the two patients illustrated who hiked, skied (low impact), and rode horses (Fig. 8.31). There were no runners, soccer players, basketball players, or tennis players.

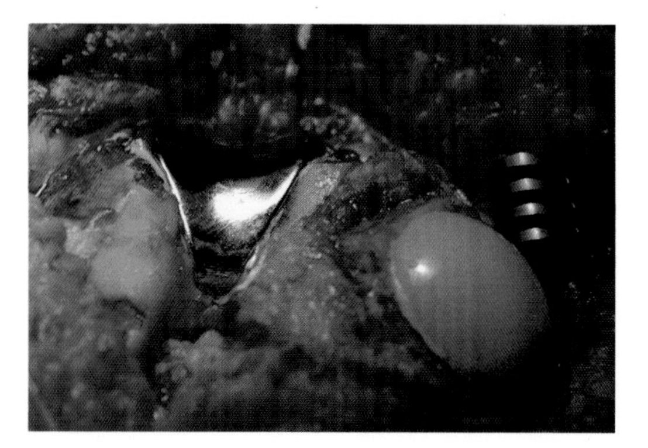

Fig. 8.28 Cemented trochlear and patellar implants

Conclusions

Sports participation after any arthroplasty remains a study in progress. There is no high level of evidence literature reports. The intermediate and long-term problems with loosening are unknown. When only the trochlea is resurfaced as with the Arthrosurface implants, obviously polyethylene wear debris as a cause of loosening is avoided. The early experiences reported are promising, yet these are a subset of PF degenerative patients (e.g., not used in severe dysplasia). As polyethylene wear is the main concern, data from TKA and UKA suggest that wear is a function of load and cycles of use. Therefore, until

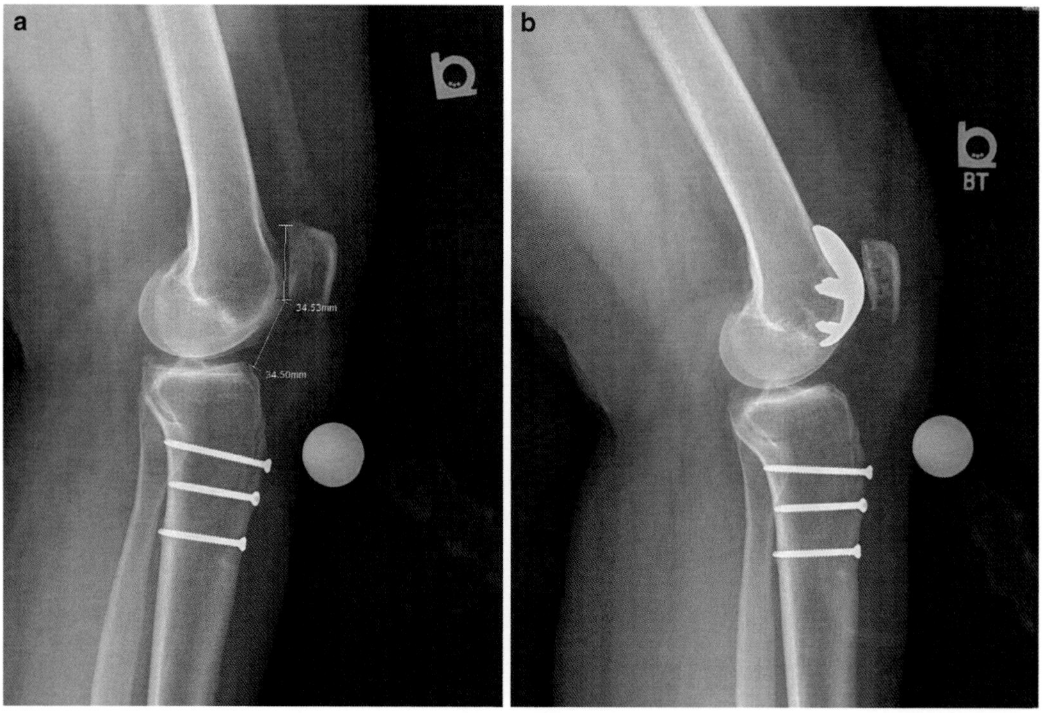

Fig. 8.29 (**a**) Preoperative lateral radiograph and (**b**) postoperative lateral radiograph

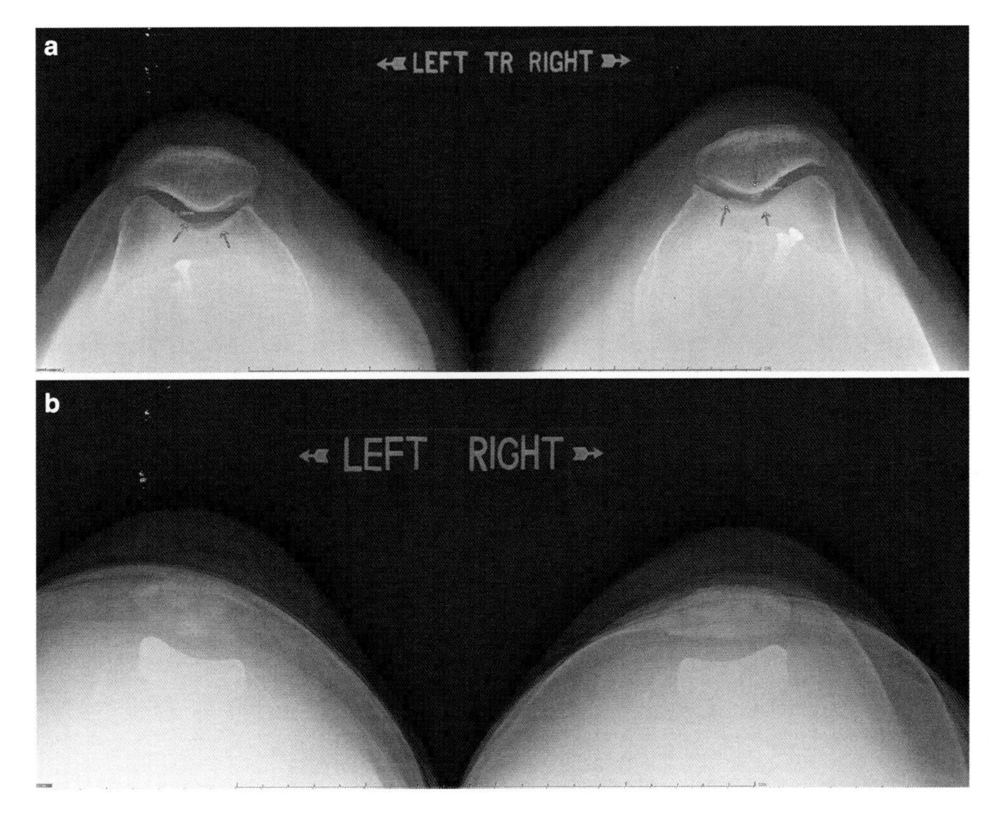

Fig. 8.30 (**a**) Preoperative merchant view and (**b**) postoperative merchant view

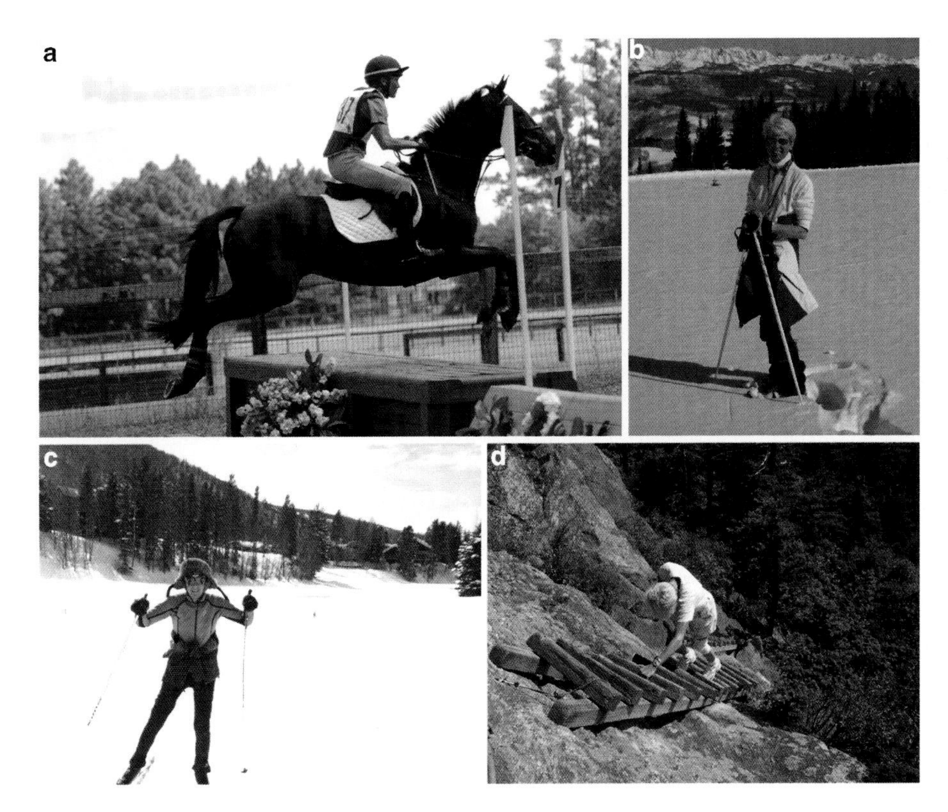

Fig. 8.31 (**a**) PFA patient riding. (**b**) PFA patient snowshoeing. (**c**) PFA patient cross-country skiing. (**d**) PFA patient on nontechnical climb

objective laboratory wear data or prospective randomized controlled studies are available, when polyethylene patella button is used in the PFA setting, it is advisable to recommend that patients participate only in low-PF loading sports and concentrate more on low-loading activities such as swimming and cycling.

References

1. McAlindon TE, Snow S, Cooper C, Dieppe PA. Radiographic patterns of osteoarthritis of the knee joint in the community: the importance of the patellofemoral joint. Ann Rheum Dis. 1992;51:844–9.
2. Maquet P. Advancement of the tibial tuberosity. Clin Orthop Relat Res. 1976;225–30.
3. Rue JPH, Colton A, Zare SM, Shewman E, Farr J, Bach BR, et al. Trochlear contact pressures after straight anteriorization of the tibial tuberosity. Am J Sports Med. 2008;36:1953–9.
4. Fulkerson JP, Becker GJ, Meaney JA, Miranda M, Folcik MA. Anteromedial tibial tubercle transfer without bone graft. Am J Sports Med. 1990;18:490–6. discussion 496.
5. Cohen ZA, Henry JH, McCarthy DM, Mow VC, Ateshian GA. Computer simulations of patellofemoral joint surgery. Patient-specific models for tuberosity transfer. Am J Sports Med. 2003;31:87–98.
6. Fulkerson JP. Anteromedialization of the tibial tuberosity for patellofemoral malalignment. Clin Orthop Relat Res. 1983;176–81.
7. Pidoriano AJ, Weinstein RN, Buuck DA, Fulkerson JP. Correlation of patellar articular lesions with results from anteromedial tibial tubercle transfer. Am J Sports Med. 1997;25:533–7.
8. Jamali AA, Emmerson BC, Chung C, Convery FR, Bugbee WD. Fresh osteochondral allografts: results in the patellofemoral joint. Clin Orthop Relat Res. 2005;176–85.
9. TorgaSpak R, Teitge RA. Fresh osteochondral allografts for patellofemoral arthritis: long-term follow-up. Clin Orthop Relat Res. 2006;444:193–200.
10. Mont MA, Haas S, Mullick T, Hungerford DS. Total knee arthroplasty for patellofemoral arthritis. J Bone Joint Surg Am. 2002;84-A:1977–81.
11. Merchant AC. Total knee arthroplasty for patellofemoral arthritis. J Bone Joint Surg Am. 2003;85-A:2253–4. author reply 2254.
12. Lustig S, Magnussen RA, Dahm DL, Parker D. Patellofemoral arthroplasty, where are we today? Knee Surg Sports Traumatol Arthrosc. 2012;20:1216–26.
13. Farr J, Schepsis AA. Reconstruction of the medial patellofemoral ligament for recurrent patellar instability. J Knee Surg. 2006;19:307–16.
14. Dejour H, Walch G, Nove-Josserand L, Guier C. Factors of patellar instability: an anatomic radiographic study. Knee Surg Sports Traumatol Arthrosc. 1994;2:19–26.
15. Pandit S, Frampton C, Stoddart J, Lynskey T. Magnetic resonance imaging assessment of tibial tuberosity-trochlear groove distance: normal values for males and females. Int Orthop. 2011;35:1799–803.
16. Bengs BC, Scott RD. The effect of patellar thickness on intraoperative knee flexion and patellar tracking in total knee arthroplasty. J Arthroplasty. 2006;21:650–5.
17. Bellamy N, Buchanan WW, Goldsmith CH, Campbell J, Stitt LW. Validation study of WOMAC: a health status instrument for measuring clinically important patient relevant outcomes to antirheumatic drug therapy in patients with osteoarthritis of the hip or knee. J Rheumatol. 1988;15:1833–40.
18. Lysholm J, Gillquist J. Evaluation of knee ligament surgery results with special emphasis on use of a scoring scale. Am J Sports Med. 1982;10:150–4.
19. Tegner Y, Lysholm J. Rating systems in the evaluation of knee ligament injuries. Clin Orthop Relat Res. 1985;43–9.
20. Sisto DJ, Sarin VK. Custom patellofemoral arthroplasty of the knee. J Bone Joint Surg Am. 2006;88:1475–80.
21. Sisto D, Grelsamer RP, Sarin V. Patient-specific patellofemoral arthroplasty. In: Fokter S, editor. Recent advances in hip and knee arthroplasty. Rijeka: InTech; 2012. p 452.
22. Grelsamer RP, Dejour D, Gould J. The pathophysiology of patellofemoral arthritis. Orthop Clin North Am. 2008;39:269–74.
23. Ackroyd CE, Newman JH, Evans R, Eldridge JD, Joslin CC. The Avon patellofemoral arthroplasty: five-year survivorship and functional results. J Bone Joint Surg Br. 2007;89:310–5.
24. Shaw JA. Patellar retinacular peel: an alternative to lateral retinacular release in total knee arthroplasty. Am J Orthop. 2003;32:189–92.
25. Zahiri CA, Schmalzried TP, Szuszczewicz ES, Amstutz HC. Assessing activity in joint replacement patients. J Arthroplasty. 1998;13:890–5.
26. Dahm DL, Al-Rayashi W, Dajani K, Shah JP, Levy BA, Stuart MJ, et al. Patellofemoral arthroplasty versus total knee arthroplasty in patients with isolated patellofemoral osteoarthritis. Am J Orthop. 2010;39:487–91.
27. Marx RG, Stump TJ, Jones EC, Wickiewicz TL, Warren RF. Development and evaluation of an activity rating scale for disorders of the knee. Am J Sports Med. 2001;29:213–8.
28. Marx RG, Jones EC, Allen AA, Altchek DW, O'Brien SJ, Rodeo SA, et al. Reliability, validity, and responsiveness of four knee outcome scales for athletic patients. J Bone Joint Surg Am. 2001;83-A:1459–69.
29. Farr J, Barrett D. Optimizing patellofemoral arthroplasty. Knee. 2008;15:339–47.

Overview of Surgical Decision Making

9

Matthew J. Salzler, Kyle E. Hammond, and James P. Bradley

Introduction

Patellofemoral pain and instability are common presenting complaints in the athlete. A prevalence as high as 16.3 in 100 in young female athletes has been reported. Specifically, an incidence of primary patellar dislocation of 5.8 per 100,000 has been noted with this number increasing to as high as 29 per 100,000 in the 10–17-year-old age group [1–3]. These complaints are often more challenging than common, as these symptoms represent a myriad of underlying and often overlapping diagnoses. However, with a careful history, physical exam, and appropriate imaging, the etiology of their pain and/or instability typically can be determined. Utilization of therapists, athletic trainers, and other specialists will aid in successful management outcomes. Although multiple surgical and nonsurgical treatment options exist, appropriate treatment often leads to successful outcomes and a high rate of return to play.

M.J. Salzler, M.D.
Orthopaedic Surgery, Sports Medicine, University of Pittsburgh Medical Center, Pittsburgh, PA, USA

K.E. Hammond, M.D.
Orthopaedic Surgery, Sports Medicine, Emory University, Atlanta, GA, USA

J.P. Bradley, M.D. (✉)
Burke and Bradley Orthopedics, 200 Delafield Road, Pittsburgh, PA 15215, USA
e-mail: bradleyjp@upmc.edu

Pain

Patellofemoral pain syndrome is a constellation of symptoms originating from the patellofemoral joint that can have various and overlapping underlying etiologies. Patellofemoral pain syndrome is a commonly used term to describe what historically was thought to be chondromalacia of the patella. Pain associated with the patellofemoral joint is specific to the patella, trochlea, and their direct soft tissue attachments. Patients presenting with patellofemoral pain are often considered challenging due to the emotional aspect of their pain, which is often chronic in nature, multiple potential etiologies of their pain, and a lack of consensus of treatment options. However, careful multimodal assessment of their pain including the history, physical exam, and imaging often leads to a clear underlying diagnosis. During the initial evaluation of the patient, it is imperative to delineate the true source of pain. Pain referral from the tibiofemoral joint can cloud the diagnostic and therapeutic decisions made by the clinician. In instances where there are concomitant pathologies, more than one treatment plan may be indicated. In addition, there are anatomic features that can lead to patellofemoral pain. An increased *Q* angle, increased tibial tubercle–trochlear groove (TT–TG) distance, increased tightness of the lateral patellar retinaculum, or lateral tilt of the patella all have been attributed to patellofemoral pain.

The patient's history can sometimes provide more clues than the physical exam, but in

R.V. West and A.C. Colvin (eds.), *The Patellofemoral Joint in the Athlete*,
DOI 10.1007/978-1-4614-4157-1_9, © Springer Science+Business Media New York 2014

conjunction, the differential diagnosis can be narrowed. Traumatic causes of patellofemoral pain include fracture, contusion, chondral injuries, and instability disorders. More chronic or overuse-type injuries, which induce pain, can be contributed to quadriceps or patellar tendinitis. Thus, it is important to obtain the patient's history as it relates to their symptoms. Further defining the patient's symptoms based on their specific complaints, such as the location of the pain, as well as factors that alleviate or worsen the pain, will aid in diagnosing their source of pain. Pain, which is located at the proximal or distal pole of the patella, worse with jumping and other impact activities, may be a clue to a tendinopathic disorder, whereas pain located at the medial patellar facet associated with a history of an instability occurrence(s) can be attributed to a chondral injury, injury to the medial retinaculum, or injury the medial patellofemoral ligament.

Isolated patellofemoral chondrosis often presents with anterior knee pain that worsens with prolonged knee flexion (movie theater sign) and activities that increase the patellofemoral pressure (ascending and descending stairs and joint loading in flexion). Also, assessment of the popliteal angle will provide an understanding of the patient's hamstring flexibility; as this angle increases, so does the concomitant stresses seen through the patellofemoral joint with activities of daily living. Assessment for flexibility of the quadriceps and iliotibial band should be performed as tightness of these structures may contribute to anterior knee pain and increased lateral pull on the patella, respectively. Patellofemoral crepitus on exam may be a normal finding, or, in combination with medial or lateral facet tenderness, it may suggest softening of or damage to the articular cartilage. This may be caused by a traumatic event and be associated with one or two isolated chondral defects; also, the signs/symptoms can be more chronic in nature with diffuse lateral trochlea and patellar facet chondrosis with little to no patellar tilt, suggestive of lateral patellar compression syndrome. Overall, assessment of the patient's lower limb alignment is required to determine if mal-tracking may be causing pain due to increased patellofemoral contact pressures or if it is causing and/or contributing to degeneration of the articular cartilage.

Imaging plays a key role in the determination of the etiology of patellofemoral pain. Standard radiographs include a standing long cassette anteroposterior (AP) view, 45° flexion posteroanterior (PA), and lateral flexion weight-bearing views, as well as a Merchant view. The AP view aids in evaluation of alignment and the PA view provides clues to early signs of degenerative joint disease and osteochondral defects. The 30° lateral flexion weight-bearing view allows for evaluation of patella alta (Insall–Salvati, Caton–Deschamps, and Blackburne–Peel ratio) and trochlear dysplasia (crossing sign). Evidence of DJD and trochlear dysplasia as well as patellar tilt, translation, and subluxation can be seen on the Merchant view. Magnetic resonance imaging (MRI) is particularly helpful in identifying and characterizing patellofemoral chondrosis, chondral defects, patellar tendonitis, and other less common causes of anterior knee pain (PVNS/tumor, fat pad impingement, painful bipartite patella). Either MRI or computer tomography (CT) can be used to measure the TT–TG distance.

Once the underlying cause(s) of pain has been determined, a generalized treatment algorithm can be utilized (Fig. 9.1). A brief discussion of the treatment options is presented as a broad overview, and further information regarding treatment, indications, and details of the various procedures can be found in the subsequent chapters.

Nonoperative Management

Nonoperative management of patellofemoral pain should be a multimodal treatment approach that aims to decrease symptoms by decreasing inflammation as well as improving deficits in strength and flexibility that contribute to pain. The utilization of certified physical therapists can be valuable, in order to provide a structured program focusing on hamstring, hip, and gluteal flexibility, in addition to a strengthening program incorporating these muscle groups, as well as the

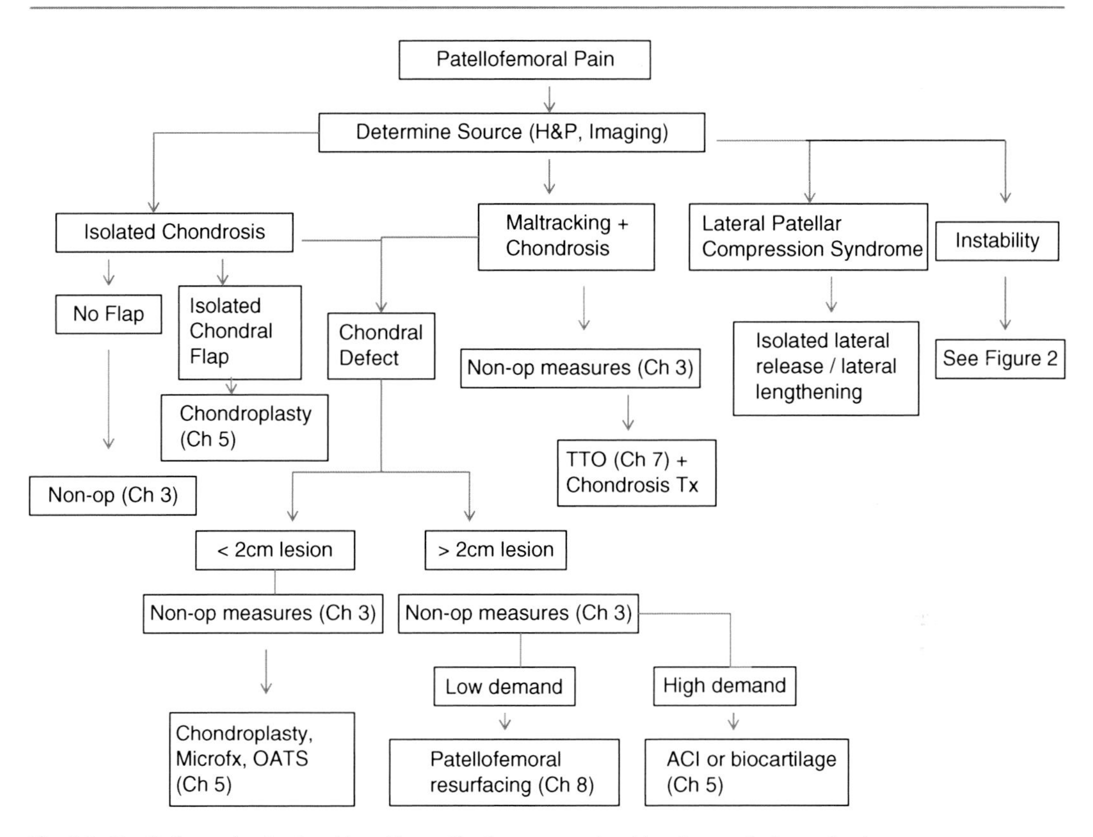

Fig. 9.1 Patellofemoral pain algorithm. Generalized treatment algorithm for patellofemoral pain

quadriceps. Nonsteroidal anti-inflammatory drugs (NSAIDs) can be used to decrease inflammation and pain globally, whereas intra-articular injections of Toradol, corticosteroids, hyaluronic acid, or platelet-rich plasma, though controversial, can be used locally. Additional extra-articular modalities used to control pain and inflammation include heat, cold, massage, ultrasound, topical medications, iontophoresis, transcutaneous electrical nerve stimulation (TENS), and acupuncture.

Lateral Release

An isolated lateral release has been shown to mix short-term and poor long-term outcomes for the treatment of patellar instability; however, it may play a role in the treatment of patellofemoral pain secondary to lateral patellar facet compression syndrome. An excessive lateral release that detaches the vastus lateralis obliquus can lead to iatrogenic medial patellar instability. One long-term study of an isolated lateral retinacular release demonstrates mixed outcomes when performed for instability or pain with only a non-statistically significant trend towards a decreased reoperation rate when performed for pain [4]. Another long-term follow-up study reports 70 % satisfaction when performed for pain and only 50 % satisfaction when performed for instability, with poorer results found in patients with concomitant chondral lesions [5]. A prospective randomized controlled trial with 86 patients comparing the results of open versus arthroscopic isolated lateral retinacular release for patellofemoral pain and mal-tracking without instability showed a slight advantage in Tegner and Lysholm knee scores with open release and a return to play at the same level or higher of 93 % in the arthroscopic group and 100 % in the open group [6].

Patellar Tendon Debridement

Patellar tendinitis is an overuse injury occurring in sports with repetitive and high eccentric quadriceps loading that commonly responds to rest and nonoperative management. Diagnosis can be made on physical exam by eliciting pain with palpation of the inferior pole of the patella with the knee in extension and improvement of symptoms with a flexed knee. Chronic patellar tendinopathy that is refractory to nonoperative management, though less common, is a cause of anterior knee pain that remains challenging to treat. Ultrasound or MRI can be helpful in determining intrasubstance tendon degeneration or partial tears of the tendon origin in these patients. Open or arthroscopic debridement of the diseased patellar tendon origin, with or without excision of the inferior pole of the patella, has shown good results with symptomatic relief but only a 50–75 % rate of return to play at the same level [7, 8].

A painful patellar ossicle can present as a sequelae of Osgood–Schlatter disease [9]. A firm and painful mass in the inferior patellar tendon that corresponds with an ossicle on a lateral radiograph of the knee is diagnostic. Conservative management is often successful, but when it fails, arthroscopic debridement has been reported to be successful [10].

Plica Excision

A medial synovial plica is an embryonic structure, which is typically asymptomatic. However, it may irritate the medial knee synovium and patellar or trochlear cartilage in sports with repetitive high-flexion activities, such as cycling. Arthroscopic plica excision is a simple procedure that can effectively treat an irritating plica, and it has also been shown to have good results in the symptomatic treatment of cartilage degeneration associated with a mediopatellar plica [11]. This procedure should be used only after all other etiologies have been ruled out and the patient has failed conservative modalities.

Chondroplasty

Chondroplasty is a technique that involves lavage of the knee and debridement of loose articular cartilage fragmentation, in order to prevent the formation of loose bodies and to remove irritating chondral flaps. It is typically reserved for low-demand patients with symptomatic small lesions (<2 cm) without evidence of generalized degenerative joint disease. It may play a role in the treatment of "masters" athletes that prefer a quick recovery.

Microfracture

Microfracture is a technique utilized to stimulate the growth of fibrocartilage from mesenchymal cells in discrete cartilage lesions. Compared with hyaline cartilage, fibrocartilage has decreased durability and wear resistance. Thus, it is more commonly used in small defects (<2 cm) and in patients with low demand due to the high pressures in the patellofemoral compartment. Several studies examining the outcomes of microfracture demonstrate good short-term results (<18 months) and with limited long-term benefits [12, 13].

Osteochondral Autograft (OATS or Mosaicplasty)

Osteochondral autografting is the transfer of one or more cylindrical osteochondral plugs from non-weight-bearing areas of the femur to weight-bearing areas with cartilaginous defects. Results of OATS in the patellofemoral joint tend to be worse than in other knee compartments, but have shown of 74 % good to excellent results [14].

Osteochondral Allograft

Osteochondral allografting is typically reserved for large lesions (>2 cm) and in lesions where subchondral bone loss is a concern. This procedure is most commonly performed in the tibiofemoral joint with effective results and, though technically challenging in the patellofemoral joint, has demonstrated good results in limited studies [15]. There is a small risk of disease transmission, as with all allograft tissue. Additionally, biologic scaffolds with or without growth factor enhancement are being developed and may be options in the future.

Autologous Chondrocyte Implantation

Autologous chondrocyte implantation (ACI) is a technique that harvests the patient's own chondrocytes, cultures them in a lab, and places them back into the defect. It is typically utilized in patients with large (>2 cm) well-contained lesions without osseous defects or in those who have failed other measures. Disadvantages to the procedure include the length of time away from sport, the requirement for two procedures, the significant rehabilitation, and the high cost. Advantages to ACI include the ability to generate hyaline-like cartilage, good short-term results, and the potential for better long-term durability than other cartilage restorative procedures.

Tibial Tubercle Osteotomy

Tibial tubercle osteotomy and combined realignment procedures can be used in isolation or in conjunction with cartilage restoration procedures to treat mal-tracking and decrease stress on the affected areas. Theoretically, anteriorization will decrease the contact pressure within the patellofemoral joint, medialization can improve the tracking of a laterally displaced patella, and distalization will improve the trochlear articulation lacking in patellar alta cases. Tibial tubercle anteromedialization for patellofemoral pain with or without mal-tracking has shown good results, though not as good as when used to treat instability [16]. Anteromedialization has also been shown to lead to improved outcomes after patellofemoral ACI as compared with ACI alone [17].

Patellofemoral Resurfacing

Patellofemoral resurfacing is a unicompartmental arthroplasty utilized in patients with diffuse Outerbridge grade IV patellofemoral lesions with preservation of the tibiofemoral compartments that have failed extensive nonoperative management and who are no longer candidates for any of the above cartilage restoration procedures. It is typically performed in order to preserve tibiofemoral bone stock in patients that are considered too young (<60 years) to undergo total knee arthroplasty. It has limited use in athletes but has demonstrated good outcomes for isolated patellofemoral arthritis [18]. Mal-tracking and patellofemoral instability are contraindications, which must be carefully evaluated before considering this procedure. The primary mechanism of failure after patellofemoral arthroplasty is progression of tibiofemoral arthritis.

Instability

Patellofemoral instability may be the result of a traumatic patellar subluxation/dislocation, or it may be atraumatic in origin. The recurrence rate after nonoperative management of a primary patellar dislocation ranges from 15 to 44 %; of those patients with a second dislocation, 50 % develop recurrent episodes of instability [1, 3]. In contrast to instability developing from a traumatic dislocation, atraumatic patients present with a history of multiple subluxations with or without atraumatic patellar dislocations and spontaneous relocations. In these patients, particularly when they are younger and without a frank dislocation, it is important to recognize that they may present with pain in addition to instability as their primary complaint. These patients need careful evaluation as treatment and correction of instability may not relieve the associated pain.

Despite varying presentations, instability of the patellofemoral joint can be separated into three sets of underlying causes that guide treatment: soft tissue risk factors, osseous risk factors,

Table 9.1 Patellar instability risk factors

Soft tissue risk factors	Osseous risk factors
MPFL rupture	Increased TT–TG distance
Medial retinacular insufficiency	Patella alta
Hyperlaxity	Trochlear dysplasia
VMO weakness/atrophy	Increased femoral anteversion

or a combination of the two (Table 9.1). Determination of the etiology is necessary to develop an appropriate and effective treatment plan, as different treatment algorithms are employed for the various underlying causes. Many surgical treatments exist for the various underlying causes of instability, and we present a simple treatment algorithm used by the senior author (JPB), which matches the surgical procedures with the underlying cause(s) of instability (Fig. 9.2).

Identifying the etiology of patellar instability is commonly accomplished through a detailed history, physical exam, and imaging. Soft tissue risk factors identified by history can include a family history of collagenous disorders (Ehlers–Danlos, Marfan, or other hypermobile joint disorders) and a history of a traumatic dislocation or of multiple atraumatic subluxations. On the global physical exam, patients should be assessed for hyperlaxity using the Beighton score that assesses elbow and knee hyperextension, ability to touch the palms to the ground with straight knees, passive thumb flexion to the wrist, and passive small finger MCP hyperextension beyond 90° [19]. Visual inspection may reveal vastus medialis obliquus (VMO) weakness or atrophy. A J-sign may be observed, which is visualized when a lateralized patella in full knee extension shifts medially in flexion as the patella engages the trochlea. The patella should be assessed for medial and lateral glide with comparison to the contralateral side with the knee fully extended and with the patella engaged at 30° of knee flexion; the presence or lack of a firm endpoint should also be assessed. After acute patellar dislocation, tenderness to palpation may be present over the medial patellar facet, over the MPFL and medial patellofemoral retinaculum, and at the femoral insertion of the MPFL. Merchant views of the knee may reveal lateral patellar subluxation and tilt MRI can demonstrate injury to the MPFL, medial patellar retinaculum, VMO, bone "bruising," chondral surfaces, and lastly the ability to measure the TT–TG distance.

Likewise, the underlying causes of osseous instability can also be evaluated via history, physical exam, and imaging. The patient may complain of painful mal-tracking or of being knock-kneed. Patients should be assessed for a high *Q* angle, femoral anteversion, and valgus alignment to the knees. Patella alta is best assessed on a 30° lateral radiograph; there are multiple measurement techniques. We prefer the Blackburne–Peel or Caton–Deschamps ratio over the Insall–Salvati ratio as they do not require identifying the insertion site of the patellar tendon, which can be difficult and lead to less reliable and consistent measurements. The lateral view can also demonstrate a double contour or crossing sign in the trochlea, suggestive of trochlear dysplasia, which can also be evaluated on a Merchant view. Because the *Q* angle can be difficult to measure accurately, we prefer to utilize the tibial tubercle-trochlear groove (TT–TG) distance as determined by cross-sectional imaging. Dejour initially defined a TT–TG value greater than 20 mm as abnormal; however, in patients presenting with patellar instability, more recent studies defined a TT–TG distance >15 mm as being a risk factor for osseous patellar instability [20–22].

Nonoperative Management

Nonoperative management of patellar instability involves many of the same modalities used in the treatment of patellofemoral pain and includes a focus on improving functional alignment via taping, bracing, improved proprioception, and elimination of deficits or imbalances in strength and flexibility. Taping and bracing can be used to unload the patellofemoral joint, pull the patella medially, and enhance muscle activation.

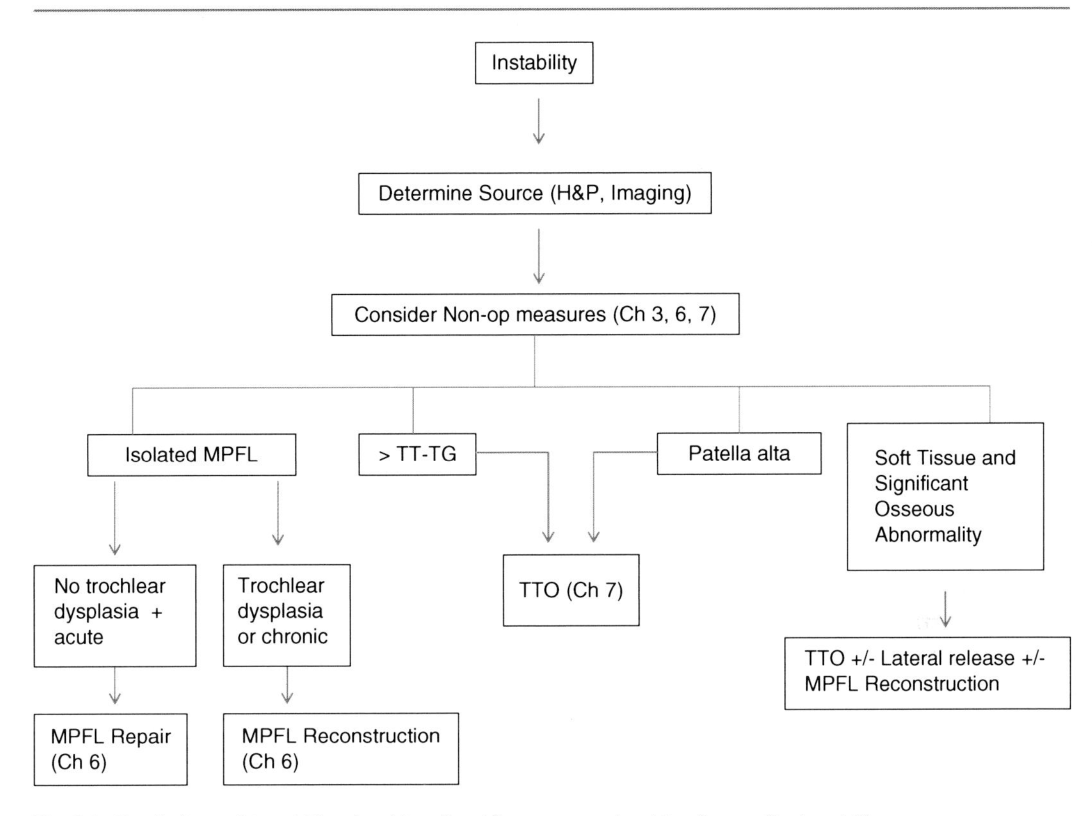

Fig. 9.2 Patellofemoral instability algorithm. Specific treatment algorithm for patellar instability

Muscle training of the VMO and external rotators of the hip as well as stretching of the hamstrings, quadriceps, hip flexors, and rotators may improve functional alignment of the patella.

Soft Tissue Procedures

There are multiple soft tissue procedures designed to treat patellar instability, many of which are performed in conjunction with osseous procedures. The goal of this section is to briefly introduce the indications and results of the more commonly utilized surgical soft tissue procedures with more detailed analysis and technical tips being presented in the corresponding chapters.

Lateral Release

Isolated lateral release, open or arthroscopic, for the treatment of patellar instability is mentioned only for historic interest. Though it may be useful, as previously described, in the treatment of lateral patellar compression syndrome, isolated lateral release for instability is associated with poor outcomes including poor patient satisfaction, persistent lateral patellar instability, and iatrogenic medial patellar instability [23, 24]. However, lateral release for patellar instability in combination with either osseous procedures or medial-sided soft tissue procedures has been advocated [25, 26].

Medial Imbrication/Reefing/Plication

Medial retinacular imbrication involves a tightening of the medial structures via a mini-open approach to the medial knee. Like a lateral retinacular release, medial retinacular imbrication is rarely performed in isolation for patellar instability. Limited data is available on the effect of medial imbrication in conjunction with other commonly utilized procedures for instability. One systematic review of lateral release versus lateral release plus medial imbrication for patellar instability shows a decreased rate of dislocations when adding medial imbrication [27]. Though the senior author (JPB) does not routinely use medial imbrication even as an adjunct to other procedures, it may play a role in conjunction with osseous realignment. One instance where imbrication may have utility in isolation is with the skeletally immature population, where injury to the femoral physis is a concern with other procedures, such as a MPFL reconstruction.

MPFL Repair and Reconstruction

The MPFL has been shown to be the primary restraint to lateral translation of the patella. Without hyperlaxity, MPFL rupture is the sign of a primary traumatic patellar dislocation. After acute rupture, these patients often present with apprehension to lateral patellar translation and tenderness at the medial patellar facet, along the MPFL, or at its insertion site on the medial femoral condyle.

Nonoperative management of isolated MPFL ruptures is often successful, with a minority of these patients progressing to patellar instability; acute MPFL repair has been advocated in cases of concomitant VMO detachment and, occasionally, in athletes with an early failure after nonoperative management. The indications for immediate surgical repair need further investigation. A recent randomized controlled trial comparing MPFL reconstruction with nonoperative treatment of acute traumatic patellar dislocations found a lower redislocation/subluxation rate and higher Kujala scores within the MPFL reconstruction group. The authors in this study utilized a patellar tendon autograft for the reconstruction of the MPFL [28]. However, two other randomized controlled trials comparing operative and nonoperative management of primary patellar dislocation failed to demonstrate any difference between operative and nonoperative management in terms of outcome scores or with the rate of recurrence, but these studies did not compare MPFL reconstruction, rather they only compared direct repairs of the MPFL [29, 30]. There have been no studies on the outcomes of operative versus nonoperative management in elite athletes, and there needs to be further studies comparing newer reconstruction techniques with ligament grafts to nonoperative treatment. Nonoperative management after MPFL rupture can also play a role with the "in-season" athlete who has patellar instability but wishes to delay reconstruction until completion of the season.

Acute MPFL repair is an option that may be helpful in treating elite athletes. A randomized controlled trial of delayed MPFL repair (mean 50 days) demonstrated no significant difference in redislocation rates or in the Kujala scores, but there was an increase in the patella stability subscore [29]. An additional study looking at failures of delayed MPFL repair identified nonanatomic MPFL repair as the only statistically significant risk factor [30]. There is little reported on acute MPFL repair; however, one recent study that included 17 patients reported no redislocations and only one patient with recurrent instability without a frank redislocation [31]. We have also had success in returning elite athletes to play after acute MPFL repair and, with attention to anatomic reinsertion, consider it to be a viable option for an acute patellar dislocation.

Reconstruction of the MPFL has shown reproducible and consistent results for the treatment of isolated soft tissues etiologies of patellar instability. There are multiple successful techniques and graft options for the reconstruction of the MPFL. However, these techniques all involve anatomic reconstruction, as nonanatomic positioning of the graft leads to decreased motion and increased patellofemoral contact pressures. One additional factor for success is appropriate graft tensioning; we recommend tensioning at 30–45° of knee flexion with the patella seated in the groove to avoid over-tensioning. Specifically, the MPFL functions as a checkrein rather than as a dynamic restraint; therefore, it remains important to allow for 1–2-quadrant lateral patellar glide to avoid over-tensioning of the grafted ligament.

Osseous Procedures

Tibial Tubercle Osteotomy

Osteotomy of the tibial tubercle is a powerful tool for realignment of the patellofemoral joint with significant changes in patellofemoral biomechanics; it has been used to off-load diseased portions of the patella or trochlea (often in conjunction with cartilage restoration procedures) and to treat painful mal-tracking, as well as instability. The angle of the cut and the amount of transfer allow for varying degrees of anteriorization, medialization, and distalization of the tibial tubercle.

Two common tubercle realignment procedures are the Elmslie–Trillat medialization and the Fulkerson anteromedialization. The Elmslie–Trillat procedure, potentially by overmedialization, can lead to increased medial patellar facet and medial compartment contact pressures and is not recommended in patients with medial patellofemoral compartment degenerative changes [32, 33]. Good results have been reported in patients without patellofemoral arthritis [34]. The Fulkerson anteromedialization has been shown to off-load the lateral patellar facet with patellar pressures being more equally distributed both proximally and medially [16, 33]. Thus, proximal and medial patellar cartilage defects represent a relative contraindication to anteromedialization of the tibial tubercle. Lastly, distalization of the tubercle is typically included with one of the above osteotomies to correct patella alta cases.

Trochleoplasty

Trochleoplasty is a salvage procedure reported with mixed results in the European literature. It involves deepening the trochlear groove in patients with dome-shaped trochlea and patellar instability. Because of the potential for serious articular and subchondral injury, trochleoplasty is rarely performed in the USA and has little indication in the treatment of athletes.

Combined Soft Tissue and Osseous Procedures

The etiology of patellar instability is often multifactorial and involves soft tissue and osseous components. A patient with patella alta, trochlear dysplasia, or an elevated TT–TG distance has a higher likelihood of patellar instability; the activation energy required for a dislocation with soft tissue disruption is lower, and the risk of recurrence is higher. Because of this, many authors have advocated combinations of soft tissue and osseous procedures. Though there are multiple successful combinations, we have had good results in combining a modified Fulkerson osteotomy and an arthroscopic lateral release in athletes with recurrent patellar dislocations [35].

Case 1

A 14-year-old basketball player sustained a noncontact valgus injury to her right knee during a basketball game. She had immediate pain and swelling, and physical examination revealed a significant effusion, ROM 0–50° (0–140° contralateral), a 10° extensor lag, symmetric varus/valgus and Lachman testing, lateral patellar apprehension, and medial facet tenderness. Radiographs reveal a shallow trochlea with lateral patellar subluxation in a skeletally immature individual (Fig. 9.3), and an MRI demonstrates an effusion with a large loose osteochondral fragment (Fig. 9.4).

The patient underwent a diagnostic knee arthroscopy with fixation of a 2×2-cm medial facet osteochondral fragment with two 3.0-mm cannulated screws and a medial reefing (Fig. 9.5). Postoperatively, radiographs confirmed the reduction (Fig. 9.6), and for 4 weeks the patient was limited to 90° of knee flexion in a brace locked in extension for ambulation. She returned to jogging at 3.5 months and basketball at 6 months. She played 4 years of high school basketball without recurrent instability.

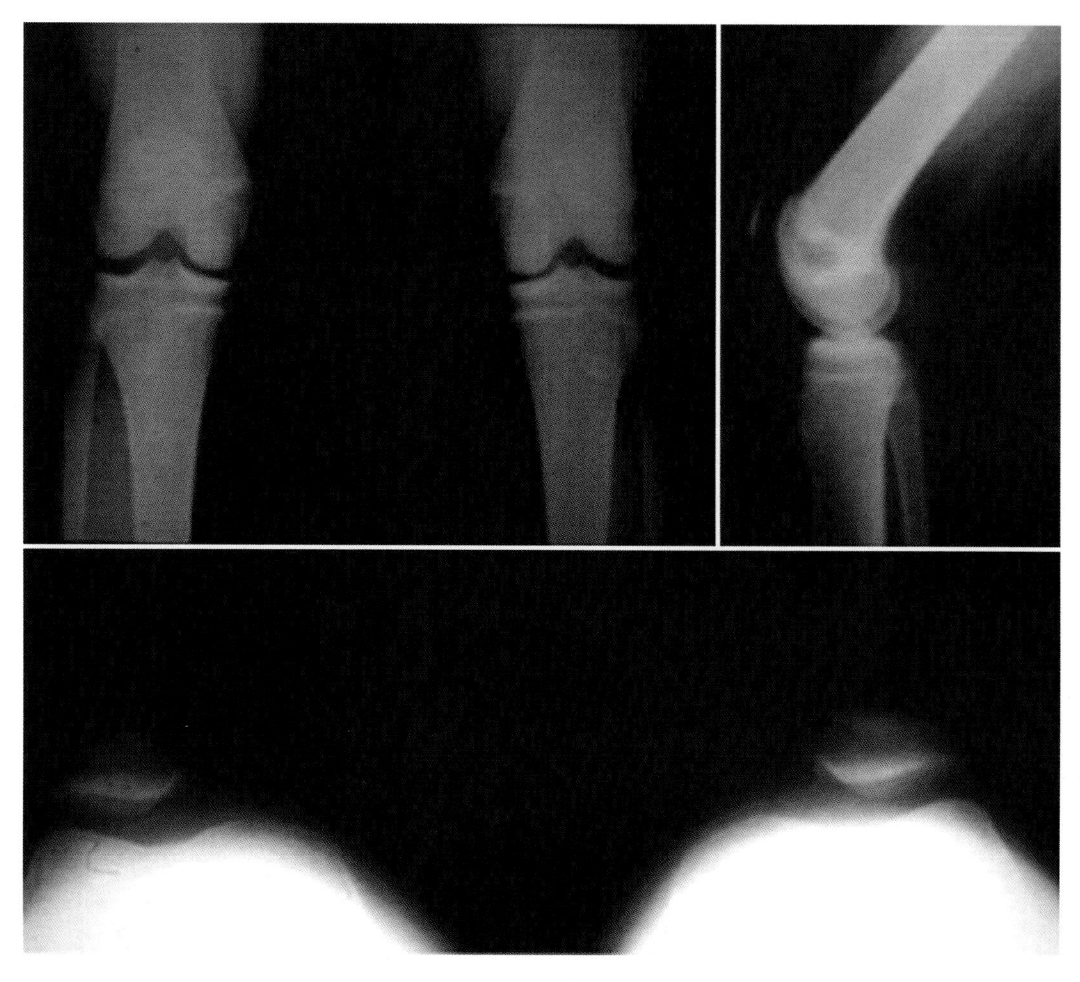

Fig. 9.3 AP, lateral, and Merchant radiographs demonstrate a shallow trochlea with lateral patellar subluxation in a skeletally immature individual

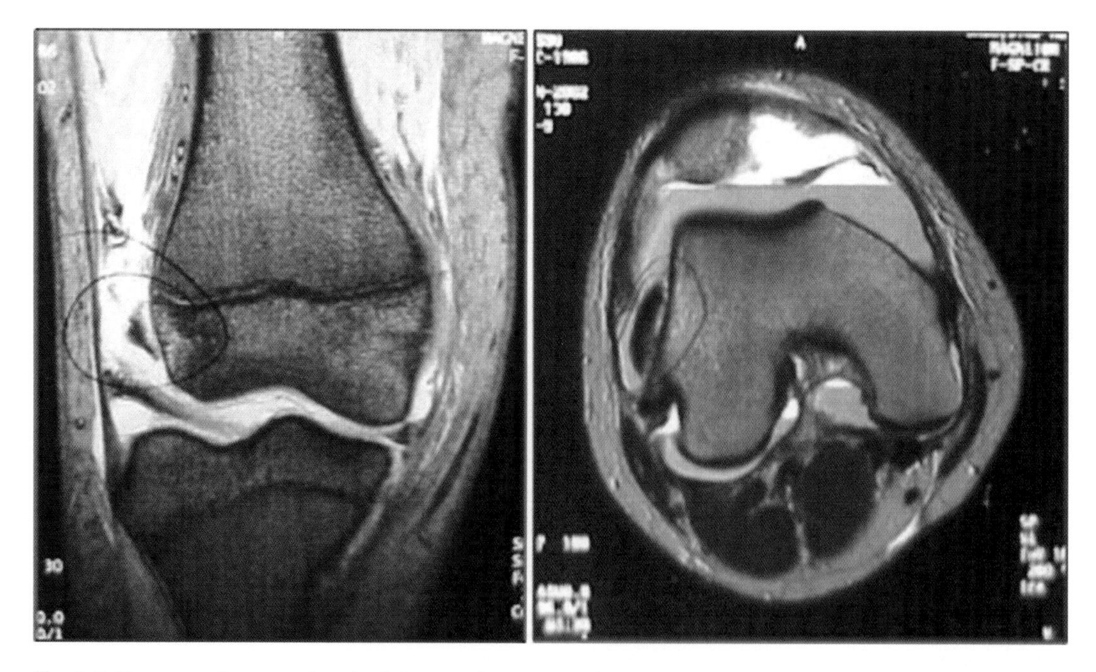

Fig. 9.4 Representative coronal and axial magnetic resonance images demonstrating an effusion with a large loose osteochondral fragment

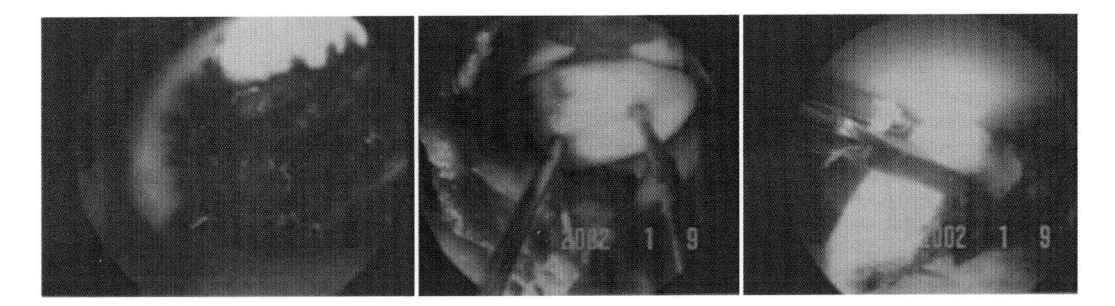

Fig. 9.5 Arthroscopic pictures demonstrating a large osteochondral fragment (**a** and **b**) reduced and fixed using cannulated screws (**c**)

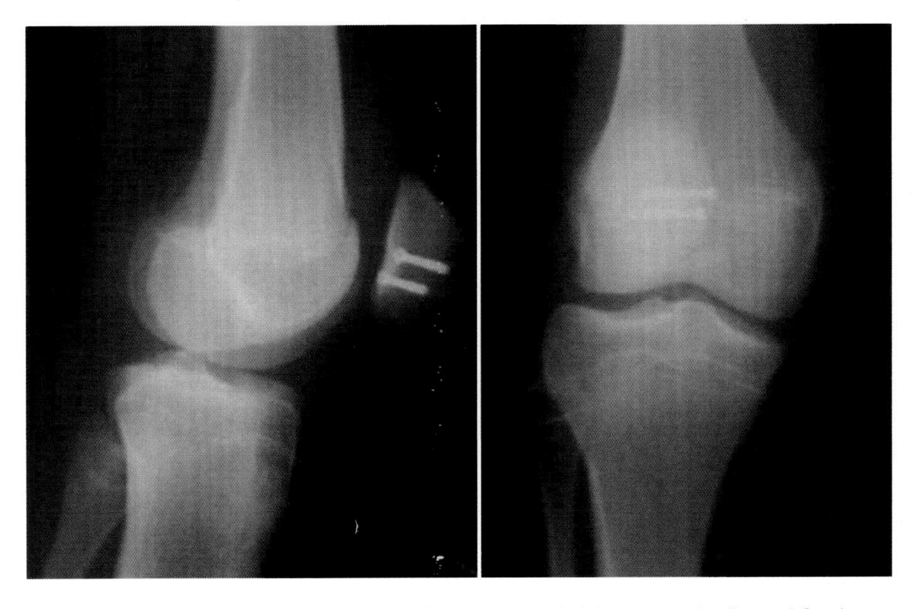

Fig. 9.6 Postoperative AP and lateral radiographs confirm osteochondral fragment reduction and fixation

Diagnosis: acute patellar dislocation with a large osteochondral fracture

Treatment: arthroscopic reduction and internal fixation of the osteochondral fracture with medial reefing

Case 2

A 17-year-old offensive lineman for his high school football team sustained a direct blow to his right knee during spring training of his junior year. Physical exam revealed a mild valgus alignment, three-quadrant lateral glide with apprehension (two quadrants on contralateral knee) in full extension and at 30° flexion, and neutral patellar tilt bilaterally in full extension. Radiographs revealed a normal sulcus angle with minimal patellar subluxation and tilt and no patella alta (Fig. 9.7). A femoral-sided MPFL rupture was seen on the MRI (Fig. 9.8).

With physical therapy and bracing/taping, the patient returned to football and completed his senior season. He sustained another dislocation in the spring of his senior year, and he wishes to play DIII college football. He opted for surgical intervention, and a diagnostic knee arthroscopy was performed with a 30° and 70° camera to evaluate patellar tracking followed by MPFL reconstruction with a doubled 6-mm

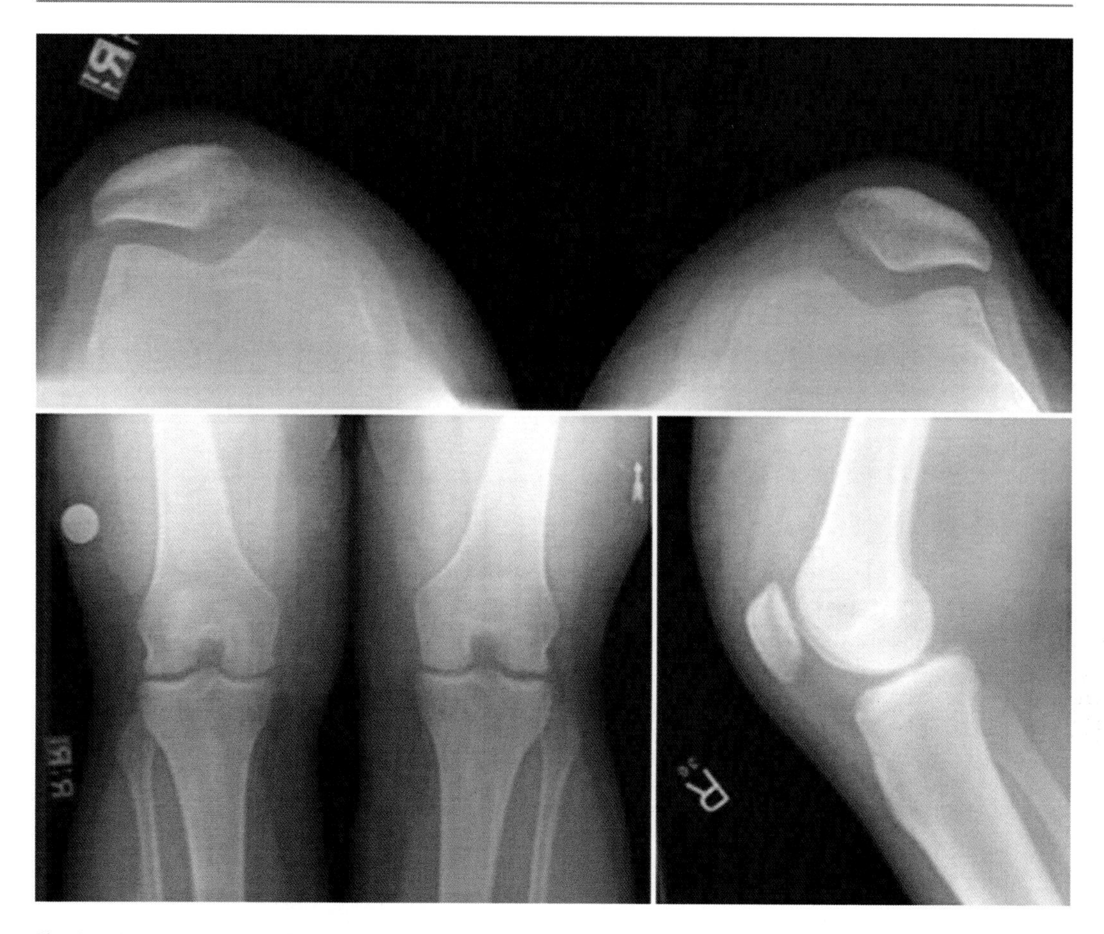

Fig. 9.7 Merchant (**a**), AP (**b**), and flexion lateral (**c**) radiographs demonstrate a normal sulcus angle (130), minimal patellar subluxation and tilt, and no patella alta (Blackburne–Peel 0.9)

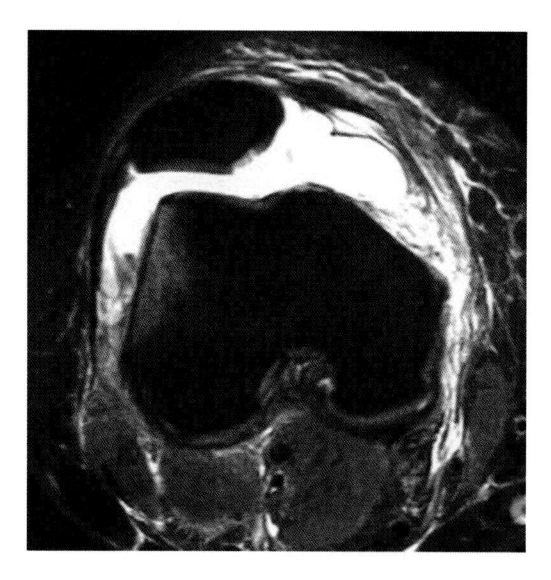

Fig. 9.8 Axial MRI demonstrating a femoral-sided MPFL rupture with shear injury to the medial patellar facet and a lateral femoral condyle bone bruise

semitendinosus allograft positioned with use of a C-arm (Fig. 9.9). A lateral release was not performed because of the neutral patellar tilt in full extension.

Diagnosis: patellar instability secondary to an MPFL rupture without osseous abnormalities

Treatment: MPFL reconstruction

Case 3

A 17-year-old girl high school lacrosse player sustained a patellar dislocation 2 years ago in a lacrosse game. She has been treated nonoperatively by a sports medicine physician with physical therapy and bracing, but she has had multiple recurrent dislocations followed by pain as well as a sense of instability playing lacrosse and basketball. Her exam is notable for an externally rotated

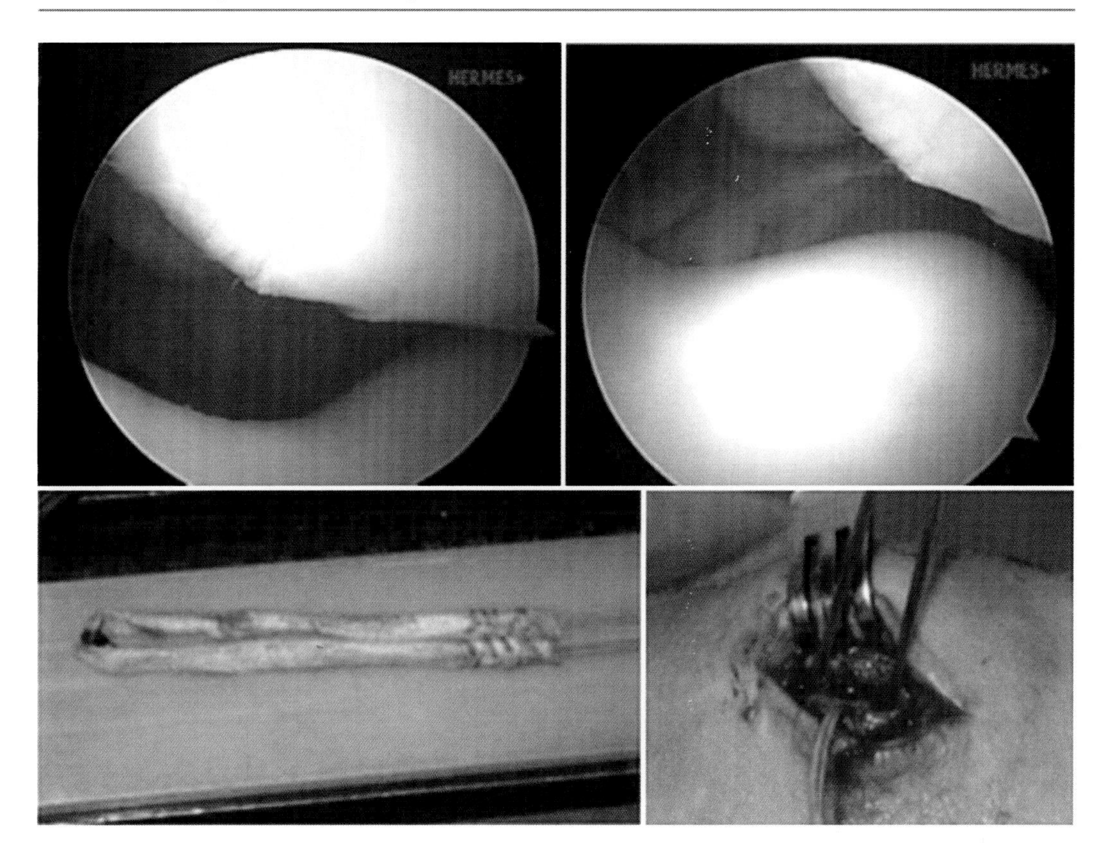

Fig. 9.9 View of the medial patellar facet from the inferolateral portal with the 30° arthroscope. (**a**) Assessment of lateral and medial patellar glide with 70° arthroscope in the superolateral portal. (**b**) Prepared doubled 6-mm semitendinosus allograft (**c**). Intraop photo demonstrating 2 biocomposite anchors fixing the looped end of the graft to the patella with the free ends passed into a femoral tunnel and fixed with an interference screw (**d**)

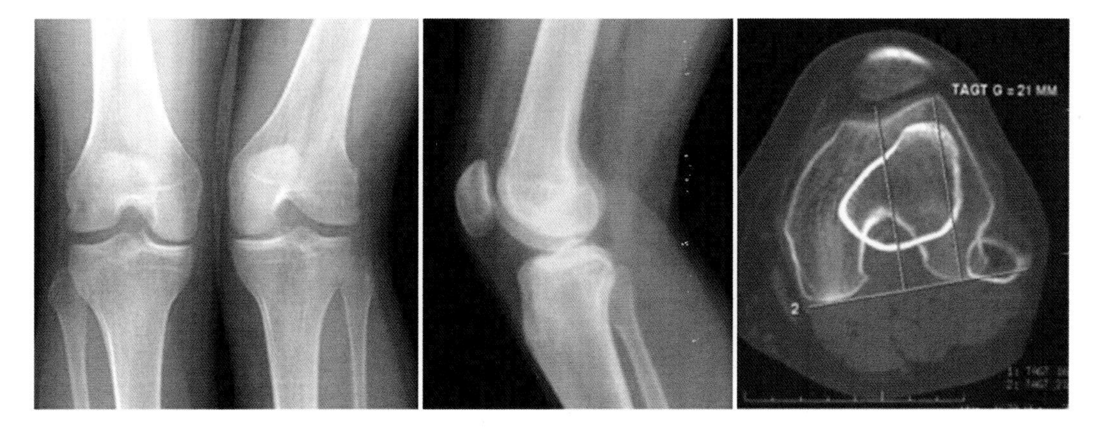

Fig. 9.10 AP (**a**) and lateral (**b**) radiographs reveal mild patella alta. An elevated TT–TG distance of 21 mm is seen on the axial CT scan

gait, a *Q* angle of 30° in full extension, a thigh-foot progression angle of 25°, and patellar apprehension. Preoperative radiographs (Fig. 9.10a, b) reveal mild patella alta, and a preoperative CT scan (Fig. 9.10c) reveals a TT–TG distance of 21 mm and normal trochlear anatomy. A preoperative MRI (not shown) revealed intact patellofemoral cartilage and an intact MPFL.

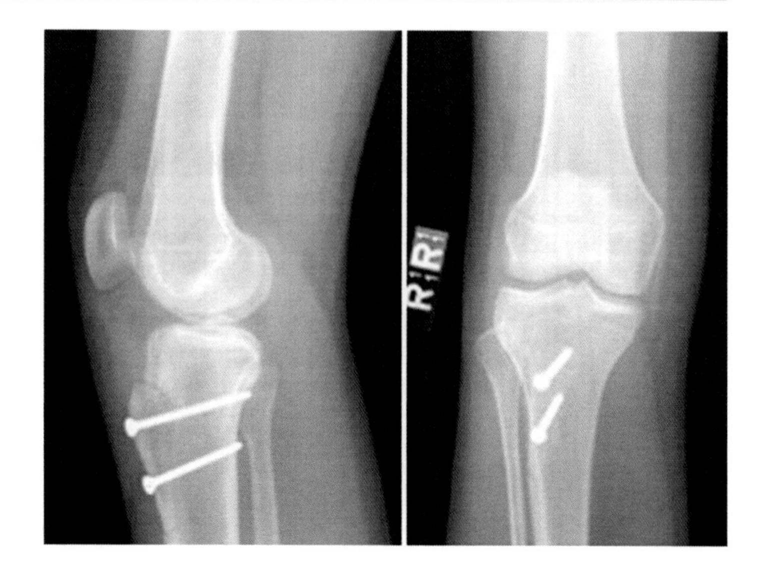

Fig. 9.11 Postoperative AP and lateral radiographs reveal a well-fixed tibial tubercle in its new location

The patient underwent arthroscopy and a tibial tubercle realignment. The arthroscopy revealed a small grade II cartilage flap in the lateral facet, healthy proximal and medial patellar cartilage, and patella-trochlear engagement at 20–30° of flexion. The tibial tubercle was medialized 1 cm as seen on the 1-week postoperative radiographs (Fig. 9.11). The patient was kept WBAT in a brace locked in extension for 6 weeks while the osteotomy healed. She returned to basketball and lacrosse at 4 months postop symptom-free.

Diagnosis: patellar instability secondary to osseous abnormalities (elevated TT–TG distance and mild patella alta)

Treatment: tibial tubercle osteotomy

References

1. Hawkins RJ, Bell RH, Anisette G. Acute patellar dislocations. The natural history. Am J Sports Med. 1986;14:117–20.
2. Myer GD, Ford KR, Barber Foss KD, et al. The incidence and potential pathomechanics of patellofemoral pain in female athletes. Clin Biomech. 2010;25:700–7.
3. Fithian DC, Paxton EW, Stone ML, et al. Epidemiology and natural history of acute patellar dislocation. Am J Sports Med. 2004;32:1114–21.
4. Panni AS, Tartarone M, Patricola A, Paxton EW, Fithian DC. Long-term results of lateral retinacular release. Arthroscopy. 2005;21:526–31.
5. Gerbino PG, Zurakowski D, Soto R, Griffin E, Reig TS, Micheli LJ. Long-term functional outcome after lateral patellar retinacular release in adolescents: an observational cohort study with minimum 5-year follow-up. J Pediatr Orthop. 2008;28:118–23.
6. O'Neill DB. Open lateral retinacular lengthening compared with arthroscopic release. A prospective, randomized outcome study. J Bone Joint Surg Am. 1997;79:1759–69.
7. Pascarella A, Alam M, Pascarella F, Latte C, Di Salvatore MG, Maffulli N. Arthroscopic management of chronic patellar tendinopathy. Am J Sports Med. 2011;39:1975–83.
8. Coleman BD, Khan KM, Kiss ZS, Bartlett J, Young DA, Wark JD. Open and arthroscopic patellar tenotomy for chronic patellar tendinopathy. A retrospective outcome study. Victorian Institute of Sport Tendon Study Group. Am J Sports Med. 2000;28:183–90.
9. Maffulli N, Longo UG, Spiezia F, Denaro V. Sports injuries in young athletes: long-term outcome and prevention strategies. Phys Sportsmed. 2010;38:29–34.
10. Beyzadeoglu T, Inan M, Bekler H, Altintas F. Arthroscopic excision of an ununited ossicle due to Osgood-Schlatter disease. Arthroscopy. 2008;24:1081–3.
11. Guney A, Bilal O, Oner M, Halici M, Turk Y, Tuncel M. Short- and mid-term results of plica excision in patients with mediopatellar plica and associated cartilage degeneration. Knee Surg Sports Traumatol Arthrosc. 2010;18:1526–31.
12. Kreuz PC, Steinwachs MR, Erggelet C, et al. Results after microfracture of full-thickness chondral defects in different compartments in the knee. Osteoarthritis Cartilage. 2006;14:1119–25.
13. Steadman JR, Briggs KK, Rodrigo JJ, Kocher MS, Gill TJ, Rodkey WG. Outcomes of microfracture for

traumatic chondral defects of the knee: average 11-year follow-up. Arthroscopy. 2003;19:477–84.
14. Hangody L, Dobos J, Balo E, Panics G, Hangody LR, Berkes I. Clinical experiences with autologous osteochondral mosaicplasty in an athletic population: a 17-year prospective multicenter study. Am J Sports Med. 2010;38:1125–33.
15. Jamali AA, Emmerson BC, Chung C, Convery FR, Bugbee WD. Fresh osteochondral allografts: results in the patellofemoral joint. Clin Orthop Relat Res. 2005;437:176–85.
16. Pritsch T, Haim A, Arbel R, Snir N, Shasha N, Dekel S. Tailored tibial tubercle transfer for patellofemoral malalignment: analysis of clinical outcomes. Knee Surg Sports Traumatol Arthrosc. 2007;15:994–1002.
17. Henderson IJ, Lavigne P. Periosteal autologous chondrocyte implantation for patellar chondral defect in patients with normal and abnormal patellar tracking. Knee. 2006;13:274–9.
18. Ackroyd CE, Newman JH, Evans R, Eldridge JD, Joslin CC. The Avon patellofemoral arthroplasty: five-year survivorship and functional results. J Bone Joint Surg Br. 2007;89:310–5.
19. Beighton P, Solomon L, Soskolne CL. Articular mobility in an African population. Ann Rheum Dis. 1973;32:413–8.
20. Dejour H, Walch G, Nove-Josserand L, Guier C. Factors of patellar instability: an anatomic radiographic study. Knee Surg Sports Traumatol Arthrosc. 1994;2:19–26.
21. Koeter S, Diks MJ, Anderson PG, Wymenga AB. A modified tibial tubercle osteotomy for patellar maltracking: results at two years. J Bone Joint Surg Br. 2007;89:180–5.
22. Balcarek P, Jung K, Frosch KH, Sturmer KM. Value of the tibial tuberosity-trochlear groove distance in patellar instability in the young athlete. Am J Sports Med. 2011;39:1756–61.
23. Kolowich PA, Paulos LE, Rosenberg TD, Farnsworth S. Lateral release of the patella: indications and contraindications. Am J Sports Med. 1990;18:359–65.
24. Lattermann C, Toth J, Bach Jr BR. The role of lateral retinacular release in the treatment of patellar instability. Sports Med Arthrosc. 2007;15:57–60.
25. Tom A, Fulkerson JP. Restoration of native medial patellofemoral ligament support after patella dislocation. Sports Med Arthrosc. 2007;15:68–71.
26. Mulford JS, Wakeley CJ, Eldridge JD. Assessment and management of chronic patellofemoral instability. J Bone Joint Surg Br. 2007;89:709–16.
27. Ricchetti ET, Mehta S, Sennett BJ, Huffman GR. Comparison of lateral release versus lateral release with medial soft-tissue realignment for the treatment of recurrent patellar instability: a systematic review. Arthroscopy. 2007;23:463–8.
28. Bitar AC, Demange MK, D'Elia CO, Camanho GL. Traumatic patellar dislocation: nonoperative treatment compared with MPFL reconstruction using patellar tendon. Am J Sports Med. 2012;40:114–22.
29. Christiansen SE, Jakobsen BW, Lund B, Lind M. Isolated repair of the medial patellofemoral ligament in primary dislocation of the patella: a prospective randomized study. Arthroscopy. 2008;24:881–7.
30. Camp CL, Krych AJ, Dahm DL, Levy BA, Stuart MJ. Medial patellofemoral ligament repair for recurrent patellar dislocation. Am J Sports Med. 2010;38:2248–54.
31. Mariani PP, Liguori L, Cerullo G, Iannella G, Floris L. Arthroscopic patellar reinsertion of the MPFL in acute patellar dislocations. Knee Surg Sports Traumatol Arthrosc. 2011;19:628–33.
32. Nakagawa K, Wada Y, Minamide M, Tsuchiya A, Moriya H. Deterioration of long-term clinical results after the Elmslie-Trillat procedure for dislocation of the patella. J Bone Joint Surg Br. 2002;84:861–4.
33. Kuroda R, Kambic H, Valdevit A, Andrish JT. Articular cartilage contact pressure after tibial tuberosity transfer. A cadaveric study. Am J Sports Med. 2001;29:403–9.
34. Barber FA, McGarry JE. Elmslie-Trillat procedure for the treatment of recurrent patellar instability. Arthroscopy. 2008;24:77–81.
35. Tjoumakaris FP, Forsythe B, Bradley JP. Patellofemoral instability in athletes: treatment via modified Fulkerson osteotomy and lateral release. Am J Sports Med. 2010;38:992–9.

Index

R.V. West and A.C. Colvin (eds.), *The Patellofemoral Joint in the Athlete*,
DOI 10.1007/978-1-4614-4157-1, © Springer Science+Business Media New York 2014

Printed by Publishers' Graphics LLC
DBT130913.15.14.6